STONEWALL
STRONG

STONEWALL STRONG

Gay Men's Heroic Fight for Resilience,
Good Health, and a Strong Community

John-Manuel Andriote

ROWMAN & LITTLEFIELD
Lanham • Boulder • New York • London

Published by Rowman & Littlefield
A wholly owned subsidiary of The Rowman & Littlefield Publishing Group, Inc.
4501 Forbes Boulevard, Suite 200, Lanham, Maryland 20706
www.rowman.com

Unit A, Whitacre Mews, 26-34 Stannary Street, London SE11 4AB

British Library Cataloguing in Publication Information Available

Library of Congress Cataloging-in-Publication Data
Names: Andriote, John-Manuel, author.
Title: Stonewall strong : gay men's heroic fight for resilience, good health, and a strong community / John-Manuel Andriote.
Description: Lanham : Rowman & Littlefield, [2017] | Includes bibliographical references and index.
Identifiers: LCCN 2017023924 (print) | LCCN 2017037565 (ebook) | ISBN 9781442258242 (electronic) | ISBN 9781442258235 (cloth : alk. paper)
Subjects: LCSH: Gay men—United States. | Gay men—Political activity—United States—History. | Gay rights—United States—History.
Classification: LCC HQ76.2.U5 (ebook) | LCC HQ76.2.U5 A53 2017 (print) | DDC 306.76/62—dc23
LC record available at https://lccn.loc.gov/2017023924

∞™ The paper used in this publication meets the minimum requirements of American National Standard for Information Sciences—Permanence of Paper for Printed Library Materials, ANSI/NISO Z39.48-1992.

Printed in the United States of America

For Doc

"It was seeing death all the time in this war got me to thinking these things. Death was so common, it didn't mean anything. That freed me to think of life. Queer, isn't it? Death made me think of life. Before that life had only made me think of death!"

—Eugene O'Neill, *Mourning Becomes Electra* (The Homecoming)

~

Contents

~

Acknowledgments

Stonewall Strong had an unusual gestation, beginning with its early represen-
tation by the Zachary, Shuster, Harmsworth (ZSH) literary agency. There I
first worked with Andrew Paulson, who was enthusiastic from the start and
up until he left the agency. Thank you, Andrew, for your input and encouragement. After Andrew, I worked with another now-departed ZSH agent,
Jacob Moore. Jacob was equally enthusiastic about the book and, before he
also left the agency, helped me conceptualize it and plot out its major sec-
tions. Finally, Maryann Karinch, with the Rudy Agency, took on the job as
agent for the book. I am grateful for an agent who understood from the start
that the stories of gay men's resilience are "human" stories, offering hope and
inspiration to many people besides gay men.

Thank you to friends who hosted me as I galavanted about the United
States doing interviews. In particular, thank you for their hospitality to Laura
Goldstein and Randy Feuerstein in New York; Greg Pappas and Imran Khan in
Washington, D.C.; John D'Emilio in Chicago; and Kitty Hempstone in Wash-
ington, D.C., for so generously allowing me to "borrow" her house in Maine.

I am deeply grateful for the friends and fans who donated to my crowd-
funding campaign for this book. Their support enabled me to do more face-
to-face interviews than I would have been able to do otherwise. I'd like to
think the material I was able to get from those interviews added greatly to
the final product. Thank you to each and all of the nearly one hundred men
and women I interviewed for the book.

Thank you to Suzanne Staszak-Silva, my editor at Rowman & Littlefield, for her patience when I blew past deadlines in my determination to

do face-to-face interviews whenever possible. My need to do "income-generating" work to pay the bills while investing tremendous amounts of time in a massive project like a book, national in scope and based on many original interviews, meant constant juggling of time and priorities. But now we have a book! Thanks to Lisa Whittington, the associate production editor who steered this book through its birthing, and to Jackie Barnes and her team for helping to let the world know about it in her publicity efforts.

To my friends Jerry Martin, Chris Smith, J. D. Donner, and Dennis Pfaff, thank you for your encouragement and the good times we certainly managed to enjoy in spite of the packed schedule.

Thank you, as always and more than ever, to my mother, Anna Andriote. She taught me to be resilient by example, and she has continued to be the most generous person I've ever known.

Finally, I have dedicated *Stonewall Strong* to Delvin L. "Doc" Covey, my college advisor at Gordon College, from the time I changed my major to English and Doc was the department chair. We have known each other for forty years, and corresponded faithfully for more than three decades. As I write this, Doc is now ninety-six years old. He, more than anyone, has modeled for me what it means to remain active, engaged, interested, and open to life. "Live while you're alive," he has admonished me over the years. That I do my best to do precisely this is in no small part a testament to the loving encouragement I've had from Doc, and my other mentors, along the way. Thank you so very much.

~

Introduction

We hear the word *hero* all the time. This one is a hero for saving a life, that one's a hero for rescuing a neighbor's pet. Time after time, heroes step out of the routine of their lives to respond to an exceptional circumstance. Time after time, the heroes say the same thing: "Someone had to do it." Nobel Prize–winning French author Albert Camus wrote in his novel *The Plague* that the essence of heroism is caring for others "as a matter of common decency." It's about doing the right thing *simply* because it is the right thing to do.

Gay men, and our LGBTQ community in general, have much to be proud of in our history of resilience and survival while vastly outnumbered by those who assaulted, condemned, disdained, exorcised, insulted, lobotomized, medicated, outlawed, and threw us out of our homes. I call it "the heroic legacy" because ours is a history of men (and women) who challenged, resisted, and undermined the prevailing notion that the world belongs to straight white men.

Early psychiatrists in the nineteenth century chalked up what we call our "gaydar" to what they considered at the time to be mental illness. Homosexuals were presumed to share the same "sickness," and extrasensory perception was apparently one of its symptoms. But while heterosexuals preoccupied themselves with trying to figure out how best to keep us on the fringe of their awareness, gay men were building networks of friends and sexual partners, the beginnings of what we call the gay community.

Even then gay men were passing down legends and lore, celebrating gay heroes from history, falling in love, working, and doing their part to keep

America going strong. They invented coded language that allowed them to carry on whole conversations with one another in a roomful of heterosexuals who hadn't a clue as to what they were saying. They adored the female divas of stage and screen because those ladies knew what Lysistrata knew way back in ancient Greece: withhold access to the honeypot and even heterosexual warriors can be bent around the daintiest finger.

The secrecy and shame we were expected to accept as our lot began to give way, at last, when the Stonewall riots of 1969 erupted like a volcano into America's awareness. The explosion reverberated loudest in the psyches of gay men and lesbians long used to living secret lives, hiding their long-time loves, and stuffing down the pain of all the trauma they had endured in their lives. Now it was out in the open, for all the world to see: Homosexuals flaunting (the preferred verb) our sexuality by—clutch the pearls!—holding a boyfriend's hand, or—coronary—a "same-sex kiss." And that disco music gay men loved in the 1970s? It was the soundtrack of the emancipation we proclaimed for ourselves. Hetero America didn't know what to do with homos who wouldn't just "keep it to themselves," stick to the shadows, and die an early and so-sad-but-you-know-how-they-are death likely as not by their own hand.

Then AIDS hit us, first, hardest, and most visibly in this country with the earliest reported cases in 1981. Those preoccupied with finding reasons we should be kept "in our place" saw AIDS as a godsend, "proof" that homosexuals were cursed by God, paying with our lives the wages of our "sin" of not being heterosexual—and, even more unforgivably, forcing heterosexuals to confront the fact of human diversity. Some were willing to suggest draconian measures. "Rounding 'em all up" was mentioned. So was tattooing gay men's buttocks to "warn" potential sexual partners of their potentially being a "carrier" of HIV. That is precisely what the erudite arch-conservative William F. Buckley Jr. proposed in 1986. Gay people responded by forming GLAAD to counter the hateful and dehumanizing lies about us propagated in the media by highly biased sources, frequently of the fundamentalist Christian variety.

But while those who crowed loudest about their religious faith continued to condemn us, we busied ourselves with taking care of sick and dying men, protesting in the streets, and demanding a voice in medical and policy decisions that affected our lives. With the help of our lesbian sisters, co-workers, neighbors, and, if we were lucky, even our families of origin, we mounted an extraordinary community response to the HIV-AIDS epidemic such as the world has never seen. Gay men with AIDS changed the world of medicine by insisting on being a partner in their care rather than a passive "patient" simply trusting that "doctor knows best." Often in the AIDS epidemic, it was the gay men afflicted by the illness who knew much more about their illness than their physicians. We knew well that information and knowledge equals power, and that silence equals death, and all our friendship and social networks crisscrossing the country shared information and forged a strong sense of a "national" gay community.

We were under siege on three fronts at once: assaulted by a deadly virus able to invade vulnerable bodies during our most intimate acts; a homophobic federal government that delayed even trying to figure out what was going on until thousands of gay men already had died; and, on what we might call the home front, the battle within ourselves. We gay men know how challenging it is to get past the shame that society has expected us to feel simply for being different, for loving and being attracted to men. The fact that AIDS hit gay men so hard, that HIV in the mind of America to this day is so closely identified with gay men, added to the struggle to break through the layers of psychological oppression and find true gay liberation in our own hearts and minds.

Gay men who lived through the darkest years of AIDS don't need to be reminded of the terrible, traumatic experiences of those years. We all went through what psychologists call an "off-time life event," forced by circumstance to deal with the mortal illness and death of our friends and lovers. We talked about growing old before our time because we lost so many friends our age within a short time and lived in a constant state of grief. Outside of wartime young men don't tend to die en masse the way our brothers did. Those of us who carry on have been forced to live into our middle years and beyond with the loneliness so many of us carried from our boyhood, compounded by the loss of friends with whom we expected to grow old. We laugh alone at reruns of *Golden Girls*, trying only to recall the happy memories of the friends we used to watch it with in the 1980s who are no longer alive.

Trauma for so many of us has been a recurring theme in our lives. It's shocking to realize, as researchers have found, that nearly half of gay men are sexually abused as children. Then there are the schoolyard bullies, and nowadays the online bullies driving vulnerable gay kids to suicide. Pile on discriminatory laws, religious condemnation, and it's not hard to understand why some of us grow up not feeling the kind of easy self-confidence that so many heterosexual men exude. Too many of us grow up into men who find ways to dissociate from our trauma. It's not coincidental that alcoholism and other substance abuse rates are higher among gay men than among heterosexual men. It's not coincidental that sex takes on exaggerated importance for men who don't have a sense of their own lovability and value beyond their ability to attract and please a partner.

But one of the most stunning findings from recent research on gay men is that the overwhelming majority of us do *not* abuse drugs or engage in high-risk sex (defined here as condomless anal intercourse), that in fact we are extremely resilient. A 2013 report from the National Institutes of Health's LGBT Research Coordinating Committee said that understanding resilience—how it develops, may protect health, and buffers against the stigma that sexual minorities risk turning upon themselves—should be a cornerstone of future LGBT health research. Dr. Ron Stall, a medical anthropologist who directs the University of Pittsburgh's Center for LGBT Health Research, has found that even gay men who had several mental health challenges did not engage in high-risk sex. He calls gay men's resilience an "untapped resource" in protecting gay men's health, avoiding HIV, and building a strong community.

I first encountered Stall's and other behavioral research when I got to thinking about my own resilience after my 2005 HIV diagnosis, at age forty-seven, knocked me for the biggest loop, ever. All of my life's traumas—the deaths of my father, "second mother," the "big brother I wish I'd had," and so many other friends and colleagues to AIDS and cancer; my own lonely boyhood as I sought escape from a dysfunctional family; the bus stop bullies in junior high—all seemed to come to a head in this singular moment when my doctor called to tell me what I, being a journalist after all, began to call "my news."

Two years after my diagnosis, I moved back to eastern Connecticut, where I grew up. I wanted a change after twenty-two years in D.C., and I thought a smaller city would be nice. So I returned to Norwich, the hometown I'd fled in 1976 to go away to college, the only person in my immediate family to do so. When I used to drive my Jeep out to the foothills of the Blue Ridge in western Virginia, I would ache inside for the hills, old farms, and country roads of the area where I grew up. I was a New Englander at heart, and I had long dreamed of returning to the region I loved so well.

Unfortunately, I returned to Norwich just as the Great Recession was unrolling in 2007. Boy did it hit hard in eastern Connecticut. Hundreds and hundreds of foreclosed homes. More and more people relying on social service agencies to help them through the hard times. There are many Trump supporters in an area that in some ways is the image of "American carnage" with its crumbling old mill buildings, ruins of America's lost manufacturing businesses and jobs, though most of the left-behind working poor are white.

I had a hard time of my own, and it went beyond "merely" living with a potentially life-threatening illness. The coffeehouse I wanted to open didn't happen because, as I discovered, even people in the area with money to invest are risk-averse, particularly in a recession. Decades of supporting myself on my enterprise and entrepreneurial drive in Washington, D.C., hadn't prepared me for what awaited. Living hundreds of miles from my consulting contacts in Washington, and providing writing and editorial services that were among the "extras" that organizations I worked with cut in the recession, I saw my income plummet to its lowest levels since I worked part time in college. My professional accomplishments and educational pedigree couldn't even get me a job interview at Starbucks or Lowes. It was astonishing how quickly I became another HIV-positive American living below the poverty line! I moved in with my elderly mother because, after supporting myself in major cities for three decades, I was unable to afford my own place back in my relatively inexpensive hometown. As Mom moved into her early eighties, our housemate arrangement became increasingly an elder-care situation as I have also become one of the growing number of middle-age gay men in this country helping to care for an elderly parent—many of them men who, like me, returned to their hometowns after years in major cities.

I realized at some point that the experience of returning to the place I started out my life, and becoming impoverished once again—after working exceptionally hard my whole life to escape the shame I felt about my family's poverty—has actually been the catalyst for my own biggest breakthrough in understanding and healing my own traumas. Being once again around family members and others I know in Norwich, the years I spent in therapy and Al-Anon groups have enabled me to clearly see the reasons I couldn't get away from there fast enough when I was seventeen years old. I see the dysfunction, threatening to pull me in if I will allow it. All around me I see people who are victims of depression yet refuse to take action to improve their lives, blaming everyone and everything except their own poor choices—particularly the choice not to acknowledge the problem and get proper help. I don't much relate to that mindset. I have always preferred to function at my highest level, even when it might mean taking medication to do so, as it certainly does for someone living with HIV. I have accepted responsibility for *all* my choices, even when they have had harsh consequences for me. As an openly gay man who has written in the local newspaper, and beyond, about living with HIV, I have never once blamed someone for infecting me because I know that whoever he was, I was a willing participant.

Judging from my financial picture, I "looked" a lot like the many other people in Norwich without much money. But inside, I *knew* I was fundamentally different—and not only because I am gay or dressed better (thanks to Marshalls's clearance rack). Yes, the difference had to do with being well educated, living in major cities for decades, and traveling many places within and outside the United States. I've lived an extremely different life from anyone in my family and everyone I know in Norwich. But I've realized that the real difference, the one that matters and sets me apart, is that I choose not to see myself as a victim.

I decided the best use of my time, energy, and talent amid the exceptionally challenging circumstances I found myself in was to do what I have always done: rely on my skills and ability to cultivate writing assignments. I wrote a weekly column for the *Norwich Bulletin*, the local daily newspaper, without any compensation. I saw the accountability I called for and the economic development ideas I introduced from "outside" experts as my contribution toward helping my old hometown's faltering efforts to reinvent itself for the postindustrial era. I convinced a couple of foundations to put up a few thousand dollars to let me update and expand my 1999 book *Victory Deferred: How AIDS Changed Gay Life in America*. I revised my 2001 book *Hot Stuff: A Brief History of Disco*. In 2014 I self-published *Wilhelmina Goes Wandering*, a "fable for kids ages 5 to 105" that has been called a "classic" in Connecticut where the true story it's based on took place. I blogged, free, for the *Huffington Post* and wrote a bunch of several-thousand-word feature articles for *TheAtlantic. com*, highly praised by my editor, which paid me a paltry $125 apiece. Twenty years earlier I was already being paid $1 per word. It didn't begin to compensate me for the time it took to develop the articles, the hours spent researching online, reading and annotating journal articles, arranging and conducting multiple interviews, writing and polishing the story to a sheen. But I accepted the low wages because I knew that affiliating my by-line with *Huff Post* and *The Atlantic* would be beneficial for my career. I hoped it would help me land a book contract. In my fifties, I was paying my dues all over again, reinventing—or perhaps refurbishing—myself. Unlike the first time I paid my dues, in my twenties, this time I was fighting to reclaim my place back in the middle class I had worked so hard to become part of since becoming a first-generation college graduate decades earlier.

Somewhere around the time I was writing "The Power of Choosing Resilience" for *The Atlantic* in 2013, the springboard for this book, I had an epiphany. It really did seem to hit me upside the head. I realized that I was extremely proud of the man I had become. I was proud that I took responsibility for myself and didn't blame others for my troubles. I was proud that I was open about being gay, right there in my old hometown. I wasn't living in a safe, urban, gay neighborhood anymore. I was proud that I wasn't simply whining about my difficult circumstances, like so many around me in Norwich, but was actively working to improve them. I can't begin to describe how challenging it has been at times to live in a place where even family members have a hard time understanding that what I do is actually work because I don't punch a time clock. I also understood, and affirmed for myself, that the choices I made along the way that eventually put me in the path of HIV were not the *only* choices I had made in my life; in fact I had made many *excellent* choices. Where inside me did those *smart* choices come from?

I began to reframe my own life story in my mind. Instead of looking back across my life and seeing only the traumas I suffered, I chose to focus instead on how I had survived them—to think of myself as a survivor. And not merely a survivor, but one whose challenges had provided what the gardener in me describes as the pruning I needed to survive the harshness of winter and blossom again in the spring. Facing a life-threatening illness, I chose not only to take care of myself, but also to squeeze every drop of joy and wisdom I can from my life's experiences, including the hard ones. I literally stop and smell roses, inhaling deeply, with my eyes closed in ecstasy.

I was taking pocket change to the Coin Star machine simply to have a few bills in my wallet. It was that tight. Yet I was savoring the simplest pleasures in my life: hiking at Bluff Point, in Groton, where I first hiked as a boy; laughing out loud as I rolled my Jetta up and down the rolling hills of eastern Connecticut; gazing out across the nearby ocean on a gray misty day. My big vegetable garden, in the backyard of one of the signers of the Declaration of Independence, kept me sane and hopeful and connected to a sense of deep, long American history during those challenging years. I did a lot of "self-talk" to silence the shaming voices in my head and to pull myself upright after feeling I'd been knocked off my Libran balance since my diagnosis in 2005.

In my journalism work I have always picked subjects I want to learn about, and then pitch an article on the subject to my editors. I like to say I have the absolute best "continuing education" because I can quickly develop a fairly high level of knowledge and expertise with focused but extensive background reading and interviewing the top people in whatever area it is I'm writing about. When I wanted to learn more about resilience—so I could share it with readers and apply it to my own life—I knew there was a book in it. I describe *Stonewall Strong* as the bookend to my earlier book *Victory Deferred*. Where *Victory Deferred* documented gay men's suffering and the extraordinary outpouring of support that built the LGBT political movement, *Stonewall Strong* celebrates what AIDS, history, and our lives' other traumas have taught us of our own power. Its dominant theme is the liberating power to be unleashed by framing our personal and community stories as tales of triumphing over the obstacles put in our way as we pursue our own heroic journey.

Part I of *Stonewall Strong*, "Growing Strong in My Broken Places," is a series of ten chapters recalling experiences from my own life that challenged me to find my own resilience. My sources for this section were my notebooks and the journals I have kept since 1980, the year I graduated from college. I felt I needed to share from my own experience of trauma and resilience if I wanted you to trust my guidance through the other gay men's stories that follow in the rest of the book. I'll admit I am a bit anxious about opening my heart and my history for public scrutiny. But I am choosing to go with a slogan I learned long ago in Al-Anon: "We are only as sick as our secrets."

The second part of the book, "The Heroic Legacy," explores moments in gay history of the last century from a very different perspective than the more common one that focuses on gay men's victimization. I found that when you look at how our gay forbears in the decades before Stonewall managed to share a vibrant, mostly "hidden" subculture—and could pick one another out of a crowd even back then—you find amazingly strong resilience. Once gay people rejected the closet as their inevitable destiny, and dared to live "openly gay" lives, we saw the emergence of what a gay community might look like. We created political clubs, community centers, hotlines, drag houses, motorcycle clubs, and even sex clubs. When AIDS hit in the 1980s, gay men and our supporters showed the world what "traditional values" look like when they are practiced rather than preached. We also showed the world that we love, cry when we are sorrowful, and celebrate our life's important moments, just as *all* humans do. Sharing our humanity, pointing out our similarities, propelled the LGBT movement for equality. Helping heterosexuals to reframe their image of us, to think of us in different terms than they themselves likely grew up with, advanced our equality movement—leading to the repeal of the military's "Don't Ask, Don't Tell" policy and, most astonishingly and significantly of all, the equal right to legal marriage.

In the book's third part, "A Home in the World," I examine the role of families and adult role models in rearing healthy young men, gay and not, and how young gay men who don't have the good fortune of a stable and loving family are being nurtured and supported by some of our community's most important organizations. Caring for our traumatized youth is a job for every gay man. We have created our own ways to do exactly that through our community centers, drag houses, HIV-AIDS organizations, and online sources of support. Many of us have even been able to reimagine our religious faith, rejecting the rejection we were led to believe we "deserved" and finding instead the healing and resilience that faith can provide.

Finally, in part IV, "At Home in Ourselves," I offer stories about gay men whose inspiring examples show what choosing a life of honesty, integration, and "outness" can look like. It makes us better and more desirable employees for bosses and companies that understand people are most productive when they are most comfortable. Even better when they can tap into the unique qualities gay men bring to our work and relationships as adding value to their business. Throughout my reporting career I've found gay men of color to be among the most resilient people I know. They—and other men I call "doubly different," including those living with physical disabilities —have *much* to teach us about the need to draw from our various sources of identity, not only our sexual identity, to find balance and strength. I discuss the latest behavioral research on gay men and the role of resilience in our mental and physical health. I suggest new, liberating ways of thinking about aging and being an "older" gay man. Then I pull it all together in the last chapter by taking you on a bicoastal tour. First stop: Portland, Maine, the old Yankee port city that knows much about resilience and proved it again in the AIDS years. Then out to San Francisco where I talk with some of the keepers of the heroic legacy, our proud history of courage, resilience, and resistance.

Please consider three key points as we now move onward into the book. First, it's important to understand and accept that trauma is not about something "wrong" with you; it's about what *happened* to you. Second, no one is *born* resilient. Resilience is something we develop over time as we experience traumatic events in our lives, and it's something we can learn. Third, we become resilient largely through the stories we choose to tell ourselves about what our trauma "means." For example, if I tell myself—as too many gay men would tell me, even in 2017—I am not "clean" because I have HIV, I would probably be quite depressed. But if instead I tell myself it means the men who would dismiss me because I have HIV aren't worth my time, it puts me in the victory stand. The more resilient we become, the more familiar we become with taking the victory stand, and being the heroes of our own life story.

Research suggests that the great majority of people who experience trauma do not become permanently traumatized. Most bounce back after a while, after they have been able to refit the puzzle pieces of their story back together in a way that lets them keep going. The experience of "living to tell" about our trauma gives us the awareness that we are able to pick ourselves up and continue on, even find happiness and love in our lives. I suggest that this awareness—what I call "conscious resilience"—can give us a powerful tool to resist the emotional onslaught that a traumatic experience can bring. Drawing consciously on our experience of survival, pulling through tough times, can help us face whatever else life may throw at us. Knowing that even when we get knocked down we have a history of getting back up makes all the difference in the story we tell ourselves *about* ourselves.

Knowing who we are, where we come from and belong, is the key to being confident, courageous, resilient men. Understanding our place in the lineage of gay men before us, sharing stories of heroic deeds, learning from our elders' wisdom—these are essential characteristics of a real community. They are equally essential for us individually, as we transform our personal stories to tales of healing and wholeness rather than woundedness and brokenness.

I am writing this introduction in Provincetown on a brilliantly sunny Monday, February 6, 2017, what would have been my father's eightieth birthday, had he not died so very young at fifty-two, when I was thirty. As you'll read in the pages that follow, it was the experience of my first stay in P-town in 1981 that led me finally to accept that I am gay. The town at the end of Cape Cod has symbolized for me the integration and integrity I try to practice in my life. It's not coincidental that this place with such meaning for me is in New England, the place I grew up, that for me is synonymous with resilience. Thinking of my dad's strong Greek spirit when he faced his final illness, the sense finally of having found my "tribe" that I first felt in P-town all those years ago, and the long history of perseverance all around me in New England, I feel my own resilience. I name it and claim it. I am very aware of where it has come from, the prices I've paid for it. That is, after all, the story behind all my stories, and the force that keeps me going.

PART I

GROWING STRONG IN MY BROKEN PLACES

~

Overview:
Part I

I am not what happened to me, I am what I choose to become.

—Carl Jung

Of my life's traumas, nothing has been more traumatic than my 2005 HIV diagnosis. The real-life dramas I described as a journalist reporting on HIV-AIDS for two decades by then suddenly unfolded inside my own life. Without warning, I was looking at the world through the eyes of an HIV-positive gay man after knowing myself as "negative" for all the years AIDS had killed my closest friends and so many of my gay brothers.

My diagnosis launched the most arduous journey I've ever undertaken: looking back across my life, sorting out how, exactly, I had arrived at this moment. I knew it was a watershed, a "before" and "after" moment in my life. I had faced similar moments before, those flashes of awareness when you realize life will never again be the same. I read my journals and recalled extremely painful experiences from my growing-up years, my college years, and the years after I came out as a gay man in the fateful summer of 1981, when AIDS first appeared among gay men.

I was reminded that I have tasted love, but only enough of it to tease my love-starved heart and keep alive the belief that real love is still possible. I revisited the painful loss of my father, when I was thirty, my "second mother," the love of my young life, and so very many friends well before I reached that life-changing day in October 2005. Because I was brought up to care for others, to put aside my fear and sorrow and need for love, I had only a vague idea of how my many traumas had affected me—how they had, in fact, led to that fateful October day in 2005.

One thing became very clear throughout my retrospective journey: It had never occurred to me *not* to press onward, *not* to take my medications, *not* to have hope. Where did my resilience come from? For giving me courage, hope, tenacity, and resilience—oddly enough—I could credit the struggles and traumas I suffered along the way. I had learned to survive, and thrive, even under duress. No wonder I felt sure that, somehow, I would pull through again this time.

CHAPTER ONE

~

Why *Not* Me?

A Medical Diagnosis Upturns My Life and Launches a Journey of Self-Discovery

I'm a reporter.

For more than three decades I've written newspaper and magazine stories, and a book, about HIV-AIDS as it has robbed the health and lives of millions of people worldwide. Many were my friends.

I decided this would be my beat back in 1986, when I was still in journalism school. By then I had already lost two friends, men in their twenties like me. It was the year that Bill, the man I loved, found out he was positive. I was afraid I might be infected myself.

All around me, I saw a terrifying event unfolding. My role would be to tell the stories of the people the pandemic touched.

I started informing myself on every aspect of HIV-AIDS, reading the literature and interviewing activists, scientists, and people living with the virus. And I reported the terrible physical and emotional suffering, the extraordinary acts of bravery and charity, and the amazing spiritual transformations I witnessed.

But despite all I knew, I never truly *knew* what I was writing about.

As a gay man, I wasn't a completely detached observer, because HIV-AIDS affected so many people close to me and in my community.

Yet the stories I told were always "their" stories. I could watch and listen and share with readers what I saw and heard. Being HIV-negative myself, though, I had only a limited understanding of even my closest friends' experiences.

Until October 27, 2005, that is. That's the day I found out I have HIV.

Now I'm not just a reporter. Now I'm a reporter living with the same lethal microbe that unleashed so much fear, sorrow, and heroism in the world—and killed so many of my friends.

I am also still a reporter who recognizes an unusual story when I see it. I knew that "Veteran AIDS Reporter Learns He Has It" was such a story. I emailed my editor at the *Washington Post* "Health" section, and shared what I started calling "my news."

"Oh, shit," he replied. That summed it up pretty well. He put me in touch with the *Post*'s "Outlook" section. They wanted the story.

My HIV "coming out" story ran in the *Washington Post*'s Sunday "Outlook" section on May 14, 2006, including a 1991 photo of Bill and me.[1] I never expected that year to mark the twenty-fifth year of the HIV-AIDS pandemic, and the twentieth anniversary of my own first articles on AIDS, by describing how my perspective has shifted, from observer to participant.

The shift took place exactly three weeks after my forty-seventh birthday, on my close and, by then late, friend Rich Rasi's October 27th birthday. My doctor called with the results of the blood work from my annual checkup. For all the years I'd been seeing him, our annual phone call began with pleasantries and the latest readings on cholesterol and such. This time was different. I could tell from the tenseness I sensed in his voice over the phone.

"I have bad news on the HIV test," he said.

I felt the ground fall out from under me. I'd probably written about this in other people's lives hundreds of times—people talking about a time before and a time after their HIV diagnosis.

Now I knew that words—the words I'd wielded like a shield against the reality of what I was seeing, hearing, and reporting—truly can't describe this moment of sickening self-awareness.

I didn't know what to think. It was when I thought of Glenn, the man I was beginning to love—and the thought "now he won't want me" hit me—that I started to cry.

I flashed back to the night I had reported on the protest at President Ronald Reagan's first AIDS speech, in 1987, when he stressed teaching "values" rather than methods of preventing the spread of HIV. That was the night my friend Gregg in Chicago told me he was positive, the night he called himself "damaged goods" that no one would want. All these years later, I felt the real weight of his words descend upon me.

When I went to my doctor's office later that afternoon for more blood work, he advised me that it was pointless to try to pinpoint exactly how "it" had happened; better to focus on dealing with this new reality, he told me. But that reality seemed surreal because I felt so well. I had no warning signs—such as night sweats or swollen lymph nodes—to tell me something was wrong. I had no clue at the time that I was one of the estimated 13 percent of Americans living with HIV who don't know they are infected.[2]

"Suddenly," I wrote in my journal, "it's all as personal as personal gets—my very person, my body, my health, my life, my sense of security, my fears of illness and death." I wrote that, but I was only beginning to grasp it. Part of me was still the dispassionate observer, looking on, writing about somebody else's life.

Then, a week later, I received more shocking news. My tests revealed a relatively low viral load, suggesting a recent infection. But the T-cells, the white blood cells that HIV infects and destroys, were also very low—only 198, compared with 600 to 1,200 in a healthy person.

I knew what that meant. It was a fact I had cited in so many stories. A T-cell count below two hundred indicates a damaged immune system and risk of life-threatening infection. I also knew that the Centers for Disease Control and Prevention (CDC) at the time considered a T-cell count under two hundred an AIDS diagnosis.[3]

I was floored. "This is so 1980s," I said to my doctor. "This isn't supposed to happen to gay men in the U.S. who get tested regularly." I thought that was exactly what I had been doing with each of my annual checkups. It turned out my doctor hadn't tested me for HIV for at least the three previous years. I was frank with him about my sexual behavior, and neither of us considered it particularly risky; perhaps that's the reason he didn't ask for the HIV test, and I didn't ask for one either.

My doctor said to forget all the images of suffering and death I had witnessed because there is effective treatment today. He assured me that living with HIV in 2005 was a very different experience than when Bill was diagnosed in 1986. He said my counts would improve once I began medication—and that if I took it properly, I could expect to lead a healthy, even long, life.

But a parade of faces passed before my mind's eye: once-handsome faces covered with lesions, atop the wasted shells of formerly muscular bodies. I had cried for so many young men as I chronicled their stories. Their stories that were now *my* story.

I recalled the last weeks of Bill's life, when I visited him at the hospital each day after work. I watched as his mind and his life slipped away in April 1994—two years before "combination therapy" and new drugs finally brought hope of living with HIV rather than dying from AIDS. I didn't think any pill could help me manage such a painful memory, or other memories like it, of friends taken by AIDS—Gregg, Ron, Allen, Fred, Bob, Louis, Billy, Eric, Michael, and Jim, to name a few.

I was afraid of the potential side effects of the medication I would now have to take for the rest of my life. I knew they could range from insomnia and diarrhea to much more serious problems, such as diabetes or heart and liver disease. I was terrified of developing the gaunt look—another possible side effect—that Gregg had the last time I saw him alive in 1998.

Despite everything I knew about HIV, I found myself rereading the most basic information, remembering what others with HIV had said about how information is power. This time I used my reporter's ability to ask questions and gather information for the biggest assignment I would ever have: staying alive.

My individual insurance policy limited prescription drug coverage to a mere $1,500 a year; the medications I needed cost $1,700 a month. Now, with a major "preexisting condition," I was locked into this insurance policy, and no other insurance company would cover me. I searched the Internet and emailed friends in Europe looking for lower prices. When I found nothing, I scoured the websites of organizations that serve people with HIV-AIDS, feeling a new gratitude for their work. Suddenly groups such as the National Association of People with AIDS didn't seem like just sources of information for a story, but sources of the kind of hope I badly needed.

I contacted several people I knew from my years of reporting to see what they could suggest about getting the treatment I couldn't afford on my own. Cornelius Baker, former director of D.C.'s Whitman-Walker Clinic, was a friend and someone I had interviewed a number of times. He suggested I look into a clinical trial at Whitman-Walker. I enrolled in a study that would provide regular checkups and free medications for ninety-six weeks.

After only four months of treatment, the medication had already suppressed the virus to the optimal "undetectable" level. My T-cells remained troublingly low. My triglycerides shot through the roof—which meant another pill to treat that particular medication side effect. But the nurses and doctor at Whitman-Walker assured me that my immune system was rebounding.

In March 2006, I asked my doctor for a sleeping pill for the insomnia that had been the main side effect of my meds to that point. I also asked for a referral to a psychiatrist to find out why I was always on the verge of tears. As a medical reporter—and former AIDS training coordinator for the American Psychiatric Association—I was comfortable with the possibility that I could have a psychiatric issue, perhaps an anxiety disorder. I was willing to take medication if necessary. My only objective was to function at my highest level.

The psychiatrist said I didn't need medication. Instead he told me I was feeling sad because my HIV diagnosis had challenged my understanding of who I am, my place in the world, and my sense of where I'm going in life. He said I was suffering, and it's natural to feel sad in the face of suffering. He told me I am extremely resilient. He also told me I was entering an "exciting" time in my life because it offered an opportunity to examine so many things and redefine what I wanted for myself going forward.

I shared my news with close friends, who affirmed my view that HIV should not define me. AIDS had overshadowed my entire adult life and all the years since I came out the summer it first appeared, in 1981. I was determined not to let it *re*-define me as I know myself and present myself to the world. I instinctively eschewed any idea of being a "victim."

Yet the thought of telling my family, particularly my beloved mother, tore me up inside. I felt as though I had let her down in some way. Clearly I wasn't immune to the shame society expected me to feel for having the misfortune of getting HIV.

I have been open with my family for years about being gay, and they have always loved and accepted me. But I am the only son, the oldest child, my two sisters' big brother, my mother's Rock of Gibraltar. Since my father's death in 1989, I felt I had to be the *paterfamilias*, always strong for others. I never learned—in fact I was taught the exact opposite—that it's okay to admit I'm frightened or that I need to be loved. I think this is the biggest reason why I was able to be detached and clinical for so long in reporting on a subject as painful as HIV-AIDS, even as it broke my heart repeatedly.

When I finally shared my news with Mom in April 2006, she said to me, "Be brave, John." I've learned that brave people—like the many I have known and interviewed—are not without fear, but they do the right thing despite their fear. I'm able to be brave, and tell my story, because I have the love and support of family and friends.

I know too well that even approaching four decades into the HIV-AIDS pandemic such openness can still get a person killed in some parts of the world. And I know there are gay men in this country who will resist believing that my story could ever become their own.

I, too, resisted believing the stories I reported would ever become *my* story. I told myself I was smart, cautious, perhaps even "spared" so I could bear witness as a reporter. But my perspective has changed. Now I understand what I've seen and heard from others. And I can only try to make those without firsthand experience understand—not by writing as a detached observer, but by writing straight from the heart.

Two weeks after the article appeared, I was a guest on Tom Ashbrook's National Public Radio *On Point* show marking the twenty-fifth anniversary of the first reported AIDS cases. Ashbrook asked several times how I got infected, "knowing all you do" about HIV. If I could get infected, was there hope for anyone else? he asked.

Alone in the NPR studio inside the Christian Science Church building at the corner of Sixteenth and I streets in downtown Washington, I squirmed. I didn't care to discuss my personal sex life on live national radio. I certainly didn't believe I was responsible for others who got infected. I was also brand new at speaking publicly about having HIV, so didn't have a response thought out ahead of time.

Ashbrook reframed his question a couple of different ways. Finally, one of my fellow guests on the show came to my rescue. Dr. Helene Gayle at the time was executive director of CARE, the global humanitarian organization. She was formerly the director of the Centers for Disease Control and Prevention's national HIV prevention program. I felt intimidated, to say the least, not knowing what she would say. But she simply explained that "knowing" the right thing doesn't mean we always do it.

The next time Ashbrook asked, I simply said I got infected because "I'm human."[4] It seemed hard to make that simple admission. I had to eat my words after saying that men my age who got infected "should have known better." I had to finally admit, at least begin to, that my sexual behavior wasn't *always* 100 percent safe.

Simply acknowledging my own human frailty launched me on a journey that eventually led to writing this book. It set me looking back through my life, sorting through my memories and journals, trying to fathom the challenges and choices that led me to become infected with the deadly virus that had already caused me so much sorrow.

I asked myself many questions: Would I have gotten infected if I hadn't lived in D.C., with its high prevalence of HIV? Would I have made different sexual choices if I had learned from boyhood that I am worthy of love and that I could marry *any*one I love? Would I have been settled down with the man I loved if AIDS hadn't disrupted our relationship when we were so young? How deeply *have* I been affected by watching most of my closest friends die while we were in our twenties and thirties? Why *me*? Why *not* me?

I *never* questioned whether I would take my medications faithfully, go for blood work, see the doctor every few months, and do whatever I had to do to stay healthy and well. I am a survivor, after all.

CHAPTER TWO

~

Survivor

The Roots of My Resilience

I first began to see what I was "made of" in the winter of 1980, during my senior year at Gordon College. I'd had several alarming attacks of intense abdominal pain and profuse sweating during the previous year, beginning one night while I was home in Connecticut on break. I was doubled over in pain, gasping for breath because it hurt to breathe. My parents rushed me to the hospital emergency room. My father practically carried me inside because I was in such pain. The doctors dismissed my mother's suggestion that the problem could be gallstones. Gall bladder problems "only" afflicted overweight middle-age females, they assured her, not slender young males. She'd had her own gall bladder removed two years earlier.

I had another attack while my roommates and I were doing an all-nighter during finals week at the end of winter quarter our senior year. With my arms draped about their shoulders for support, they took me to the emergency room at Beverly Hospital. Hours later I underwent emergency surgery for a ruptured gall bladder.

I spent more than two weeks in the hospital, including several days in the intensive care ward. By the time I was released, I had lost twenty pounds off my then-slender 150-pound, 5'10" frame. I had missed the first week of spring quarter. As senior class president, I was responsible for organizing three major class events in the short few weeks before graduation. I was overloading on my courses and had papers and exams to wrap up the four incomplete classes from winter quarter that my hospitalization forced me to put aside. I was also interviewing for airline flight attendant jobs—inspired by my friend, and unrequited love interest, Jim.

Jim was a few years older than I, and a year ahead of me. He had taken off a couple years between the first and second half of his college career to work as a flight attendant for American Airlines. He looked like an L.L. Bean model: dark blond hair, blue eyes, khakis, and Bass Weejuns. I was drawn even more strongly to the brooding sadness that hung about him. We met during the summer of 1978—after I returned from a choir tour in England and spent a week or so back in Connecticut during Mom's gall bladder surgery—when we both worked on campus, painting dorm rooms to make money for school. I was going into my junior year, and Jim was a senior at the evangelical Christian liberal arts college on Boston's North Shore. Although I wasn't raised in an evangelical tradition, I'd wound up at Gordon College after singing for a couple of years with a group called the New Life Singers in my midteens. We traveled throughout New England performing at a variety of mostly evangelical churches. I'd joined the group mainly as a way to get away from home every weekend, and I enjoyed wonderful times with the group of about twenty-five and the adults who managed the logistics. There was a good deal of "kidding" among some of the guys in the group, myself one of them. I was too terrified to act on it. Homosexuality was an official abomination in this crowd. I learned years later more than one of my male friends had done more than kid about having sex together.

Meanwhile, Jim and I talked about, and wrestled mightily with, what we called "our problem," hoping and praying to end our anguish and guilt for being attracted to our own sex. My own struggle was complicated by the intensity of my feelings for Jim. Although I had plenty of other friends, I only had eyes for Jim. Applying the label *immoral* and *sinful* to the self-immolation I experienced in adoration of Jim was beyond cruel; unrequited love was painful enough. Winning his love became an obsession, almost a contest in which I had to "prove" my own lovability.

Years and repeated heartaches later, therapists would help me understand that I was so attracted to Jim because I was emotionally programmed to try "rescuing" men like him from their sadness and self-loathing. In a real sense I was trying to "rescue" my father—to save him from his own self-destruction. As I did with my father, I tried futilely to "prove" my value, my worthiness of love, by twisting my insides into knots to accommodate the rejection that lay just below the surface of the relationship.

My father had become an alcoholic by his thirties, and, when he was drunk, regularly became angry and violent toward my mother, two sisters, and me. He was funny, easy-going, and loved music when he was sober. But his demons drove him when he drank and vented the pent-up anger I later came to believe he felt about his life. Missed work and lost jobs dimmed the prospects that already were limited for a man with a tenth-grade education. We mostly got along well when he wasn't drunk. One of our closest times was the summer of 1979, when we worked third shift together at a local mill. I don't know any other guys who have had the experience of actually working with their dad. The mill paid me a dollar or two an hour more than they paid Dad because I was a college boy. I didn't understand what that had to do with operating a wire-winding machine, and I didn't tell Dad. For his part, Dad couldn't understand why his son didn't like "normal" boy things like football, and more than once in my growing-up years said I "need to see a psychiatrist."

Mom was the classic enabling wife. She choked back the tears and rolled with the emotional and verbal blows, Dad's latest infidelity or DUI arrest, and even the occasional physical blows, too. She was already used to making do, and doing without, having grown up in what most would consider deprived circumstances during the Great Depression and World War II years. Her family's house in Montville, Connecticut, had no electricity or indoor plumbing. Water was fetched from the outdoor hand pump, and the outhouse was a short walk up a stone path. There was a bucket on the back porch for nighttime necessities. There was no telephone until Mom was old enough to work and pay for it. When I asked Mom how she explained to her friends why her family didn't have these common household conveniences, she told me she didn't; she simply never invited friends to her house. She bought her own clothes at yard sales, but Mom made sure her three kids never lacked for food or Christmas presents—even as Dad's drinking got him fired from jobs, and he drank away his pay when he had one. For thirty-seven years, she punched in at 6 a.m. to work in a cafeteria until retiring at age seventy. Along the way she gave each of her children down payments for their homes and saved for her own retirement, too. In our home state of Connecticut—nicknamed "the land of steady habits"—one of Mom's steadiest habits, unfortunately for me, was to use emasculating shame to "harden" her son to be the caregiver who "never complains," just like her.

I was trained at a young age to stuff away my feelings, needs, and pain, to be "strong" and take care of everyone else—just like Mom. I was cast in the role of the "good child" who is never believed to need anything because he simply doesn't talk about it, exactly as he's been trained. Being told at age ten or eleven you are the "man of the house" while Dad is in jail for another DUI (or was it domestic violence that time?) doesn't leave a boy much room to enjoy being a boy. It certainly didn't provide *this* boy with a healthy and responsible male role model.

As if things at home weren't unpredictable enough, there were the bullies at my junior high school bus stop. Sissy. Fag. Queer. I heard it all, like so many other gay kids. I didn't understand as a thirteen-year-old the "difference" about me those boys picked up on. They didn't know about the sex play I had engaged in with the boys next door when I was an eight- to twelve-year-old kid living in "the project," the World War II–era housing development we lived in during my elementary school years in Groton, Connecticut. I never saw it as "abuse"—even if the oldest boy was five years older than I. I always saw it, still do, as just a part of our friendship, along with our hikes to Bluff Point, on Long Island Sound, and neighborhood kickball, baseball, football, and foursquare games. Besides, I enjoyed it a lot. I took the bullies' insults, name-calling, and spitting with a strained smile. I didn't know how, exactly, but I knew I was going to make something of myself that would "show them." I certainly did not tell my parents; I felt ashamed of *myself* for being bullied. I was sure it *must* have been my fault because I was the oddball kid—odd, that is, if the norm is poor, white trash boys from a low-income housing project.

I spent a lot of my free time in my early teens reading books, hiking in the woods behind our house with an axe and my camera, and imagining other lives; anything to escape the unpredictability and unhappiness at home. I sought solitude because I could be alone with my thoughts of brighter possibilities. Left to myself I was a happy kid with a powerful curiosity and vivid imagination, and the joyful spirit I inherited (ironically) from my dad. But it seemed others around me, including my own parents, were determined to pull me into their unhappiness.

By the time I turned eighteen during my freshman year of college, I had gotten away from my bullies, my family, and the decaying old mill town where my father and his parents had grown up. I wanted to escape, and thought of it as exactly that, an escape from a place, people, holding me back from the life I wanted. I felt something compelling me—to "better" myself, see the world, and live a bigger life than I would have had in Norwich.

I didn't think about it in terms of survival, but in fact I had already survived a great deal of trauma even before that all-but-overwhelming spring of 1980, when I was only twenty-one years old.

Besides my medical crisis, massive academic workload, class responsibilities, and out-of-state interviews for airline jobs, I had a constant inner ache over Jim's lack of interest in me. "What is wrong with *me?*" I wanted to know. On top of it all, I was becoming friendly again with my closeted professor. He had taken a shine to me my junior year after I revealed to him I was in love with Jim. Married to a woman, father of two, and a nationally known speaker in evangelical circles, he invited me to accompany him to church services and, eventually, a ski trip for two in New Hampshire. That was the first time he came on to me sexually. I didn't want sex with him; I really just wanted an older man to care for me.

He was quiet the morning after he climbed in bed with me on that ski trip. For the next several months guilt cooled his ardor and there were no more invitations. Later I would recognize that he had "groomed" me for seduction and abused my trust. At the time I was a very innocent young man basking in the attention of a man my father's age who showed interest in what I think and feel. Much later I would also learn I was only one of his conquests at our evangelical college, where homosexuality was grounds for expulsion *and* condemnation to hellfire. At the time I was simply confused and sad that another man I trusted had abandoned me.

Somehow, despite what felt like a cosmic pig-pile-on-John, I completed all the work for my nine courses, planned and executed the senior class events, and survived a "no confidence" vote after some student government association leaders tried to force me to resign as class president, allegedly for missed meetings. I even landed the job I wanted, and left for Dallas a week after graduation to train as a flight attendant for American Airlines, following in Jim's footsteps and one of my few classmates who had a job lined up after graduation.

"My last term at Gordon," I reflected in my journal the following year, "is, to me, probably my greatest (and most strenuously attained) achievement to date." After the extraordinary ordeal of my last few months of college, I felt my efforts to meet and rise above my challenges "really do, I think, speak for themselves."

Learning to speak for *myself*, to tell the world "this is me and I am happy about it," would prove to be an even greater achievement.

CHAPTER THREE

∼

Normal

My Gay Liberation

I called Allen Satterfield one evening in November 1980, after returning home from Manhattan on the Long Island Rail Road to Greenvale, Long Island. Allen was a friend of my closeted professor, who had lived in New York years earlier. He co-owned a prospering fabric and wallpaper company in the Decoration and Design Building on the Upper East Side, diagonally across Lexington Avenue from Bloomingdales, his favorite store. He was a season subscriber to the Metropolitan Opera, and a firm believer in the power of ball fringe and chintz to cover a multitude of decorating faux pas.

A friend of Jim's family had helped me get a clerical job at Merrill Lynch at One Liberty Plaza, after American Airlines furloughed me and the hundreds of other new flight attendants hired for what turned out to be a summer job. For eight months I commuted into the city early in the morning, took the A train from Penn Station to the World Trade Center, and hated my dreary job. Over those months I spent many weekends at Allen's duplex on Barrow Street, in the West Village.

With brown hair going to gray and the gracious manners of his southern upbringing, Allen was a mature and civilized guide to a magical world I had only imagined—and couldn't afford on my $12,000 salary: Broadway shows. Brunches. Dinners in "gay" restaurants. Allen's friends were other upscale gay men who owned nice condos in Manhattan, rented or owned houses on Fire Island in the summer, traveled to Rio in the winter, and regularly visited the Mineshaft, the everything-goes BDSM bar and sex club in the Meatpacking District.

Allen was a romantic. He didn't go with his friends to the Mineshaft. Instead we went to church together, at St. Mary the Virgin ("Smoky Mary's") in Times Square and Grace Church on lower Broadway. He read to me from Edna St. Vincent Millay's poetry, and wrote his own poems for me. Although I didn't share his romantic interest, I would be forever grateful to Allen for giving me a tremendous gift I would come to value far more than the snow-white sweater from Bloomingdales he gave me for Christmas. He showed me for the first time, up close and over time, what a gay man looks like who believes he isn't broken. The stepson of an Episcopalian priest lived out his integrity before my eyes. Not only that, but he told me in a letter that he believed I had "everything anyone could want"—the first time anyone had said something like that to me.

I didn't immediately recognize the value of Allen's gift. I resisted the idea that I was gay and had no chance for a family—the prevailing experience of "out" gay men at the time. I felt a strong desire to become a father. I also asked myself, "Am I condemned to a life of celibacy and restraint?" After all, the church declared—and my closeted professor admonished me, despite his own hypocrisy—that there were only two options for homosexuals: celibacy or marriage to a woman, and likely celibacy there too. Were there other options I hadn't yet seen?

Three days in Provincetown, Massachusetts, August 10 to 12, 1981, answered *that* question.

I moved from New York to Boston in June 1981, still working for Merrill Lynch. Boston was the first major city I got to know while I was in college, and I was happy to be living there after a year in New York. In my first overnight visit to Provincetown, just across Cape Cod Bay by ferry from Boston, I found an entire town, at the tip of the Cape, full of men who were gay and seemed unabashedly happy about it.

Foggy mornings at The Captain and His Ship, our charming and impeccably restored Victorian guesthouse on Commercial Street, stand out among my memories of that trip. "It seemed that we, all the guests, would rise at the same time, around eight in the morning," I wrote in my journal. "Speaking in hushed tones, sipping the coffee provided by our hosts, we chatted mostly about our homes and what we did. Being gay, for the first time in my life, was not an 'issue,' it was an assumption."

In the decades since, I have always said my coming out as a gay man was about wanting to preserve the feeling I had in Provincetown on those August mornings in 1981. That's when I felt normal for the first time in my life.

"My vacation has been quite an inundation of gayness, of homosexuals, and homosexuality," I wrote in my journal on the evening of Tuesday, August 11, 1981.

I would only realize in 2016, as I connected the dates in writing this book, that even as I was writing those words in P-town that evening three and a half decades ago, the writer Larry Kramer was hosting the world's first AIDS fundraiser at his Manhattan apartment. A July 3 *New York Times* article, "Rare Cancer Seen in 41 Homosexuals," had alerted those paying attention that something frightening was beginning to unfold, the deadly epidemic the Reagan administration a year later would declare "the greatest health threat of our time."

For this moment, at the plague's start—the beginning and end of my own innocence, as it would turn out—my gay liberation was filled with relief and revelry. I felt like a man freed from prison for a crime he did not commit. On the dance floor at the Boatslip in P-town I danced like a maniac to Kelly Marie's big hit "Feels Like I'm in Love." That's exactly how I felt! Because I always have a song to capture a mood, Joey Scarbury's "Believe It Or Not," peaking at number-two the week I was in P-town, gave words and melody to the exuberance rising in me. "I never thought I could feel so free," I sang along at the top of my lungs when I didn't think anyone could hear me. "Flying away on a wing and a prayer, who could it be? Believe it or not it's just me."

Even after accepting my homosexuality, bigger issues remained: What did I really believe about God? Love? How could I have a healthy relationship with my family? How did being gay fit in with the other things about me that also give me a sense of identity—including my education, my faith, and my strong sense of being a New Englander? What would I do for a career? What happens when I get old?

A college friend had chided me our senior year about how I have always created an image in my mind of what I want to do or be, and then set about making it real. I expect it goes back to my years of hiking the woods by myself, snapping photos of trees and sunsets, trying to picture a better future. It turns out that "visioning" is actually a powerful tool to shape one's future, but I am getting ahead of myself. At the time I had no vision to guide me about what kind of gay man I would be. I knew I didn't feel comfortable in Allen's social circle. What were the possibilities? Where did *I* fit into the gay world?

And what about sex? Not long before P-town, I wrote in my journal about living in downtown Boston. "I find my head revolving and my heart doing somersaults as I pass these kindred faces on the streets. I feel such a desire to have one of those faces smile at me with a smile that says, 'I like you. I find you attractive. Can I get to know you?' And how I want to say 'Yes. Yes. YES!!'" After P-town, and before I knew it, I was saying yes to a *lot* of men. In a city full of college-age men, I was a twenty-three-year-old kid in a candy store. I was a regular at the dance club Buddies near Copley Square. I inherited my father's love of music and dancing, and had been going to dance clubs since they were actually called "discos" in the 1970s. Now I not only went to dance but also frequently left with a "date." I quickly discovered that, besides good dance moves, a young man's cute face and other prized physical attributes are hot commodities in the gay world.

Directly across Boylston Street from my apartment, I found another aspect of gay life I didn't know existed. The Fens is a lush park that encompasses both the Boston Victory Gardens and the tall, dense reeds along the edge of the narrow, aptly named Muddy River. At night, it becomes the most popular gay cruising area east of Central Park's Rambles. Until I saw it with my own eyes, I had no idea there were such places, outdoor places, where men—strangers—meet to have sex together. I was actually quite innocent and unaware of such things while I was wrestling with my sexuality at an evangelical college.

The curious part of me found the Fens utterly fascinating. The pleasure-loving part of me loved the rush of outdoor sex in the dark, and the abundance of attractive and willing young partners. A year after my first visit to the Fens, my vow of "no casual sex" long since broken, I wrote in my journal, "I have been frequenting the Fens at night lately, becoming a veritable 'regular' there." I continued, "It is habitual, addicting." It troubled me that I was so drawn to the anonymous sex in the Fens. I hadn't yet figured out why it seemed so strongly compelling to me—besides the obvious: the masculine thrill of the hunt and sheer carnal pleasure.

Of course my coming out wasn't *only* about sex; it was at least as much an intellectual and spiritual transformation. John Boswell's National Book Award–winning *Christianity, Social Tolerance, and Homosexuality* came out in 1980, the year before I did. It became the intellectual springboard for reconceptualizing my faith. Citing documents in their original languages, the gay Catholic Yale historian who read and spoke seventeen languages demonstrated how antigay prejudice had become Catholic Church dogma when the homophobes took power.[1]

A lapsed Catholic who'd come by way of evangelicalism to the Episcopal Church, when I attended church, I could no longer accept religious condemnation of homosexuality as anything more than prejudice. "Sanctity isn't the denial of things we are afraid of," I wrote in my journal. I also noted the scripture verse saying that we must each work out our own salvation. It seemed clear to me that meant figuring out how to live out our faith through our own unique experience.

It was apparent I had changed when I went to confession at the Church of the Advent, the Anglo-Catholic ("high-church" Episcopalian) parish at the foot of Beacon Hill I attended at the time. I hadn't been to confession since I stopped attending the Catholic Church I was raised in. "I didn't mention anything about my being gay or the fact that I have had sex with men," I wrote afterward in my journal. I didn't feel guilty about it, so didn't consider it worth confessing. I did, however, feel guilty about exploiting men for my own pleasure.

I was certainly on the receiving end of exploitation and manipulation, too. I quickly realized the men I was meeting in the bars expected sex and emotion to remain separate; expressing more than desire could lead to being labeled "needy." It was a hard lesson for someone who tends to engage and connect with people. It hurt deeply to realize I was being reduced to nothing more than "dick." It also hurt, when I thought about it, as I did at confession, to realize I too was learning to treat other guys as little more than living sex toys. The posture I tried to project was to feign apathy, not show feelings that suggested I was interested in someone or that I was hurt by his detachment. I thought a cynical, nonchalant attitude might shield my easily bruised heart. Growing up with the need to hide tender feelings because it was unsafe to be vulnerable, I had plenty of experience wearing this particular mask.

But a phone call from Allen Satterfield brought me up short. He gave me one of what I called his "wonderful little sermonettes" after I told him I was starting to date a guy named Danny, and I didn't know how to handle it because I had never dated a guy. He told me not to rush into anything, but at the same time not to shut myself off to the possibility of a relationship before giving it a chance. He said he wished he had real relationships to remember, rather than a blur of sexual experiences. He reminded me that playing the field too much may leave you, finally, alone—just like Malone, the protagonist of Andrew Holleran's 1978 novel *Dancer from the Dance*. Allen had given me the book as part of my education in being a gay man. Clearly he intended it to be a cautionary tale.

CHAPTER FOUR

~

Destiny Calling

How a Lonely Boy Became a Professional Outsider

Like so many college graduates today, I started my adult life thousands of dollars in student loan debt because I had to pay for everything myself. I was the only person in my immediate family to go to college. Loans, grants, work-study, I did whatever I had to do because I saw my education as the ticket to the life I wanted.

A year after I graduated, a major car repair bill charged to my Amex card, without having enough money to pay it all off at once, was a rude first lesson on how easily derailed are the best intentions to live within a budget. But then no one had taught me how to manage, let alone make, money. I didn't acquire those skills in my family where conversations about money revolved around "how expensive everything is," and my parents regularly argued about their own unending financial worries.

Moving among urban gay men with nice apartments and summer beach house shares, I suddenly felt I "needed" at least a smart new shirt for each party I was invited to. Then there were the colognes, skin creams, sweaters, and shoes. Fancy stores my family never shopped in, that intimidated me at first, became regular stops. Jordan Marsh. Filene. Brooks Brothers.

I didn't understand then that credit card companies, and our materialist culture, thrive on people like me—people ashamed to have grown up poor, wanting to give the appearance of prosperity; those who don't have a proper sense of our value apart from our appearance, clothing, and other possessions.

Living beyond my means caught up with me pretty fast. I started falling behind on the credit card payments. Financial worry was now a regular part of my life, depressing me and undermining my self-confidence. "I feel over-whelmed with anxiety about finances," I wrote at the beginning of 1983. "I find myself incapable even of saying 'I love you' to Arthur," I wrote of the boyfriend with whom I had moved into an apartment on Union Park only two months to the day after we met at the Napoleon Club. "I feel that saying it seems to express a kind of 'need' love, a dependence on his strength . . . I don't feel terribly good about myself right now."

In a similar frame of mind a few months later, I realized it had been during earlier anxious times like this that I became sexually hyperactive, picking up guys at bars, cruising the Fens. "I transferred my feelings of inadequacy into a physical sphere," I wrote in my journal, "and attempted to validate my *self* by having my physical/sexual appeal and attractiveness affirmed. All the nights in the Fens, for instance. There was much more to my behavior than mere sexual desire. It was more the symptom than the actual cause of my actions."

I came out to my mother on Easter Sunday of 1983, when she and my sister Sue and Sue's boyfriend visited me in Boston. Mom said she suspected I was gay since I stopped dating girls. She also said she just wanted me to be happy. It was just one example of Mom's amazing generosity. Not long afterward, my parents' divorce became final. Nearly twenty-five years of sepa-rations and reconciliations done. I was relieved to be out to Mom, but now I also had to deal with sadness over my parents' divorce. That was just the stuff in my head. Then there were the graduate-level writing and publishing classes I was taking at Emerson College, my full-time waitering job at Ciro & Sal's restaurant, and escalating tensions at home with Arthur. He wanted to see other guys; I wanted to be a couple. One night we'd lie in bed, arms and legs entwined, singing love songs to each other. The next night it was tears and separate rooms. My stomach was in constant knots. I don't think it was coincidental I smoked pot for the first time that summer.

I escaped the tension for a few days that July, joining Allen Satterfield for a visit to Fire Island. I indulged in all the fun the Pines offered in 1983: swimming and sunning at the spectacular beach, dancing until dawn at The Pavilion, gourmet dinners prepared by the men in the house Allen was shar-ing, strolling through the "meat rack," and even a late-night hook-up with Paul, the tall, handsome, blond houseboy across the walkway.

I was able, on a surface level anyway, to fit in. I had started working out at the time Arthur and I moved in together in the fall of 1982, and my gym-toned body was among the many like it at Fire Island. But even as I participated, I also felt detached. One moment I blended in with the other attractive young men on the beach or at the Botel tea dance. The next mo-ment I'd sit back with my arms crossed and a puzzled look as I attempted to understand the self-consciousness of gay beauty, the "attitude," vanity, and hedonism. "As much as I might feel in it," I wrote as I lounged naked by the pool, "I never fully feel 'of' it. I am perpetually aware of there being something more out there, some voice speaking in the waves that crash around my tanned, virile body."

Could that voice have been my destiny calling? Telling me to prepare for the life of a perpetual, professional "observer" and outsider?

It surely felt like it a few months later as magazine editors began to echo the compliments on my writing I'd had from a couple of my college professors, particularly the closeted one. "Wonderful news!" I wrote in my journal on November 8, 1983. "I got a phone call yesterday afternoon from Mark Thompson, at the *Advocate*; they're going to publish my review of [a new translation, by Richard Howard, of Andre Gide's] *Corydon*. I just about hit the ceiling I was so elated. At last, I break into print! And for money! Dear GOD!"

My first published articles lifted my spirits and boosted my self-esteem. They "proved" to me that my faith in my writing talent was well founded. A door was opening at last to see myself as possessing value beyond the physical qualities that attracted men and got me the attention I craved. A few visits with a therapist also "helped me to begin, at last, to assess my 'true worth,' so to speak," I wrote in my journal. I decided the Emerson writing and publishing program wouldn't provide the launch pad I needed for the career I envisioned, so I applied to the country's top journalism schools and chose Northwestern University's Medill School of Journalism. I would begin my master's program in January 1985.

While I waited to start, I arranged an internship in the newsroom of the *Christian Science Monitor* to get some practical experience, and continued waiting tables at Ciro & Sal's. "I'm feeling something akin to elation," I wrote in April 1984. "I am so busy, so occupied, that I have little time to sit and think about how lonely I might, on occasion, feel."

Not even a Memorial Day weekend gay-bashing attack, in Provincetown of all places, could deter me. I required surgery to repair a fractured eye socket after my seventeen-year-old assailant punched me, hard, in the face on a jam-packed street outside the A-House. I pursued my basher in court for the next six months, driving and taking buses back to the Cape to serve as a state's witness against him. I was uncomfortable discussing my sexual orientation publicly for the first time, but I was determined to counteract my basher's brutality with my own civility by pressing as hard as the law would allow for him to be justly punished.

I was proud of myself for having the integrity to be honest and stand up for myself, even when it meant acknowledging that I was gay in a public courtroom. My courage was bolstered by Rich Rasi, my friend and roommate that last year in Boston. Rich was a Melkite (Eastern Catholic) priest and psychologist I met at the Napoleon Club in the fall of 1980, after my layoff from American Airlines, when I lived briefly in Marblehead, Massachusetts. The night of my attack, Rich arranged for friends of his in Hyannis to pick me up at Cape Cod Hospital and let me stay overnight at their house until he could drive down from Boston to get me the next day. Ultimately, I agreed to settle the case for the cost of my medical bills after my attacker appealed the judge's guilty verdict to a jury. The trial date was set for the same day I was starting at Northwestern. I was not about to miss the first day of my future.

As I turned twenty-six that October, I took stock and looked ahead. In two months I would leave Boston—the city "where I grew up," as I thought of it—for a new adventure in another big city, Chicago. Counting the days until I left, an unexpected phone call one evening confirmed the good choice I had made to pursue a writing career.

"Hello, John? This is Armistead Maupin."

The *Tales of the City* author was calling me! We'd had coffee and an interview in Boston earlier that fall after he read from the series' newest installment, *Babycakes*, which I was reviewing for the *Advocate*.

"Somehow," I wrote in my journal, "I managed to sound casual and calm, but I was thrilled." He was calling me, from San Francisco, to tell me how much he had appreciated my favorable review in the *Advocate*. He told me that I write very well. I gallantly accepted his compliment. "Well, thank you!" I said. We chatted a bit, and I told him I was moving to Chicago to do a master's degree in journalism. "You definitely have a career ahead of you," he said, again praising my writing. He gave me his address and phone number in San Francisco, and offered to show me around if I found myself in the city some time.

My journal reminds me that after I hung up the phone, "I screamed and jumped around, shouting, 'I can't believe it! I can't believe he called!'" I was so eager to tell someone. I tried phoning Mom, but no answer. I couldn't think of any of my friends who'd be as excited as I, so I calmed myself down as best I could until Rich came home. He was about as excited as I was. I went out and bought a bottle of champagne to share with Rich and celebrate what I expected to be "only the beginning."

That is how good it felt to be encouraged by a man I admired for something about myself that *I* greatly valued.

CHAPTER FIVE

~

The End of Innocence

How AIDS Became My "Beat"

I had been in Chicago only a few months when a letter in May 1985 from my former beau Arthur brought the shocking news that our mutual friend Michael, in New York, had died from AIDS four months earlier, around the time I left Boston. Michael was twenty-five years old. I had last spoken with him the previous summer, after my P-town bashing.

Less than a week later I had a call from Frank, the sexy Italian American podiatry student from Boston's North End with whom I had enjoyed a number of good times since we met at Carol's Speakeasy. He wasn't calling this time to arrange a hook-up. Instead he told me a mutual friend of ours in Boston had recently died from AIDS, thirty-year-old Jim.

AIDS was now real for me. I was twenty-six years old.

I walked the streets of Evanston, glad for the sunglasses that hid my tears. I pictured my dead friends: walking with Michael in Manhattan, proud to be seen with such a tall, handsome, brilliant man, chatting about German philosophy. Riding the swan boats in Boston with Jim only months before I left the city.

I was scared, too. I had slept with both Michael and Jim. Like many gay men's friendships, ours had included a sexual phase at the start, before we settled on being friends. I tried to recall precisely what I had done with each of them. I had once bottomed for Michael without a condom.

Even as I absorbed the news of my friends' deaths, I was reviewing for the *Advocate* Paul Reed's novel *Facing It*, the first novel ever to address AIDS. In that summer of 1985, one of the epidemic's darkest years, screaming magazine covers fanned America's hysteria. *Newsweek*'s blood-red cover featured an image of actor Rock Hudson's AIDS-ravaged face. *LIFE*'s cover proclaimed, "Now No One Is Safe from AIDS."

I began to think about what my role as a journalist could be, how I could help. My professors at Medill told me I was "well on my way" as a writer. So *which* way to go? "What can I *do?*" I wondered in my journal. "Somehow it doesn't seem adequate to simply grieve for my dead friends. Some kind of action seems in order."

I arrived in Washington, D.C., in mid-September, to spend the fall quarter as a "real" reporter for Medill News Service, the journalism school's news bureau staffed by graduate journalism students. Beyond my career, I pondered three things that fall. I wanted to come back East after I finished at Northwestern. I wanted to fall in love. And on a grander, but deeper, scale, I also wanted to find a noble cause to give my life meaning and purpose.

Then I met Bill Bailey, and it all seemed to come together in one handsome, blue-eyed package. "He's bright," I wrote in my journal a few days after we met Sunday night, November 3, 1985. "He's attractive. He's hot in bed. He seems gentle-spirited. And he seems very interested in me." I had never known a man as passionate about anything as Bill was about AIDS. He volunteered as a "buddy" with D.C.'s Whitman-Walker Clinic, helping out a gay African American man living with AIDS, and with his family, in the predominantly black Anacostia area of the city. He made it clear he thought it was my duty, as a gay man who was also a journalist, to use my skills to chronicle our community's suffering and valiant efforts to address the epidemic.

I had to return to Chicago in January 1986 for my final quarter at Northwestern. Bill and I kept the U.S. Postal Service busy that winter, sending cards and letters between Chicago and Washington overflowing with mutual professions of love. We cheered each other on, shared our dreams of finding a mission and purpose in life, and confided our insecurities. "I believe in you, Bill," I wrote in a letter on the twenty-fourth. "I believe that with your sense of compassion and justice, and with your smooth, confident style and eloquence, you will be an invaluable asset to gay people—and, by extension, to all people—who are now, by quirk of birth and nature, disenfranchised by our American society. You are a gifted man, my love, and I think you'll use your gifts well."

I put aside my fear of being hurt and trusted in Bill, and in love. Within days after I turned in my last papers at Medill in March, I loaded up a rental car with my recently acquired Russian Blue cat Misha and all my worldly possessions, minus the twenty boxes I had already shipped ahead on Amtrak.

Driving out of Chicago I aimed in a southeasterly direction. Even after being stopped by a state trooper for speeding across the cornfields of Indiana, I was determined to sleep with Bill in Washington that night.

Bill broke up with me four days after I arrived. For another month, as I "temped," looked for a job, and saved money for my own place while staying with Bill, I felt as though I was repeating the painful summer of 1983 with Arthur. We slept together one night; the next night Bill didn't want to be with me. It tore me apart inside. When I could finally afford my own apartment, I moved into the English basement in D.C.'s Mount Pleasant neighborhood where I would live for the next five years.

Bill called me at 11:30 Tuesday night, July 1, 1986, to tell me his doctor had diagnosed him as having swollen lymph nodes. It was potentially nothing serious. But it was also potentially very serious, deadly serious, because lymphadenopathy was often a precursor of developing AIDS. Bill had been sick a few times in the spring. He was going to get tested the following week to see if he had the virus.

He was positive. The man I loved, in spite of his ambivalence about "us," had AIDS, the hunky, confident man who curled up in my arms like a baby as I sat on his red butterfly chair, asking if I would protect him when he got scared. We both knew that in 1986, with no effective treatment, it would be only a matter of time until Bill got sick and then died. "I want him to *live!*" I wrote in my journal. "And I want to live, too. My God, that young men like us should even have to think of things this awful."

I spent August doing interviews for my first major feature article on AIDS, one of the first articles anywhere to explore the subject of "gay bereavement." I spoke with men whose partners had died from AIDS, bereavement therapists, behavioral scientists, and even the only funeral director in D.C. at the time who would accept the remains of people who had died from AIDS.

After returning from an interview with a man whose partner of twenty-four years had died New Year's Eve, I hurried home because Bill was supposed to call. I found a voicemail message from him saying we shouldn't be in touch.

By the time "The Survivors" ran on the cover of *Washington City Paper* at the end of September, Bill and I were back together again. But Bill had changed. Only two months after his diagnosis, the rather closeted "socially liberal, fiscally conservative" Republican U-VA good old boy had plunged into AIDS full time. Besides his volunteer work, Bill threw himself into his new job as a lobbyist for the American Psychological Association. He focused his passion on pushing the federal government to engage psychologists' behavioral expertise in creating effective HIV-AIDS prevention interventions.

Bill Bailey had found the mission he wanted, the brilliant, though tragically brief, destiny he was made for.

I wasn't nearly as enthusiastic about focusing so exclusively on AIDS. I was emotionally wrung out after writing "The Survivors." Even before it, I was already in enough pain from losing my friends the year before and living with the reality of Bill's diagnosis. Allen Satterfield was diagnosed with AIDS that September, too. I told Bill I couldn't live and breathe AIDS twenty-four hours a day. "I can't bear this constant confrontation with death and illness," I wrote in my journal. "There's so much more to life, to my life, and I refuse to be that consumed with the issue."

But the accumulated injustices against gay men that I witnessed, together with the grief I felt for my friends' and my community's losses, began to fuel a growing activist spirit in me. I was moving beyond simply reporting on HIV-AIDS as a journalist, viewing my role as not merely a reporter but also as an advocate and educator as I shared with others what I learned and observed.

Bill and I continued our push-pull for the next year. Round and round we'd go with the breakups and reconciliations. But something happened to *me* during one of our breakups in early 1987. I'd already been seeing a therapist—Paul Van Ness, the psychologist who led the gay men's bereavement group I described in "The Survivors." I was determined to stand on my own apart from Bill, and not get sucked back into our tangled web of love and rejection, the pattern of my relationships with men that began with my father.

I finally read the book another psychologist, my friend Rich Rasi, had given me. *Adult Children of Alcoholics*,[1] by Janet Geringer Woititz, changed my life. I had never read such an accurate description of my family and childhood. Now I finally began to understand how my family history was undermining me. For the first time I found assurance that my instincts about people were actually quite astute, but that I had been conditioned from childhood not to trust my own gut when it warned me of emotional turmoil to come.

I read more books. I joined an Al-Anon group specifically for adult children of alcoholics, and got a sponsor. I used Al-Anon's *One Day at a Time* daily readings as affirmations. I came to understand that I was a classic "enabler," precisely what Mom had conditioned me to be. I allowed myself to be treated like someone who doesn't matter, mistreated because I essentially didn't value myself enough to insist on better, or to leave the relationship. I also learned to use "self-talk," the voice in my own mind, to help reframe the story I tell myself about my experiences—especially the challenging ones.

All this introspection was far from my mind as I reported for *Washington City Paper* on the Third International AIDS Conference, held in D.C., during the first week of June 1987. In "AIDSweek" I described the protests outside the tent in Georgetown where President Reagan gave his first speech on AIDS at an AmFar fundraiser, the first national protests by ACT UP, the mass arrest of LGBT community leaders in front of the White House by D.C. police wearing rubber gloves, the scientific presentations inside the conference, and the colorful HIV-AIDS educational posters and other paraphernalia in the exhibit hall.

It all hit home for me that day. I recalled my friend Gregg in Chicago, terrified of losing his dental practice and the lover he was devoted to, calling himself "damaged goods." I'd spoken earlier in the day with Allen Satterfield in New York. He was blind from Cytomegalovirus (CMV) and undergoing chemotherapy to treat the Kaposi's sarcoma in his throat.

Even more intimately, I reflected on how it felt to talk with Bill, who was also attending the conference. We were "off" at the moment. "Hearing the angry shouts," I wrote in the newspaper, "considering all I'd heard in symposia that day about gay sexuality and seropositivity, I looked at the man who had shared my bed for a year and a half, and remembered the fear and pain we'd borne together. I realized again how personal an issue AIDS really is."[2]

CHAPTER SIX

~

Tribulations

Perpetual Grief Fuels My Budding Activism (and Self-Defeating Sexual Behavior)

A phone call from New York on July 11, 1987, brought the expected, dreaded news: Allen was dead. His friend Alfie told me that he and Allen's family were by Allen's side when he died. The first man to show me how to live with dignity and integrity as a gay man was gone. He is buried in the graveyard of St. John's Church in Hampton, Virginia. I weep three decades later as I read what I wrote in my journal the day Alfie called: "I hope my life and my attempts to contribute energy and talent to helping us all through this goddamned AIDS crisis, and my attempts at being honest and expressing love to others, will be an appropriate tribute to Allen's memory."

All too soon that same summer I was stunned by the strong likelihood of an even more singular loss when my father was diagnosed with throat cancer. After undergoing a laryngectomy to remove his damaged voice box, he amazed even his doctors by how quickly he learned esophageal speech, a way for laryngectomees (as survivors of the operation are known) to "speak" by inhaling air into the esophagus and controlling its release to produce sound.

Even cancer and radical surgery couldn't defeat Dad's strong Greek spirit.

Spirits and anger were both riding high a few months later, during the National March on Washington for Lesbian and Gay Rights and the first national display of the AIDS Memorial Quilt, on Sunday, October 11, 1987. It was an extraordinary experience—from the powerful sensation of openly venting anger at the Reagan administration for its neglect of AIDS as we marched down Pennsylvania Avenue, to the pain and pride of seeing very ill gay men with AIDS in wheelchairs leading the parade, to the shock and sorrow of seeing all those coffin-size quilt panels laid out on the Mall.

The activist spirit burned in me that fall. "I find myself feeling very proud to be part of the gay community," I wrote in my journal just before the march, "as I've seen the charity and sheer love gay people have shown one another, taking care of one another in this horrible AIDS crisis." Not long after the march I began volunteering as a writer for the National Gay and Lesbian Task Force (NGLTF) newsletter. I was also interviewing mothers and fathers of gay men and lesbians for an article about parents of LGBT children for the *Advocate*.

Bill and I couldn't stay away from each other. A tearful phone conversation at the end of the march day sparked the last big flare-up of our romance. But it was doomed to fail because Bill wanted me to be the strong, stoic man he could lean on without being held too close—precisely the familiar role I was determined *not* to play—and I wanted equity, for the two of us to be both strong *and* vulnerable, as warranted by whatever each of us needed from the other.

After a magical holiday season together, and just after the New Year in 1988, Bill and I agreed we should no longer be a couple. I felt sad that we loved each other, and were so strongly attracted to each other, yet couldn't make it work. But I also felt a great sense of relief, as though a weight had been lifted off me.

Much too soon afterward, I had a new boyfriend. Scott and I met in Boston when I was there the day after Christmas to shop. I was still "with" Bill, but I reasoned that we were probably on our way out again, and, well, Scott's dark hair and eyes, and warm, winning personality grabbed my interest pretty fast. He made me laugh, something I had not done so freely during my time with Bill. After three months of back-and-forth visits, Scott was sharing my apartment in Washington after landing a job with a D.C. law firm.

I also had a new job, as the writer and publicist for the National AIDS Network, a sort of trade association that provided "TA" (technical assistance) to community-based AIDS service organizations across the country. I interviewed and wrote stories about men and women doing pioneering work in those early years of the epidemic to care for people living with HIV and prevent new infections. My journalist's soul and youthful energy fueled my work. I felt proud that I had skills that were helpful both for my community *and* my country's efforts to address the epidemic.

I was extremely anxious when Scott and I each had our first-ever HIV antibody test in June 1988. We both tested negative. I knew I'd had unprotected sex, as both top and bottom—even with Bill *after* he tested positive.

To celebrate our good news, we bought a bottle of Dom Perignon, "only" fifty-eight dollars at the time, and enjoyed a romantic dinner at Tout Va Bien, an aptly named French bistro in Georgetown.

But our relationship wasn't going well. The fact is I wasn't ready for another serious relationship after the emotional roller-coaster ride I'd had with Bill, I was frightened of losing myself. But instead of acting wisely and heeding Rich Rasi's advice to stay single, I tried to allay my fear in the most self-defeating ways while I was with Scott, causing both of us tremendous grief. He found out soon enough about my "dalliances" with men in the YMCA steam room. Sex was easy enough to explain; so much of it goes on in such places. But how to explain my own rationalization of these infidelities (we had agreed to be monogamous) as "necessary" to keep myself distanced from Scott? Somehow it made sense to me that keeping a kind of "reserve" sex life meant I wouldn't lose myself in the relationship or be devastated if it didn't work out. And what man, gay or otherwise, is going to admit he seeks out sex to feel better about himself?

The relationship limped along into the fall with recriminations and a stifled feeling that I should have ended it sooner. As unhappy as I was, though, I still left it to Scott to break it off. I could feel like a victim that way, didn't have to take responsibility for my feelings. It was a familiar role at the time.

Even as I tried to move on and nurture a healthy self-image, Dad's health deteriorated. When I arrived home from an ACOA meeting at 8:20 p.m. on Tuesday, January 17, 1989, there was a message from Mom on the answering machine. Call her by 8:30. She said the doctor told Dad he had at most another month to live. The cancer was spreading rapidly, and there was nothing more they could do for him other than give him morphine to ease the pain.

Mom tried to calm me down as I cried on the phone. I resisted. "All my life I've been told not to show my feelings," I said to her. "I've tried to be strong about all this. But my father is dying and I'm allowed to cry about that." I told her that I am a very strong person. "All the shit I've been through in my life has made me strong," I said. "But even strong people break down sometimes."

I traveled up to Connecticut that weekend knowing it would be the last time I'd see my father alive. I was determined to talk with him, father to son, man to man. It was the hardest single feat of my life. "After sitting in a chair close by his bed," I wrote in my journal the next day, "I finally got up and sat on the edge of Dad's bed, buried my face in his shoulder and cried. My father—Dad, Daddy—is dying. He knows it; we know it. There's no denial or wishful thinking or prayers whose answer is anything less than a divine

intervention. I sat with him, one hand on his arm, the other serving as a support. It was the most physical affection I think we've ever had."

Dad told me to be brave. I assured him that I *am* brave, even as I cried.
"As we talked," I wrote, "I was a boy again. I trusted this man, that there
were never again to be hurtful words or uncontrolled bouts of hostile drunk-
enness. I poured out my heart as I've never done with him before. I told him
I wanted to have this talk with him, that I'd come home expressly for this
reason. All the arguments or hard feelings we'd ever had would now be put
aside. I thanked him for the good things he's given me, especially for his
stubbornness and tenacity."

He said he was hurt that I would never give him grandkids or carry on his
name. I said I understood that hurt because I'd heard it from other parents I
interviewed that fall for my *Advocate* story. I told him I wanted him to know
how important it was to me to make him proud of me, how I always felt I
somehow needed to prove myself to him—and that the life I was building
for myself would do him proud. He told me he was very proud of me. He said
he will always love me. I pointed out to him how, the older I get, the more
I resemble him. I had been looking at his face in profile as I sat on the chair
and observed how much my forehead looked like his. He put his hands on
either side of my face and looked at my forehead, smiling, obviously pleased.
He called me his "Number One Son"—a la Charlie Chan. I called him my
Number One Father.

He was getting tired and choked-up, I could tell. "You'd better get out of
here," he said gently. That's when I knew he was feeling the weight of our
exchange. I hugged him, kissed his forehead, and rose to leave. I was crying
again as I said goodbye. I told him I'd phone. "I got in the car and out the
driveway onto the main road," I wrote later, "pulled over and leaned my head
on the wheel, sobbing. And sobbing some more. Wailing, really."

Despite the excruciating pain in my heart, I also felt a sense of serenity. I
felt I made my peace with Dad and that I had said everything I hoped to say.
"I can't help but think last night's visit, leave-taking, will be a comfort to me
for the rest of my life," I wrote. "How odd it seems to know that my actions
and words will have consequences forever. In this case, I believe they'll be
good consequences—maybe I'll finally find some peace and wholeness in
myself."

He died on March 13, 1989, exactly five weeks after his fifty-second
birthday. The Greek Orthodox service, on St. Patrick's Day, was hauntingly
beautiful, though I could only pick out a few words in the liturgy conducted
in Greek. I mostly went through it in a daze. I didn't remember later the
pallbearers carrying out the casket from the church after I went up to it to

pay my last respects, leaning over to place a final kiss on Dad's forehead, as I had done the last time we saw each other two months earlier. I had a strong awareness that the waxen figure before me was *not* my father; he had departed this body. I walked to the back of Holy Trinity Church in tears. When I attempted to hug Mom, she pushed me away. "Your sisters need you," she said.

Fulfilling the old adage "bad things come in threes," I was told a week after Dad's funeral that as of April 14, I would be unemployed. The federal funding supporting my job was being cut. Now I could add the loss of my job to the loss of my dad and my relationships with Scott and Bill. "I'm sure I'll pull through because I'm a survivor," I wrote in my journal. "Fake it till you make it," I told myself, quoting the slogan we used in Al-Anon. Even if I didn't yet feel like a survivor, I could try to *behave* like one.

~

CHAPTER SEVEN

The Cruelest Month

Watching the Man I Loved Die

It was still seventy-seven degrees as I sat in Dupont Circle on Wednesday evening, March 23, 1994, reflecting on recent events. "I am greatly disturbed at what seems to be Bill Bailey's declining health," I wrote on my notepad as daylight slipped into night.

Bill and I had reestablished our friendship in the summer of 1989, after I was able to begin healing from my father's death, my breakup with Scott, and my lay-off from NAN. By then Bill was dating David. Only three years after his HIV diagnosis at that point, Bill's T-cell count had plunged to only forty, and he was about to go on AZT, aerosolized pentamidine to prevent pneumocystis pneumonia, and possibly acyclovir to prevent the CMV that had made Allen Satterfield blind.

I had seen Bill and David only two days earlier for their third annual Oscars party. Like many gay men and their ex's, I had become friends with David, too. Besides being handsome and sweet, I understood that David could offer Bill the security of a nice home and reliable income that a struggling writer like me couldn't. Bill had looked frail, was obviously fatigued, and clearly was not himself. He wept bitterly during Tom Hanks's eloquent and moving acceptance speech for his "best actor" role in the AIDS film *Philadelphia*. I had only seen Bill cry like that once before, at a memorial service. I couldn't hold back my own tears knowing he felt so sad.

By the next week, I reported in my journal "Our Billy Bailey isn't doing so good." He'd been admitted to the hospital soon after our Oscars party.

In many ways it was remarkable Bill had survived even this long. He had virtually no immune system to speak of. He'd had pneumocystis pneumonia, Kaposi's sarcoma, and, most recently, had an IV permanently implanted in his arm to treat CMV retinitis. Now he had brain lymphoma. When David called me with this particular news, we agreed Bill's seemingly rapid decline could ultimately prove to be a "severe mercy," to borrow C. S. Lewis's words, if it meant less pain and suffering and deterioration. Bill had told David the one thing he could not bear would be to become demented.

So we kept our vigil. I visited Bill nearly every day after work while he was at George Washington University Hospital during those tough weeks. Because I arrived around suppertime, and Bill became unable to feed himself, I fed him his food. I brought in my electric razor and shaved his face; I knew Bill would want to be clean shaven.

The clashing images of those April days jarred my soul. Evenings, I sat with a young man slowly dying. By day, bright happy daffodils smiled in the sunshine and danced on the breeze. I felt sad and frightened at the thought of what horrors might yet lie ahead for the man I still loved, even after all this time. Yet I was also aware of a strength within me that enabled me to go to Bill's hospital room each day after work and simply be there, even when he was mostly asleep.

Witnessing Bill's decline was the closest I have been to anyone at that extremely advanced stage of HIV disease. I was struck by how terribly grown-up I felt during this ordeal. I knew from my experience of so many losses by then that, awful as it feels, I had to go on anyway. I wrote in my journal, "There's something almost refreshing about thinking of Bill's comfort, something that takes me out of my self-interest and self-pity. This is love, I recognize it, and I am serenely happy to know that after eight and a half years of knowing Bill, I am at this place where I love him in such a way as to have no expectations at last, and want only to give of my strength and life to him in his direst hours."

During his last good weeks Bill and I talked about everything that seemed to be important between us. One evening he kept repeating over and over, "I really do love you." Was his mind still intact? I wondered. I chose to believe that he was rolling over the thought in his mind, coming at it from different angles, and trying to convince me, at last. Or maybe he was astonished that in the end it was, after all, true. Either way, we were making our final peace with each other. Our tumultuous years were far behind us.

I often thought that spring of a conversation with Bill one June night the year before. Coming from a coffee date on Seventeenth Street NW, I ran into him as he left JR's Bar and Grill. He looked disheveled and rather drunk. I asked what was wrong, and was startled by his answer. He and David were on the verge of splitting up. We went to People's Drug so he could buy cigarettes. Bill hadn't smoked in a long time, so I knew he was really upset. At the Fox & Hounds, we settled into a corner outside table, ordered Rolling Rocks, and *both* lit up cigarettes even though I wasn't a smoker.

Bill was clearly in a lot of pain, breaking into tears, talking about how vulnerable he felt, how afraid he was to reenter the market of "sex and the single man" because he had AIDS and felt extremely undesirable. He told me he was embarrassed talking with me about this because part of his motivation for staying with David was to prove to me that he was capable of sustaining a love relationship. "David was my rebound from you," he said. "Scott was my rebound from *you*," I replied.

We spoke a lot about values. Bill told me he admired my "working class" values of strength and loyalty. This was a 360-degree reversal from a cutting remark he'd made not long after we met about our families' class difference. He told me then it would never work between us because his father had been a diplomat while mine worked in grocery stores and textile mills. He even called me "My Stanley Kowalski" a time or two, and not because I was told more than once back then that I "oozed sex" and looked like "a young Marlon Brando" in *A Streetcar Named Desire*; it was more about being a fantasy of the rough-hewn blue-collar "type." I hadn't taken it as a compliment.

On this night, years later, Bill told me, in a somewhat rambling, drunken flurry of words, never to forget where I came from, to find strength in identifying with my family and my upbringing. He also said I probably didn't belong in Washington because of my discomfort with the pretense and posturing that too often passes for relationships there. He saw me as one who needs more genuineness and less of what I referred to as "this city's political power-grubbing bullshit." It wasn't the first time I thought about how out of place I felt in D.C., but it was affirming to hear from someone who knew me as well as Bill did that my discomfort came from something *positive* in myself, the value I place on authenticity.

As Bill's days waned, back home in Connecticut my maternal grandmother was also in the hospital, and not expected to live much longer. Mom told me her mother had stopped taking the medications for her various ailments, and her heart and kidneys were failing. Only a couple months earlier, my other grandmother—my father's mother—had also died. It seemed I was about to experience another rash of bad things happening in threes as I lost within a short time both of my grandmothers and the man I had loved best.

David called me on Saturday, April 23, to tell me Bill died that morning at 8:35. Now it was over. The inevitability, the feelings of resignation, concern, fear, and despair would all merge into a sense of great loss. I cried, but only a little, when I called Mom to share the news—and to receive her news that Grandma was close to death herself, now on a respirator. She was eighty-one years old. It felt profoundly wrong that a thirty-four-year-old man would be robbed of his life at what should have been only the beginning of its prime. Mostly I felt calm, even numb. I was glad to know Bill died peacefully and not in pain, that he didn't suffer a long decline.

"But goddamn it!" I wrote that day. "This was a man I loved a great deal—more than I've ever loved another man, in a lot of ways." He was the "icing on the cake" when I decided to move to Washington. He vexed me by breaking up with me regularly and keeping me always guessing what he felt for me. He hurt my feelings greatly at times with unchecked comments. But we also became great friends and colleagues who delighted in each other's successes. He told me while he was sick how proud he was that we were colleagues. Coming from a man so highly regarded for his hard work and effectiveness, I took it as a high compliment.

Two days after Bill's death, I gathered with David and Bill's other close friends at our friend Curt Decker's for what we called Shiva. Like the Jewish mourning ritual, ours included plenty of food and wine, stories about Bill, anger about his fate, laughter, and tears. I learned that Bill had told David, after that unusual conversation we'd had the year before, "John Andriote is the only one who understands me." Besides sharing our grief we also began to plan what we called a "tribute" to Bill. A memorial seemed too final for a soul we knew would live on through the impact of his work and those of us he had touched.

In the grand lobby of the American Psychological Association's office building on Capitol Hill, on Tuesday, May 17, 1994, men and women in dark suits gathered to pay their respects to "the father of the HIV prevention lobby in Washington," as Bill was described. It looked for all intents and purposes like another Washington cocktail reception—like the many Bill had attended in his roles as a cofounder of the National Organizations Responding to AIDS (NORA) coalition and as a board member of the National Gay and Lesbian Task Force.

Everyone was there to honor Bill: members of Congress, Hill staffers, scientists from the Centers for Disease Control and Prevention and the National Institutes of Health, the national LGBT political groups, and a range of national organizations. Rep. Nancy Pelosi spoke for many when she said, "I can't find words to say what a loss it was. He was such a happy soul, and persistent. So many lives have been saved because of his work."

I stood off to the rear of the crowd, listening to the tributes to Bill Bailey the gay activist and brilliant HIV-AIDS lobbyist. I shook hands and exchanged hugs with friends and colleagues, some I had known for years, most who likely didn't know my history with Bill. In my mind I sorted through mental snapshots of Bill in earlier, happier times—times like our first visit to Waterford, Virginia's, annual house and garden tour on my thirty-third birthday in 1991, captured in the photograph of the two of us that ran with my *Washington Post* HIV coming-out story fifteen years later.

I remembered a Bill Bailey few of these people knew. A gentle soul who loved folk music and *A Prairie Home Companion*, and in his best Garrison Keillor voice would call me "you wonderful man." A man-boy curled up in my arms asking if I would protect him when he was scared. A man who left a mark on others and whose belief in me I still strive to live up to. "Billy," I thought to myself. "You broke my heart all over again."

CHAPTER EIGHT

~

Hard Ways to the Stars

Romantic and Professional
Rejections to Overcome

I started seeing a new therapist, Gene, in early 1995 just as I got seriously underway working on my book *Victory Deferred*. My two earlier therapists in D.C.—first Paul Van Ness, then Tripp Van Woodward—both died from AIDS. I had taken these shocking losses in stride, as though losing therapists and friends in the prime of their lives was normal. I tried hard not to feel that every man I trusted would abandon me, or that every gay man I got close to was going to die long before his time. I fought mightily with my lifelong fear of being left behind.

The isolation of my work—long days and nights at the computer, preoccupied thinking about the book when I wasn't working on it—kept me out of circulation to the point that one friend in Washington told me I was getting a reputation as a hermit. During a visit to Boston, Rich Rasi told me he had never seen me like this in the fifteen years we had known each other. He said I seemed very lonely. My journal reminds me I felt "profoundly alone."

I didn't kid myself about the reason for my singleness—and busy sex life. "I know why I've been 'unattached' for so long, even as I've had lots of sex," I wrote in my journal. I was terrified of opening myself to another loss. "It's easier to have anonymous sex with men at the Men's Massage Party, in the Black Forest, and in the sauna," I wrote. It seemed better than risking another rejection, usually because I was "too serious" or "too intense." And it beat the hell out of watching another young man I love die.

During my visit home to Connecticut at Christmas 1995, I had an enlightening conversation with Mom. She recalled incidents from my boyhood that validated my recollections of always being expected to be the "strong" one in the family, the "good child" no one has to pay much attention to because he doesn't appear to need anything. She told me how much she had relied on me, when I was a boy, to get my two sisters up and dressed and all three of us to the babysitter before school because she was already at work and Dad was often sleeping off the night before. "I don't know what I would have done without you," she told me. Mom recalled a time when I was a boy when we'd all gone to the beach with our next-door neighbors, the boys who introduced me to sex. When it was time to leave, all seemed accounted for. It was only when they got home that they realized they had left me at the beach—the good, unmissed child. When they drove back to the beach, they found me—walking, crying, "You left me alone!"

"Is there any doubt," I wrote in my journal after that conversation, "about why I have these fears of abandonment—and difficulty expressing my needs?"

To my great dismay, the anonymous reviewers my original editor at the University of California Press chose to critique the draft of my *Victory Deferred* manuscript ripped it to shreds. Historian and friend John D'Emilio told me that in all his years of reviewing book manuscripts for university publishers, he had never seen such vitriolic "reviews." It was evident these people had an agenda. John and I suspected it might have had to do with wanting to extend the reign of Randy Shilts's *And the Band Played On*, his dramatization of the first six years of the AIDS epidemic, as "the" book on the subject. My editor at Berkeley loved the book but suggested I find a literary agent who could sell it to a commercial publisher.

It was a huge blow. I felt angry, confused, sad, and extremely disappointed. After the thousands of hours I had put into the book, the anguish I suffered as I poured myself out for it, I was devastated. I couldn't escape the too-familiar sense of abandonment that ran so deep in me. Being a writer and a longtime journal-keeper, I confided in my journal, "Sometimes I just want to be held and told it's okay to feel sad or disappointed."

Two weeks later I was on a train to New York City to meet Warren Frazier, the agent I was referred to by a mutual friend. He called the draft of *Victory Deferred* "wonderful" and suggested minor adjustments in the text to better move the narrative from beginning to end. "I have had to learn to listen to the praises of my work," I wrote in my journal, "not just hear the criticisms." Riding a new wave of hope fueled by Warren's confidence in me and the book, I made my annual pilgrimage to Provincetown in August. I was hoping to meet a guy there, someone who would explore P-town's quieter pleasures together, the sunset beach strolls and kisses under the full moon shining down on Cape Cod Bay.

I met Brian on the Boatslip deck just before I left for the ferry back to Boston. We stared at each other as I walked by him. "What the hell?" I told myself as I turned around, walked back to him, and we shook hands. He lived just outside of D.C., grew up on a big potato farm in Wisconsin, drove a Jeep Wrangler (I wanted one), and had a PhD in economics. Our eyes were locked the entire time we spoke. Clearly he felt whatever it was that had grabbed my attention, too. I was startled by how strongly he reminded me of Bill. Even his lips.

In the weeks that followed an all-afternoon bike ride in Rock Creek Park, hours of talking, a sushi dinner on Perry's rooftop, and our first (sexless) overnight together, Brian told me about his best friend Lynette. He said he would have married her if she were a man. He told me I was "just like" Lynette, and, besides her, only the second person in his life to treat him with loving tenderness. He kissed me with passion, held my hand in front of his friends, and held me tight when we were alone—yet didn't want to have sex with me, even when we slept together. He told me he was haunted by memories of his abusive ex-boyfriend shaming him about his looks and body. I couldn't comprehend how a man I found so handsome, masculine, and smart could be so crippled—or why he would have stayed with someone so loathsome.

It seemed all my life's sorrows poured out in tears for Brian. My eyes streamed as I rode my bike along Rock Creek Parkway to Memorial Bridge, listening on my DiscMan to Madonna singing "You Must Love Me," from the soundtrack of the just-out film version of *Evita*. I was afraid of frightening him away by my need for love. I was afraid of loving him and having him die young. He told me he was frightened of losing himself, as he had done with the abusive boyfriend. His mixed signals upset my Libran need for balance, and I felt very confused and anxious. "I want to be the confident man Brian was attracted to," I wrote in my journal, "not a clutching insecure wreck."

In the entire sixteen years to that point since I had come out as a gay man, I had never laid off of sex for more than the usually short time it took to have it again, whether I had a steady boyfriend or not. For the first time in all those years I didn't have sex with anyone. Despite my anxiety and sadness because of Brian's ambivalence and my own fear, I wanted to "feel my feelings," however hard it might be. I thought a lot about needing to love myself. I realized that although my other good friends loved and esteemed me, I didn't let their love *matter* deeply enough to prevent me from allowing Brian to become the latest rejecting father figure.

All too soon Brian's haunted memories of his abuser, on top of the older pain of his father on their big, isolated farm calling him "runt" and putting him down, pushed him to tell me I "expected too much." So ended yet another attempted relationship with an unhealed, wounded man who couldn't love me because he didn't love himself. Gene actually told me I handled the relationship well, but now it was time to focus on taking care of myself and detach from Brian. I did a lot of self-talking about my value and my power to rise to this latest challenge. "I am not a victim," I told myself in my journal. "I am a grown man who has been lonely and eager to give and receive love. I never did anything to hurt Brian; I was wonderful toward him."

I thought about needing to give myself permission to have a different experience as a gay man. "I have relied on sex and my sex appeal rather than building up real self-esteem," I wrote. Either I had to learn to also value my capacity to *give* love, and believe that I am worthy *of* love, or there would be an endless string of Brians. I admonished myself to "rejoin the living and stop walking in the gloom of my ghosts, especially Bill's." I was certain that if I could finally value myself and the love I offer, "I will attract a man who also values me."

I went to a few Adult Children of Alcoholics meetings to be reminded again by others with a similar background that I don't have to be controlled by the "old tapes" in the recesses of my mind, the endless loop of pernicious messages: "You are a failure," "You don't deserve love," "You should stay single so you don't wind up divorced like your parents and sisters."

My friend Sandra Jacoby Klein, a therapist in Los Angeles who created the earliest AIDS bereavement groups there for gay men, recommended I read psychologist Alice Miller's brief, profound book *The Drama of the Gifted Child: The Search for the True Self*. Miller looks at highly functional adults whose self-image has been warped by childhood trauma. She makes clear that the only way we can shake the power of this early conditioning is to mourn for our stolen childhoods—and to recognize that the strange, sad "gift" of being able to turn off our feelings in the face of even terrible pain was nature's way of shielding us and letting us survive.[1] The implications of Miller's insight were profound for me, though it would take years to really understand that perhaps I wouldn't have survived my life's many traumas were it not for—ironically—the ability I developed as a boy to put aside my own fear and pain to be strong for others I love. I hadn't thought of it as a gift, but I could at least have a new way to frame my story as one of strength and survival rather than weakness and defeat.

I also started going back to church after being a Christmas and Easter churchgoer for years. St. Thomas's Parish in Dupont Circle is a small Episcopal church housed in the gray stone Church Street building that used to be the parish hall before its grand nineteenth-century Gothic sanctuary was destroyed by arson in 1970. After checking it out over a few Sundays, I auditioned for, and spent the next eight years singing first tenor in, St. Thomas's outstanding choir. The rehearsals and new friends—particularly other gay men, who accounted for a good share of the congregation—helped to get me back in circulation. I had wanted to find a faith community where the particulars of my beliefs were less important than sharing in the spirit of community itself, and I found it at St. Thomas's.

As 1998 got underway, Gene encouraged me to love myself as a "wounded masculine man" with the same commitment and devotion I showed to Brian and Bill. I resolved to internalize the love of those in my life who cared about me. My new mantra for the year was, "I have survived a lot; now it's time to thrive." Over the next three months, I lurched from the depths of disappointment about the book and heartache over Brian to the dizzy heights of potentially great literary and financial success. At least that's what my agent and editors thought. Warren arranged meetings and luncheons in Manhattan with several editors. Hamilton Cain, then at Dutton, told me he "stands in awe" and that *Victory Deferred* was "extraordinary." Michael Denneny, Randy Shilts's own editor, told me over lunch in a Greek restaurant he hoped that for my sake I would make hundreds of thousands of dollars on the book, but for his own sake, he would like to publish it. "I'm on the verge of a breakthrough," I wrote in my journal. "I'd like it to be internal, too, to esteem and value myself as a loving, lovable man." I linked my self-esteem to the responses I got for my work, hoping the positive feedback would "sink in."

Jump forward to January 1999. Excitement is building at the University of Chicago Press. When the New York publishers backed off, senior editor Doug Mitchell wooed me with long email messages praising my writing and promising strong marketing for the book. Now *Victory Deferred* is going to be the lead nonfiction title in the spring catalogue. Publicist Erin Hogan tells me it "could take off big time," as she enthusiastically promotes the book to her contacts in the news media across the country. The editor of *Lambda Book Report*, whose offices are right around the corner from my apartment, tells me she has never seen as much buzz about a book.

My snowballing good news that winter includes a message from my doctor after my annual checkup. "Everything is normal," he says. Blood pressure and heart rate are lower than normal; a sure sign, he says, that my cardio and aerobic work in spinning classes and rowing are paying off. My prostate is fine. I don't have a varicocele in my left testicle, as I thought I did. "For a forty-year-old dude I'm in really good shape," I write in my journal. Most importantly, as I see it, I am still HIV-negative. The anxiety of testing never goes away, particularly as I find it easier all the time to rationalize why I am not using condoms if my partner doesn't insist. I reason that, since I am negative I am not going to infect anyone, and my own risk on top is marginal even if he is positive. At least that's what the medical literature suggests.

Library Journal is the first to review *Victory Deferred*, even giving it a star. Doug calls it a "real boon" and says I have "replaced Shilts." *Kirkus Reviews* echoes his assessment when it calls *Victory Deferred* "the most important AIDS chronicle since Randy Shilts' *And the Band Played On*." For good measure *Kirkus* calls *me* a "voice of conscience for the gay community," and says the book has "captured the love shown in the gay community." Other excellent reviews, the stuff of writers' fantasies, follow in major newspapers, magazines, and journals.

My dream of being recognized for my writing is coming true. And it makes me feel good about myself. "I'm feeling such gusto about my life," I write in my journal, "really confident, though barely yet asserting my 'right' to be taken seriously, the very thing I've wanted since I was a child, what has driven me as a writer. I've finally become a man, able to value myself—and, as importantly, with a new expectation that I will be valued by others I let into my life."

After the summer of traveling from coast to coast to give talks and read from *Victory Deferred*, I am back in Provincetown for Labor Day weekend, eighteen years after my first overnight visit in 1981. This time I am in town to give the homily for the P-town chapter of Dignity, the gay Catholic group, which holds its services at the Provincetown Inn. My Boston friend Rich Rasi, still a priest, founded the chapter, and he invited me to be the guest speaker for their Eighth Annual Healing Liturgy. Posters around town and ads in *Bay Windows* and *Provincetown Magazine* promote the service and my participation in it. What a rush it is to think people are actually interested in what I have to say!

"Those of us who have survived the AIDS epidemic have certain obligations as the price of our survival," I tell the group in my homily. I look out the windows of the inn, across the stone breakwater, toward the dunes of Herring Cove, the place I feel freest in this world as I lie, nude, on the sand by the shore of Cape Cod Bay. "We have to put our love into action," I continue. "This means loving ourselves and one another well enough to protect ourselves and our partners against HIV. We must share with one another and with non-gay people our stories of struggle, suffering, loss, healing, survival, and strength."

I swallow a hard lump in my throat more than once.

"These stories," I say, "comprise our history and heritage and bind us together in community. Each of us must do our part to nurture and build a gay community and a society that embraces all its young people, that gives all of us the freedom to be who God has intended us to be, and that cares for all those who are sick and suffering."[2]

As I speak about sharing our stories, I am keenly aware that my *own* story includes dreams-come-true as well as a great deal of loss and pain, so many false starts with loves I hoped would last, so many times I settled for being *desired* when I really wanted to be *loved*. It feels so very right to speak here, in Provincetown, about "healing the broken places." It was here, after all, in this special place at the end of the world, that I felt normal for the first time in my life.

CHAPTER NINE

~

Struggling Writer

Trying to Stay Balanced as
Losses Mount and Risks Increase

By St. Patrick's Day of 2000, six years after I began to write the book proposal, *Victory Deferred* was either nominated or a finalist for six prizes and
awards. I found out that day the Lambda Literary Foundation was going to
give the book its "Editors' Choice" award. I felt a growing sense of pride and
satisfaction as I "absorbed" the accolades for *Victory Deferred*. I tried taking to
heart others' positive regard for me and my work, trying to convince myself,
at last, that I was entitled to respect and consideration by any man I might
get close to.

I focused on the positive things going on in my life—including the
purchase of my condo in D.C. from my landlord that April. Mom gave me
the down payment, demonstrating once again why I consider her the most
generous person I've ever known. Rich Rasi helped arrange the mortgage.
Overnight, the "low-rent" apartment in desperate need of renovation that
embarrassed me for nearly eight years was transformed, in my mind anyway,
into a "fixer-upper." It struck me as a more respectable status.

Although the eighty-year-old wood floors looked awful after I tore up the
hideous gold nylon carpeting—with their gouges, black linoleum tar, and
whole areas patched with what looked like scrap lumber—I began to envision what the place *could* look like. All my life I had brought about change
and achieved my goals by "visioning" what I wanted the outcome to be and
then working to bring about circumstances that would make it real. "I love
the feeling of tearing down to build up," I wrote in my journal, "seeing a

vision of how something could look, knowing it will be beautiful, and then doing the work needed to bring out the beauty in it."

Adding to the good things happening that spring I got my biggest article assignment yet for the *Washington Post*'s "Health" section. The three-thousand-word cover story would focus on an innovative support program for people with cancer run by an organization then known as Smith Farm, and today as Smith Center for Healing and the Arts, a Washington offshoot of California-based Commonweal. I was happy to expand my health reporting beyond HIV-AIDS, but it was hard to do this particular article. Interviewing people living with cancer or in remission dredged up painful memories of Dad's illness and death. I thought of his suffering, what he must have felt inside, how painful and terrifying it must have been to face cancer without a Smith Farm to support him.

I felt extremely gratified to think of the people who would read the story and be inspired to get the support they might need in dealing with their own or a loved one's illness. I was also excited to think people could even learn valuable lessons about life from the survivors whose stories I shared in my article. "I have come to realize," I wrote in my journal, "that a great part of my calling in life, my role as a writer, is to pass down wisdom gleaned from those who have been at the edge of life's experiences."

I tried to apply in my own life the wisdom I learned from the men and women I interviewed. One woman in particular, Katherine, made a huge impression on me. Katherine had breast cancer that had spread to her brain. She was traveling regularly to Chicago for an experimental treatment. We talked about the colorful profusion of flowers and grasses outside the front door of her house. Katherine called it her "Garden of Life," and spoke about finding hope and meaning in the exuberance of nature.

Katherine helped me finally to reject the bullying that gay men casually inflict on one another ("Of *course* you like flowers, dear!") that I had allowed to become a feeling of embarrassment about something I had loved since my first garden when I was only five years old. I embraced my lifelong love of gardening as something joyful and sustaining, a source of resilience. Katherine also helped me understand the wisdom of accepting that our own lives have seasons and cycles, as in all of nature.

Just before my forty-second birthday that October, as we wrapped up the Smith Farm story, I finally saw my doctor after having night sweats for two weeks. I felt achy and fatigued. I was nervous about a puncture wound on my penis, an injury I sustained from one of my buddies' overzealousness. I prayed there was no connection between my illness and the two regular buddies of mine who recently found out they were HIV-positive. I had topped both of them without condoms. "I would be shattered if, God forbid, I were infected with HIV at this point," I wrote in my journal. Fortunately, an antibiotic knocked out whatever it was making me sick.

I started 2001 frantically gathering photo permissions for my next book, *Hot Stuff: A Brief History of Disco*—and worrying that the phone would be cut off because of a $201 bill. The mortgage check bounced and my gym membership was suspended because I was late with the payment, again. Unfortunately *Victory Deferred*'s critical acclaim wasn't matched by big sales, and the book didn't become the financial salvation I'd hoped for. It would be years before I understood that authors are best advised to regard their books as platforms rather than moneymakers.

"THIS IS FUCKING CRAZY!" is how I described the tug-of-war within me between the excitement about my work and gut-wrenching anxiety about my finances. I had plenty of contract work, but the erratic payments wreaked havoc on my cash flow. I never seemed able to accumulate a re- serve to tide me over between unpredictably spaced paychecks, the bane of consultants and freelancers. I paid my bills on time when I had the money, but when I had a compelling opportunity that required me to choose how to allocate a limited amount of money, I frequently opted to delay bills and seize the opportunity. I was aware even then that my experience of losing friends at a young age made me hypercognizant of "living in the moment." But my inability to manage money in the face of the unpredictable income made me feel badly about myself. I couldn't escape the feeling that there was something fundamentally flawed in me, that I was unworthy of love because I didn't have it all under control.

I smoked more pot than ever and carried on like a sexual glutton. "Pot helps me focus and is sexually disinhibiting," I wrote in my journal. "It's a buffer against my own feelings of sadness and anxiety. Sadness about feeling alone and lonely." In fact I felt lonelier than ever. "I am acutely aware of the fact that days and days and weekends pass and not one friend calls me," I wrote. Was it the outcome of all my isolation while writing *Victory Deferred*? Or was it because so many of the friends who used to call had died? I knew that more than just a quest for pleasure, my sexual hunger was fueled by stress and panic as I worried about my finances. Really, I mostly wanted *someone* to reassure me I was okay.

I was about to do twenty radio interviews the week of March 12, when *Hot Stuff* was officially published. The *Washington Post* was keeping me busy, writ- ing about a new rapid PSA test, the state of HIV vaccine research, and what was expected to be another "Health" cover story on the medical benefits of fun and laughter. Whitman-Walker Clinic hosted a book launch party for

Hot Stuff at Lizard Lounge, a dance club on what was then up-and-coming Fourteenth Street NW.

Rich Rasi flew down to Washington from Boston to spend the weekend with me and come to the party, as he had done for the *Victory Deferred* launch party two years earlier. We blasted Grace Jones's "La Vie en Rose" as we drove about D.C. in my Jeep. We laughed uproariously about the fun times we had shared over the years, reminding each other why we were still such good friends after more than two decades.

A week later I was off to New Orleans, joining comedian Bob Smith and New Orleans author Chris Wiltz (*The Last Madam: A Life in the Underworld*) on an author panel called "Hot Stuff, Hookers, and Humor" at the annual Tennessee Williams Literary Festival. People wanted to know why I had gone from writing a "heavy" book about AIDS to writing a book about disco music. When David Swatling interviewed me during the festival for a Radio Netherlands show focused on disco, I told him that, far from offering only an escape from life's harshness, disco music in the 1970s reminded us to celebrate life's good times even *amid* the hard times. And no city knows better than New Orleans that we can laugh and live and love even in the face of death. That's why death masks are part of every Mardi Gras revelry.

There was no laughter, but too many thoughts of death, when I called Mom just after getting back to D.C. from New Orleans. Her closest friend in the world, Joan, had just been diagnosed with stomach cancer. There was also involvement with her lymph nodes. Joan's mother had died of cancer, too. Joan's being diabetic and taking insulin meant she was a poor candidate for the surgery that would be needed to remove the baseball-size tumor in her stomach. Of course Mom also brought up Dad's death from cancer. To top it off, Mom and Joan's good friend Charlotte—they were like the Three Musketeers in high school—was also in the hospital, her kidneys failing and on dialysis. Charlotte's own husband was dying of cancer and not expected to live much longer.

Only months after my Smith Farm story, and all it stirred up in me, cancer was once again stalking people I love. AIDS, at least, had slowed down for a while.

Mom was clearly shaken, a rare event for a woman who kept her vulnerable feelings locked up. A question or two revealed that she wasn't only upset about her friends, but worried by these painful reminders of her own mortality. I was sad for Joan and her husband, Joe, and their daughter Susie. I was sad for Mom. I was sad for me, too. From the time I was a boy, I had loved Joan and Joe for their lighthearted attitude toward life. They thought nothing of heading out for a cup of coffee and winding up on a road trip hundreds of miles away, spontaneously and joyfully turning something ordinary into something memorable. Joan understood what it meant to celebrate life even in the face of illness and death. Mom and I talked about Joan's amazing spirit and humor. Joan had already made a joke about the chance to lose weight if they had to remove half her stomach. Freud considered that kind of "gallows" humor the *highest* coping mechanism, *precisely* what is most needed in such a frightening situation.

Of course I thought of the parallels between Mom's experience with her friends and mine with my friends' deaths from AIDS. I spoke to her from whatever wisdom I had developed as a result of my own losses. She said she had hesitated to call Joan because she didn't know what to say. I knew this was one of the times I needed to be strong for *her*. I told her she would need to put aside her fear and sadness, and be there for Joan. It was a much-too-familiar experience for me. In fact I had been doing it all my life, just as Mom had trained me to do. I found out later Mom called Joan right after we got off the phone.

Rich Rasi called me two weeks later to share his own shocking news. He had gone to see his doctor a few days after returning to Boston from his recent visit to Washington. He figured the pain in his back was from pulling a muscle in a workout. Instead Rich found out he had cancer on his right kidney. There was a history of cancer on both sides of his family. Two months later, what seemed good news after surgery to remove the diseased kidney became terrible news when Rich learned he had a rare form of cancer involving the lymph nodes near the kidney.

As the dark cloud of death once again shadowed my life, I actually had a major stroke of good fortune when Family Health International offered me a job as senior editor in its D.C.-based global AIDS program. I would split the full-time position with a longtime friend I recruited to join me in what for the global public health consulting company was a novel job-share arrangement. I was excited to have a steady income again, and glad the half-time job would pay well enough that I could continue my freelance writing. I've always seen my by-lined published writing as the real core of my career.

Two months later, our supervisor was moved to another position in the organization. My job-share colleague and I bumped up to full time and now split the role of directing FHI's information programs unit. My salary doubled. I also filed for Chapter 13 debt reorganization, hoping that now, with a good income, I could finally pay off the old debt that had weighed me down for so many years. A court-appointed trustee would take $1,000 a month from my pay, deducted before I ever saw it. Rather than feel embarrassed about it, I chose to see it as an empowered step. I focused on being grateful finally to have enough income that I *could* pay off old debt. In fact I felt extremely relieved.

I was home from the office the morning of September 11 for an appointment at eleven with Dr. Fred Finelli, a colorectal surgeon, at Washington Hospital Center. After watching in horror as the twin towers collapsed on live television, I drove across town as tens of thousands of people in downtown Washington scrambled to get out of the city as fast as possible. Every road out of the District was jammed with bumper-to-bumper traffic. When I got to Dr. Finelli's office, I found out he had gone to pick up his three daughters from their schools. Our discussion of anal warts would have to wait a while. They showed up in the anal Pap smear my doctor routinely, and wisely, gives all his gay male patients. This time mine tested positive for HPV.[1] Human papilloma virus, the most common sexually transmitted infection in the United States, is so infectious I could have spread it there myself. Chances are good, though, it was passed along by one of the rare men who had topped me in the previous couple of years.

Not long after the surgery to remove the warts, I was at Washington Hospital Center for a follow-up visit and had a disturbing little moment. When I stepped out of the elevator, I suddenly couldn't remember where Dr. Finelli's office was located, though I had been there several times. I felt discombobulated, unsure which direction to head in the corridors. It was bizarre, as if my mind was blocking out something really awful. Then I realized: I was terrified. I had convinced myself the doctor was going to tell me I had anal cancer. All the talk about cancer had rattled my nerves. Fortunately the treatment worked and there were no further problems.

"Requiem eternum, Joan," I wrote in my journal after Joan died on May 16, 2002. "We will look forward to seeing you again 'on the other side.' I know you'll be laughing because you are a happy soul. Thank you for showing me how to be adventurous and curious and for helping to inspire me to pursue my dreams. I hope I can have half your sense of humor when I am forced to deal with whatever will be my own final battle. I am grateful to you and to God for letting me know you for forty-three-and-a-half years. Not as long as Mom, but long enough to know you were the real thing—a truly joyful spirit."

Six months later I spoke with Rich's partner Jeb as I was driving to Dulles Airport, heading to Nigeria for my job with FHI. Rich's prognosis was bleak. He had exhausted every traditional and experimental treatment he could find. I had visited him in his room at New England Baptist Hospital, in Boston, on October 28, the day after his birthday. It ripped my heart out to see Rich so frail. He was such a physically vibrant, joyful man—his big brown eyes, long Syrian nose, and (back when we met in 1980) dark curls the image of a Byzantine icon. He called me "Moosie," his pet name for me, and I called him my "Sitto," Arabic for grandmother, the nickname he had chosen for himself many years earlier when he was helping care for me after my bashing in Provincetown. I couldn't hold back my sobs as I sat on his bed, lay my head on his chest, and we hugged each other for what I knew was likely the last time. I could tell. Rich was even more frail than Dad or Bill had been. I had so much experience by now.

I cried on my sister Sue's shoulder when I got outside the hospital. She had driven up to Boston with me. "I've lost so many friends," I sobbed. "I just can't bear to lose Rich, too." My closest friend in the world, the big brother I never had, the priest-shrink who first opened my eyes to the insidious effects on me of my father's alcoholism, celebrated with me over breakfast at the Ideal Diner when I got my acceptance letter from Northwestern, came to my book launch parties, and encouraged me every step of the way.

I found out when I returned from Nigeria that Rich died while I was away.

I was "living to the point of tears," as Albert Camus put it. I craved intense and exhilarating sensory experiences—opera! sex! travel!—inversely proportioned to my intensely painful ones. You might say I was living out Newton's Third Law of Physics, responding to every trauma I suffered with an equal and opposite reaction aimed at celebrating life and defiantly shouting at death. Take, for example, my forty-eight-hour layover in Amsterdam on the way back from Nigeria.

David Swatling, who had interviewed me in New Orleans about *Hot Stuff* for Radio Netherlands, also interviewed me while I was in Amsterdam for his radio show *Alien*. We spoke about what I had observed in Nigeria, my conversations at the hotel bar in Lagos with "female sex workers," as we referred to the beautiful young women I befriended in my two weeks there. I asked them about their lives and whether they used condoms. I bought them drinks and dinner, even handed them cash simply because I knew they needed it more than I did. They had warmed my heart with their honesty, and broken it with their sad tales of needing to support younger family members back in their home villages so they could avoid a similar fate.

Besides the interview, I had only two objectives in Amsterdam. The first was to visit one of the city's famous coffeehouses so I could enjoy the experience of smoking weed without feeling like a criminal or psychological weakling, the only reasons I'd ever heard in America someone could possibly like cannabis. The second objective was to check out the city's famous leather bars. I've never been a leather man per se, but have long enjoyed the bars' music and masculine energy. I was also intrigued by all I'd heard about the bars' busy darkrooms where all *sorts* of things are known to occur.

I paid about $13 for a large bud of White Widow at Route 66, a coffeehouse on the Warmoestraat, the main street in the red light district, and I enjoyed the sensation of freedom it gave me to partake matter-of-factly while sipping my cappuccino as others around me did likewise. After my evening interview with David Swatling, I went to the bars Argos and then to the Eagle. "There, in the basement darkroom, I met my match," I wrote two days later on my flight from Amsterdam to Washington. He was one of the youngest, hottest men there. He strutted around with his shirt open and a kind of warm-up suit. In one dark corner we were standing directly across from each other in a doorway. I reached out my hand to his hard abdomen, and we were off and running.

"He didn't cum inside of me," I wrote later. "In fact he kind of pushed me away when it was time to pull out and get off." I wince reading what I wrote next: "I didn't even have to feel guilty or worried about taking a real risk—though I'd just had the kind of barebacking that even I can read in Dutch is completely discouraged and/or forbidden."

I had won an award and acclaim for my history of the AIDS epidemic. I had helped ease friends to their deaths. I loved life and reveled in its beauties and pleasures. I was excited about my future. Yet more than two decades after I discovered the anesthesia of anonymous sex in Boston's Fens, I was willing potentially to risk my future, my health, even my life, in a hot, anonymous encounter "where it was only about energy and not about exploiting knowledge of personal makeup," as I described it in my journal. It was a hot scene and we were two hot guys having fun together. Simple, right? I didn't understand, perhaps chose not to believe, that placing myself in that moment had anything to do with anxiety, loneliness, or the grief that haunted me. As a writer I connected dots for a living, yet I didn't connect how I had sex with the traumas of my childhood, or the heaped-on trauma of all my losses.

Through strange office politics my job-share friend had become my supervisor at FHI, and he was a compulsive micromanager. Calling him abusive would not be overstating it. My stomach twisted in knots when I saw him because he was so volatile. Behind closed doors in our weekly check-in meetings he told me more than once I was "not worth" what FHI paid me. He seemed to watch my every move, waiting to pounce. After returning from what everyone else considered my second successful trip, this one to Haiti and St. Kitts, to advise FHI's country office directors on their communication strategy, he put me on a "PIP." I couldn't say it without thinking of Gladys

Knight, but the performance improvement plan wasn't a laughing matter; it was a vengeful micromanager's way of eliminating a perceived threat.

On February 4, 2004, I was called into a meeting with my supervisor, his boss, and the human resources director. My by-now former friend, the one I'd recruited to job share with me, told me I would "no longer fit" in the organization. I reminded those assembled that there was nothing in my resume to lead any reasonable person to conclude I was either a book editor or a webmaster, yet those roles had been laid on me without training or support. I had often told my supervisor I felt I was being set up for failure. Perhaps that was the intent.

I had to lick the wounds inflicted on my ego by the now-former boss's incessant nitpicking criticism of my writing and just about everything else I did. Some friends encouraged me to contact an employment lawyer to protect my good reputation. I comforted myself by rereading the reviews of my books and the comments about talks I'd given. I needed to reabsorb the good things others said about my work. I wanted to remind myself of who I am and what I had accomplished in my life. I had to remind myself I have value even if my former friend did his best to devalue me.

Shortly after all this upset, I attended St. Thomas's Ash Wednesday service. Rev. Elizabeth Carl, one of the Episcopal Church's first openly lesbian priests and our interim rector, spoke in her sermon about how the day was a reminder of death, our own death in particular, but why it's a good thing. She said death could be seen as a sort of friend hovering nearby to remind us that our time is short and precious, and to do all we need to do in the time we have. She said that as long as we are still alive, "we aren't dead yet." We are able to make choices about *how* to live our lives. The question, then, is what do we want to do with the rest of the time given us?

It wasn't long before I was already moving on after FHI. In my journal I wrote of the former boss and ex-friend as "a mere blip on the screen, a splattered insect on the windshield of life." I was excited about the communication consulting services I was planning to offer other international public health organizations. I paid an attorney to get me legally incorporated as a one-man operation, Health & Science Reporting, Inc. I hired a graphic designer to help brand me with a business card, brochure, postcard, and website. "The time has come to really rake in the big bucks!" I wrote in my journal.

Within a few months I lined up thousands of dollars worth of consulting projects. At the same time, D.C.'s overheated real estate market spiked my condo's value to more than four times what I paid for it only four years earlier. I refinanced the mortgage, took out tens of thousands of dollars from the equity, and proceeded to do a complete, bottom-to-top renovation, from the restored antique heart pine floors to new crown molding. I put in a spa-style bathroom with black slate tile, a glass-bricked shower, and a pedestal sink. The once ugly little kitchen became a solo cook's highly functional galley with granite countertops, natural cherry cabinets, mirrored backsplash, and stainless appliances. I even bought new furniture to complete the transformation.

I had chosen the dragonfly tattoo I got on my left bicep in Ft. Lauderdale, on the way back from the Haiti trip, as the perfect symbol for how I now thought about the condo and, even more importantly, about my life and being a gay man. The insect that metamorphoses from an ugly underwater nymph into a marvel of flight and beauty perfectly represented how I had transformed the condo from a shabby fixer-upper into a "stunning renovation," as realtors would later describe it. More than anything, my dragonfly reminded me of the long, frequently hard, journey I had already made to arrive at this moment in my life, and how grateful I was that through it all I had never lost sight of life's beauty and grace.

CHAPTER TEN

~

Wounded Warrior

How AIDS and a Shame-Filled
Man Taught Me to Value Myself

I was on top of the world as I sat on the sand at Race Point Beach on New Year's Day 2005, bracing myself against the cold wind blowing off the Atlantic on Provincetown's ocean side. In spite of the snow piled high on the streets, I wanted to start the new year in my sacred place. I'd had dinner New Year's Eve with my friend Greg Pappas, at Ciro & Sal's, the P-town flagship of the long-demolished restaurant I worked at in Boston two decades earlier. In my little black moleskin notebook I reflected on recent events, and looked ahead. More than a quarter of a million people had just died in the Indian Ocean tsunami the day after Christmas. It was beyond comprehension, so many deaths at once, such a dark cloud of sorrow cast over the world during the most joyous time of the year.

My overwhelming feeling was one of gratitude. "Grateful for life and health," I wrote, "and the chance once again to spend time in this place still sacred to me. Grateful for the chance to feel optimistic about my life despite the world's disasters, horrors, and wars. Grateful for my loving (through it all) family, the friends who remain (and the strength to cut loose those who have proved they aren't made of the stuff real friends are made of), the work I do." Above all, I was grateful for life. "That is the operative principle, and the attitude, I will cultivate, again, in 2005," I wrote.

By the time I returned to Provincetown in August, my new kitchen was finished and the condo renovation was done. I felt enormously pleased with my success in starting with a vision and then actualizing it. I was also working on another big health story for the *Washington Post*, on the epidemic of crystal meth use wrecking a lot of gay men's lives in D.C. I had already seen its impact firsthand on a couple of men I knew.

I burst into tears as I drove across the Sagamore Bridge onto the Cape, listening to Josh Groban singing "You Raise Me Up." I thought of Rich, and Joan, and Bill, and Dad, all the people in my life I had lost to terrible illness and premature death. As my tears ebbed, I actually felt a new serenity thinking about how my dearly departed had, each in his or her way, contributed to the building of my life. Their love had truly raised me up. Even their deaths had made me wise beyond my years. I had the oddest sensation as I came into P-town. It felt like back in the fall of 1985, when I moved to Washington and met Bill Bailey. It was as if my departed loved ones were giving me permission to carry on with my life, telling me it was time to love again.

I met Glenn as we both sat on a step across from Spiritus Pizza after the bars closed and everyone came to get a slice and people watch. I don't remember what we talked about, but we kept talking for a long time. We walked to his car, a big old Ford, and smoked some weed. A guy walking by popped his head in my passenger-side window, obviously flirting with me. "I'm with *him*," I told the man, motioning toward Glenn. Glenn told me later what a good impression that made on him. I liked that he lived in my home state of Connecticut, and that he was tall, handsome, and, judging from his stories, obviously kind and compassionate. He was a nurse, after all.

We made plans to meet up in Manhattan the first weekend of October, just before both our birthdays. "Magical" was the word Glenn used to describe it. We "flowed together," he said. "We fit like a hand in a glove." Those were exactly the kinds of words I dreamed of hearing from a man. In the following weeks we talked for hours on the phone. We planned another visit, over Thanksgiving, in Connecticut. "This one has a lot of potential," I wrote in a letter a week after my forty-seventh birthday to "Doc," my then eighty-five-year-old college advisor with whom I had been corresponding for more than twenty years. I had visited Doc in Harlingen, Texas, in 2000, to interview him for a book I wanted to write on aging. He had admonished me many times in our letters over the years to "live while you're alive!" It became my mantra. "In fact," I told Doc, "I don't recall ever having anyone among my paramours who told me how much he misses me, how attracted to me he is, etc., etc. I could get used to that. Stay tuned!"

Keeping up on the news, as Doc and I did in our letters, I commented about the devastation of Hurricane Katrina the last week of August. I had cried watching TV images from New Orleans, recalling my last visit to the city for the Tennessee Williams Literary Festival in 2001. An article I had just read in *Rolling Stone* about New Orleans music confirmed what I had also sensed there, the city's ability to celebrate life in the face of death. It called New Orleans the nation's most "African" city, culturewise, and cited the city's famous jazz funerals as an example. "Of course jazz funerals are basically the same as traditional African funerals," I wrote to Doc, "with the somber dirge on the way to the graveyard and the festive dancing on the way back, giving death its due but *defying* it *joyfully* anyway." I thought that attitude offered a terrific basis for a well-lived life: "being mindful of how precious and brief our time is, recognizing our mortality, and then living deliberately and exuberantly in spite of it."

I wrote to Doc again a month to the day after that letter. "Doc," I said, "I'm afraid I have some bad personal news to share with you—though I hope you will see (as I am trying to see) it isn't necessarily as bad as I first thought. My doctor told me two weeks ago that I have tested HIV-positive." I told my mentor and pen pal that my doctor assured me I wasn't likely to die from AIDS, and that current medications were easy to take and had minimal if any side effects. "Still this has been shocking news," I wrote. "After having my annual checkup and accompanying blood work, I fully expected to hear 'negative' when Ben, my doctor, gave me my various test results. When he said, 'I have bad news on the HIV test,' I began to tremble. I simply couldn't believe it."

I told Doc that I had cried a lot. "But overall," I said, "I've been very calm and rational about it. I have a great advantage over most people learning this news because I have been immersed in it for twenty years. Of course it's still challenging because it is forcing me to rethink some fundamental things about myself, my sexuality, my future. I haven't told my family, and won't until I have a clearer sense of what our course of action is going to be. I don't want them to worry, as they will do, and (as friends have pointed out to me) I don't want to take care of them at this time when I am trying to learn how to let others care for me. The curse of being the eldest is that my mother taught me all too well to suppress my own needs and fears and take care of everyone else but myself."

Only a couple of weeks after my diagnosis, I was already realizing that writing about other people's experiences with HIV-AIDS, even for as long as I had been doing it, was a *whole* different experience than talking about my own story. I was clear about a few things, though. "My new situation," I wrote to Doc, "confirms, underscores, boldfaces, italicizes and glows in large, red all-caps what I believe to be true: I must live while I am alive, as you put it. Life is precious and brief, no matter how many years we are on this earth. I will do my best to make the most of each day given me. And I will not let HIV define me."

The first person I phoned with what I called "my news" was my friend Dennis Pfaff. We had known each other about fifteen years by then, and Dennis and I had shared some of our wildest times—late-night dancing at the Frat House for one, riding together a hundred and twenty miles from D.C. to Rehoboth, Delaware, on his motorcycle was another. Dennis was also the only person I had ever let see me at my most wretched—sobbing "What is *wrong* with me? Why doesn't he love *me?*"—back when Brian told me I expected too much after I took the bait when he led me to believe the romantic interest was mutual. Dennis was the only friend in whom I fully confided about my sex life because he never judged me. He is from a working-class background like me, and we understand, lift up, and celebrate each other's triumphs and share our tragedies.

I trust Dennis with my life—and did, literally the very day after I got my HIV diagnosis. I had long planned to fly out to Phoenix for Dennis's annual Halloween party, and was scheduled to leave D.C. on what became my "day after." Dennis was afraid I would cancel. But I went, and told him it was "just what the doctor ordered." Riding on the back of his motorcycle, without a helmet, wasn't my idea of smart. I told him I wanted a helmet because I felt very fragile. He insisted I face my fear and challenge it—as I needed to do in my life. We sped through the streets of Phoenix, tears flying from my eyes, my heart pounding, feeling so very *alive*.

When I shared my news with Glenn later in the afternoon on the first day of knowing I was HIV-positive, he told me my new status didn't bother him. He told me his previous partner had HIV, too. I visited Glenn often during the winter of 2005 to 2006, and came to think of his little white house in Connecticut as a refuge, a place—in my home state, no less—that wasn't haunted by ghosts, the way D.C. had become for me. We drank cocktails, smoked weed, and danced together all alone in the house. It was easy to think HIV was far away, back in Washington, not lurking within my own body. We slept together every night I was there. But Glenn always turned his back to me in bed, I was the "outside spoon," and he didn't want to have sex with me.

I lavished gifts upon him that Christmas, including a beautiful faux Tiffany dragonfly lamp. I even had L.L. Bean ship him a wreath from Maine. I mustered the courage to take the chance and sign the card, "With love at Christmas, John." The *L* word was fraught with so much pain for me, but I was determined not to be held back by fear. If I could face the microbial monster that had killed so many of my friends, I could risk using the word *love* with a man I thought loved me too.

Glenn gave me nothing for Christmas. Not even a card.

We each saw *Brokeback Mountain*, separately, when it came out that winter. I had never seen a movie so powerfully portray the kind of love I had experienced with men. I instantly identified with Jack Twist, the risk-taking bull rider who is ready to give his all for love. And I recognized in the emotionally crippled Ennis Del Mar the men I was so powerfully drawn to, the men who couldn't love me back because they are trapped in their own fear. Glenn even took to sometimes calling me "Jack Fuckin' Twist," as Ennis did in the movie. Talk about life imitating art.

One day Glenn took me around his house, pointing out the dents in doors and chinks in wood moldings where his former partner of eight years had shoved or hit him in one or another of the partner's violent outbursts. Glenn already had experience dealing with violent men even before that. He told me about the time his father, a tall, husky Tony Soprano lookalike, knocked him to the ground in a fit of anger. Glenn was twenty years old at the time. He couldn't understand why he had "let" these men abuse him or why he'd stayed with the violent ex for so long.

Glenn pushed me away as hard as he held me tightly when we slow danced together in the dark. The powerfully conflicting signals he put out had me nearly consumed with anxiety. He played "Come What May" from *Moulin Rouge* ("Come what may . . . I will love you till my dying day") and told me he wanted to fall in love with me, then treated me like someone he was punishing for crimes I never committed. "You don't know what to do with me because I treat you like a prince," I told him.

I was trying to understand who I was supposed to be with the new "person with HIV" tag hung on me. I was terrified of the great uncertainty I felt about my health and future. I was trying to practice what the psychiatrist told me about being gentle with myself and present to my own suffering. Yet here I was, once again, anguishing over another messed-up man—as if *he* was the most important thing in my life. But the psychiatrist had also told me that the true measure of a relationship is its degree of reciprocity, and *this* should be the standard to measure my relationship with Glenn, or with anyone else for that matter.

When Glenn finally responded to the email I sent him with my *Washington Post* HIV coming-out story, his two-line message said he was proud of me "for putting yourself on stage for the entire nation." His comment rang hollow for me. It had taken him eight days to answer my message. He hadn't called in weeks. "He simply has not acted like someone who is proud of, or proud to know, me," I wrote in a letter to Doc. "Maybe it gives him bragging rights to have a 'friend' who does the sorts of things I have been doing in public places. But that is not the same as acting like someone who cares about me."

I strung myself along until summer. Well, a late-night text from Glenn—
"Missing you tonight"—and ensuing phone call with a drunk Glenn, kept
my torch burning. The drunk part was familiar enough; he drank pretty
heavily and on a regular basis. But the forthrightness about his feelings had
been *un*familiar since the earliest weeks of what he insisted on calling "our
friendship." As I had done during the Brian affair, I had abstained from sex
with anyone else—this time for seven months—because I wanted to feel my
feelings rather than hide from them by having sex with a man I didn't love,
as excruciating as it got (and as horny as I got!) at times.

I visited Glenn for what became the last time in July 2006. We sat behind
his secluded house one night, staring into the flaming logs in the fire pit. We
slow danced in our boxers in the muggy air. He told me more about his former partner, the one with HIV. He had been extremely sick and was rushed
to the emergency room more than once. I knew it had been very trying for
Glenn. I assured him it was unlikely I would ever become sick like that because my medication was working exactly as my doctor told me it would, I
was taking very good care of myself, and the chances were good I could even
live a normal lifespan.

"I don't want to be Florence Nightingale," said the nurse.

I was stunned. I felt as though I'd been kicked in the gut. I had never
felt such a sense of total rejection and abandonment. For good measure he
told me he never loved me and only slow danced with me because he "felt
comfortable" with me; it didn't "mean" anything. Once again, another man
I loved threw all he could into telling me my instincts were wrong, that I
shouldn't trust my gut and definitely shouldn't believe my lying eyes.

It was the kick I needed to push myself beyond Glenn. In a way it was another "before" and "after" moment. I knew I had to reject the fear and shame
that paralyzed Glenn and led him to drink too much, too often, and held *me*
back as long as I held out for him. I had to acknowledge that there had been
very little reciprocity in this relationship. I decided to stop being a victim to
an abused man who had become abusive himself. I had worked on my own
mental health far too long to settle for this kind of treatment.

All my life I had put aside *my* needs, *my* pain, *my* suffering, to care for
wounded men. I *finally* understood that *I* was also a wounded man, and that
I had to care for myself. I *let* myself get angry, and stopped trying to justify
Glenn's rejection. I also *let* myself feel truly proud that I had managed to be
loving and generous toward Glenn in spite of my own pain, confusion, fear,
and sorrow.

For the first time in my life, I understood that my love and loyalty have
great value, and that I simply have to trust my instincts about people. It was

time to heed, not reason or wishfully think away, the warning signs when men show and tell me things about themselves that portend trouble. I understood I needed to reframe my story, make *myself* its hero. I needed to draw *consciously* from my resilience when I faced future challenges, not be knocked down by them. I wanted my story to inspire others who might read or hear it some time. "It's a wonderful, forward moving story," I wrote in my notebook, "of surviving and thriving after painful suffering—HIV, Glenn, all my life's losses. *That's* the story I want to tell."

I wanted *my* story to be worthy of the other gay men whose stories I had helped to report. I wanted to be a man who cares more about honesty, integrity, and freedom than about others' disapproval, judgment, or rejection. I wanted to be worthy of my community's heroic legacy, the men and women to whom I would look for inspiration and hope as I pressed forward on my *own* heroic journey.

PART II

THE HEROIC LEGACY

~

Overview:
Part II

Greatness, in the last analysis, is largely bravery—courage in escaping
from old ideas and old standards and respectable ways of doing things.

—James Harvey Robinson, American historian (1863–1936)

Gay men don't tend to grow up learning in school about our community's
history. Until the last forty years, when our own historians have begun to
document our existence, we learned what we could from other gay men.
In fact one of the more remarkable aspects of gay life is the way gay men
have always been able to recognize, encourage, and support one another in
resisting the physical and psychological blows of oppression. How we loved
one another in the AIDS epidemic didn't surprise us, but it stunned the
world—and it propelled the relatively rapid achievement of marriage equality in 2015.

We often smile with bemused condescension at the quaint euphemistic
names—"friends of Dorothy," for example—and adoration of strong female
divas common among our gay forbears before the 1969 Stonewall riots.
In fact, however, those names and even diva worship were actually well-
developed tactics for survival in a hostile world. If history pivots on the
timely actions of "great men" (and women)—the right person in the right
place at the necessary moment—then gay history just before, and within,
our lifetimes has pivoted on great men such as Harry Hay, Frank Kameny,
Rev. Troy Perry, Arnie Kantrowitz, Mark Segal, Dr. Howard Brown, Dr.
Richard Pillard, Rev. Carl Bean, Larry Kramer, Peter Staley, Cleve Jones,

Paul Boneberg, and Evan Wolfson. These are men who rose to meet the challenges they were presented, and did what heroes do: Standing up and being counted when it counts most. Keeping alive the stories of their struggles and triumphs offers a powerful heritage of *real* gay pride. Indeed, our heroic legacy of proud gay men can inspire, motivate, and sustain us—*if* we claim it for ourselves.

CHAPTER ELEVEN

~

Subversives

How "Gaydar" Helped Gay Men
Survive in the "Old Days" Before Stonewall

Stephen Sondheim, Broadway's reigning composer of the day, called it "the shot heard round the world." Leonard Bernstein, conductor of the New York Philharmonic and Sondheim's collaborator on *West Side Story*, jumped to his feet and screamed "Bravo!" *New York Times* theater critic Clive Barnes called it "by far the frankest treatment of homosexuality I have ever seen." Neil Simon, the new hotshot playwright after winning the 1965 Tony Award for *The Odd Couple*, said it was the most honest thing he'd ever seen on stage.[1]

Mart Crowley's play *The Boys in the Band* opened at New York's off-Broadway Theater Four on April 14, 1968. The revolutionary show dared to show gay men "at home." The story centers on a group of friends at a thirty-second birthday party for Harold, hosted by Michael, when Michael's supposedly straight college roommate, Alan, unexpectedly shows up. Anxiety, depression, guilt, and self-loathing fuel the free-flying insults as the men verbally flay each other and themselves.

Birthday boy Harold, who describes himself as "a thirty-two-year-old, ugly, pock-marked Jew fairy" castigates his friend Michael for not fully embracing his own homosexuality. "You're a sad and pathetic man," Harold tells him. "You're a homosexual and you don't want to be, but there's nothing you can do to change it. Not all the prayers to your god, not all the analysis you can buy in all the years you've got left to live. You may one day be able to know a heterosexual life if you want it desperately enough. If you pursue it with the fervor with which you annihilate. But you'll always be homosexual as well. Always Michael. Always. Until the day you die."

What may be saddest of all is the friends gathered in Michael's apartment actually *do* care about, and even love, one another like the "gay family" they are. But after lifetimes of being told men who love men are sick, sinful, and second class, it's small wonder the pain they carry inside boils over regularly with the only people with whom they feel safe enough to vent. "If we could just learn not to hate ourselves so very much," says Michael in the play's final scene, before speaking the show's most famous line: "You show me a happy homosexual, and I'll show you a gay corpse."

That line hurts even today because it still rings true for too many gay men. The hatred of gay people we grow up hearing and seeing, frequently from our own parents, still sinks in and undercuts our self-esteem. That hatred—and gay men's ability to survive and thrive in spite of it—has been around a *long* time. "The main reason why the characters in *The Boys in the Band* are miserable is because the straight world of old made them that way," said theater critic Peter Filichia. "If people in the forties, fifties, and sixties had been tolerant, these guys wouldn't have turned out as they did."

Only twenty-two when the show opened, Filichia said, "I saw *The Boys in the Band* countless times way back when, and, believe me, plenty of men in the audience were weeping openly." He added that although it might not be the story of most gay men today, it certainly resonated with gay men of the time. "How could the 1968 production have set a then-record-high ticket price of ten dollars (when Broadway plays were still charging six dollars and ninety cents), and run one thousand performances, if it weren't telling a story that resonated and rang true?"

The play was an important milestone in gay history—and one of the events that fueled the Stonewall rebellion only a year later. "After gays saw *The Boys in the Band*," said Filichia, "they no longer would settle for thinking of themselves as pathetic and wouldn't be perceived as such any longer. Now that Michael and his friends had brought their feelings out of the closet, this new generation would dare to be different."[2]

Before *Boys* in 1968 showed the world our pain—and the Stonewall uprising the following year began to show us our power—most gay men lived essentially "straight" lives. They were often married to women, fathered children, and kept their "gay life" a secret. Yale history professor George Chauncey, in his landmark book *Gay New York: Gender, Urban Culture, and the Making of the Gay Male World, 1890–1940*, says it was easy for gay men in the vast and multilayered city to lead double lives in the earlier decades of the twentieth century "because they did not consider their homosexual identity to be their only important identity." It's important to remember that keeping their gay life hidden was also a strategic choice because hostile heterosexuals could see to it that jobs and families would be lost and lives wrecked.[3]

It's remarkable that gay men managed, quite well, to find one another over the centuries and in the decades immediately following Oscar Wilde's famous 1895 trial and conviction in London for "gross indecency." Even medical researchers of Wilde's day were continually astonished at gay men's ability to pick one another out of a crowd. They attributed it to a kind of sixth sense. Gay men usually call it "gaydar." At a time when homosexuality was considered a mental illness, this perceptiveness was dismissed as further proof of aberration. "Sexual perverts readily recognized each other, although they may never have met before," wrote one doctor in 1892, "and there exists a mysterious bond of psychological sympathy between them."[4]

Of course gay men viewed that mysterious bond quite differently. In the early twentieth century, gay men had all sorts of interesting ways to find one another. The risks of being visible in the streets led them to resist and undermine their marginalization by developing their own tactics and lingo to identify and communicate with one another without alerting hostile outsiders to what they were doing.[5] Most interesting of all was the fact that gay men had to do this on their own; these were not survival skills learned from their families.

House parties were a popular, and safe, way for gay men to meet one another. So were many cafeterias and restaurants. Chauncey says gay men in New York "turned many restaurants into places where they could gather with gay friends, gossip, ridicule the dominant culture that ridiculed them, and construct an alternative culture." The men created safe spaces for themselves where they could discuss opera or the latest Broadway show, talk about art or a favorite singer, and "laugh collectively about the morning paper's picture of the sailor with his arms wrapped around the cannon he was cleaning." These restaurants served as de facto social centers. They provided an important entry point into the gay world for men just beginning to identify themselves as gay, and offered a way to disseminate useful information about police activity and community events.[6]

In New York, Central Park was a favorite gathering place for gay men to meet their friends and "cruise," a term already used in the 1920s to describe the public search for sex partners. In fact, says Chauncey, "in the 1920s so many men met on the open lawn at the north end of the Rambles that they nicknamed it the Fruited Plain." Throughout the 1920s and 1930s, hundreds of men would gather for an evening in the park. Chauncey says, "The greatest concentration of men could be found (packed 'practically solidly,' according to one account) on the unbroken row of benches that lined the quarter-mile-long walk from the southeastern corner of the park to the mall, a stretch nicknamed Vaseline Alley by some and Bitches' Walk by others."[7] Gay men recognized the homosexual pantomime for the mating game it was; that, of course, is why they were there. Meanwhile, most nongay observers hadn't a clue. They only noticed the "nance element," the most femme of men known even among other gay men at the time as "fairies." All the gay men, says Chauncey, were "fully aware of their numbers on such evenings and exulted in transforming Central Park into a gay park."[8]

Bathhouses were another popular place gay men met one another. One of the oldest and the most famous baths in New York was the Everard. Prominent financier, brewer, and politician James Everard converted the former church into a bathhouse in 1888. The Mount Morris Baths, located in Harlem, was the only baths in New York to admit African Americans from the time it opened in 1883 to the 1960s, when other baths finally admitted them, too. The baths offered a safe, secure place for gay men to have sex with other gay men, rather than to service "normal" men. But they were more than that, too. They fostered a sense of connection among men who shared the same stigmatized "differentness." Chauncey says, "The experience of men at the baths highlights the way gay men built social ties on the basis of their sexual ties and created a social world on the basis of a shared and marginalized sexuality."[9]

No matter how a man might first connect with the gay world, he usually needed guidance in exploring it. Often it was an older man who introduced him to community institutions and to friends, and even helped him figure out how to live as a gay man. They taught newcomers the gay slang, passed on famous stories, and, as Chauncey puts it, taught them "how to survive in a hostile world."[10] Chauncey makes clear that "gay culture was more successful in helping men resist others' negative judgments than is generally imagined." As antigay attitudes came at them from every authority figure in their lives—doctors, clergy, the U.S. government—many gay men resisted the natural tendency to internalize all the condemnation. More than one physician was astonished to find male patients he considered mentally ill because they were homosexual who actually felt quite well. Some even believed they were specially gifted precisely because of the unique sensibility their homosexuality gave them.[11]

Associating with one another was key to counteracting the negative images of gay men. Chauncey says they "also developed cultural resources and subcultural strategies that allowed them to undermine the authority of the dominant culture more directly and to create more affirmative conceptions of themselves."[12] Gay men created histories and claimed their own heroes from the past, gay or at least rumored to be, including not only Oscar Wilde but also Shakespeare, Michelangelo, Julius Caesar, and Alexander the Great.

As early as the 1920s gay men called their most distinctive cultural style "camp." Chauncey describes camp as "a style of interaction and display that used irony, incongruity, theatricality, and humor to highlight the artifice of social convention." It was also an important component of gay men's resilience. Camp humor gave them a way to express their anger at their marginalization and the loss of their male status that came from being grouped with women. Camp also showed that some gay men recognized the artificiality of social and gender roles. "The social order denounced gay men as 'unnatural,'" says Chauncey. "Through camp banter gay men highlighted the unnaturalness of the social order itself."[13]

Nothing embodied camp humor, and turned both the social order and gender roles on their heads, more cleverly than drag. Borrowing and claiming as their own the long tradition of masquerade balls, gay men by the 1890s had already begun to organize their own "drags." Hundreds of heterosexual slummers attended the Greenwich Village drag balls of the 1910s to see the "homosexualists." The balls' popularity and social cachet grew tremendously during Prohibition. In the 1920s, drag (or transvestite) balls drew thousands of participants and thousands more spectators, straight and gay, including the cream of New York society. The biggest, most popular drag balls of all were the ones in Harlem. It was also in Harlem that more men were willing to venture into public in drag. "Drag queens appeared regularly in Harlem's streets and clubs," says Chauncey.[14]

The drag balls were a source of pride, particularly for the fairies who were usually derided by the more traditionally masculine gay men referred to in the day as "normals" or "queers." Gender inversion was central to gay culture, the reason Chauncey says the balls and their organizers occupied an honored place in it. Like ethnic parades and festivals, the balls helped establish a sense of community by bringing people together to share a common culture. In the balls even butch queers could acknowledge their affinity with the femme fairies because they were *all* stigmatized as non-men. "In a world that disparaged their culture," says Chauncey, "it was at the drag balls, more than any place else, that the gay world saw itself, celebrated itself, and affirmed itself."[15]

One of the most important steps gay men took to subvert and survive society's prejudice was in choosing the word *gay* to represent themselves. *Gay* was a coded term that began to catch on in the 1930s and became the choice of white homosexuals in the 1940s. The black gay men who turned Harlem into a homosexual mecca referred to themselves as being "in the life" or "the sporting life." Chauncey points out that as early as the seventeenth century "gay" was used to describe a life of immoral pleasures and dissipation. By the nineteenth century it referred to female prostitution. Of course it also referred to something brightly colored, someone showily dressed, or simply cheerfulness.

Not all homosexuals liked the term, but it provided a way for them to identify themselves to one another without alerting those not in the know. Certainly most gay men, then and now, would agree that embracing their homosexuality as a natural part of themselves made them feel gay in the cheerful sense. Most importantly, Chauncey says, "In calling themselves gay, a new generation of gay men insisted on the right to name themselves, to claim their status as men, and to reject the 'effeminate' styles of the older generation."[16]

The days were passing when gay men felt a need to live vicariously through female divas to provide them with courage and a socially acceptable outlet for the pain and rage they felt at their marginalization. Banter about movies, musical theater, opera, and other cultural and aesthetic subjects would in time come *not* to be the shared reference points for men calling themselves gay the way sports are for many straight men. Gay men would no longer need to refer to one another with winks and euphemisms about being "musical" or "horticultural," discreetly inquire about being "friends of Dorothy," or drown their pain in pills and booze like the real-life Dorothy, Judy Garland herself.

John Clum, professor emeritus of theater studies and English at Duke University, was seventy-four when I interviewed him for this book in early 2016. He's well positioned in time to reflect on gay culture from the age of divas to the era of legal same-sex marriage. In 2000 I reviewed Clum's book *Something for the Boys: Musical Theater and Gay Culture* for the *Washington Post*. In it he looks at pre-Stonewall gay culture from the point of view of what he calls "show queens"—gay men, like himself, who collect and discuss the minutiae of musical theater and its stars. You might say he wrote the book on diva worship.

Clum understands what strong leading ladies represented to many gay men, particularly in the decades before Stonewall. It made perfect sense that a wounded diva like Judy Garland appealed so strongly to gay men back then. "To closeted gay men," writes Clum in *Something for the Boys*, "the diva heroine was a figure of identification. Where does one find magic if one is different and must try to hide one's difference? The ideal is escape from the provincial, where one is hated, and fabulousness, an antidote to grayness and the strong sense of entrapment."[17]

Divas offered both escape and fabulousness in equal measure. Their gay fans identified with women like free-spirited and glamorous Katharine Hepburn, shrewd yet vulnerable Bette Davis, talented and tough Barbra Streisand, and, above all, tragic and triumphant Judy Garland. "Garland was a wreck, but she went on," said Clum.

That is what gay men saw on stage and on the screen: *resilience*. The grit to go on in spite of everything that wants to hold us back. For the divas of screen and stage, the struggle was to be independent women in a world dominated by men. Even today gay men frequently struggle to be true to ourselves in a world dominated by *heterosexual* men. "We were like the divas," said Clum. "We go on and on, but underneath we're hurting." He added, "Divas are survivors. We loved them because they were survivors."[18]

CHAPTER TWELVE

~

Gay Power!

Seizing Control of the Discussion About Gay Lives

While gay men in New York were creating culture and naming themselves, one man in Los Angeles was asking the most fundamental questions of all about us: Who are gay people? Where do gay people come from? Where have gays been throughout history? Harry Hay founded the Mattachine Society in Los Angeles in the fall of 1950 for gay men to gather and ponder these questions. Hay didn't intend the Mattachines to be a political organization per se, but a group that would come together to enhance their self-understanding and explore the contributions gay people had made to the human race through the ages. The group was named after the secret male societies in France that in the Middle Ages dressed as jesters and used dance and comedy—a kind of camp humor—to mock the king and ridicule society's false pretenses.

In a 1988 essay titled "A Separate People Whose Time Has Come," Hay described homosexuals as "spirit people," who, throughout the ages, had served society in their roles as "messengers and interceders, shamans of both genders, priestesses and priests, imagemakers and prophets, mimes and rhapsodes, poets and playwrights, healers and nurturers, teachers and preachers, tinkers and tinkerers, searchers and researchers."[1] Hay believed that gay people had something special to teach nongay people about human life, and for that reason should be nurtured, rather than reviled, by society. He postulated that "gay people represent a genetic mutation of consciousness whose active fostering is now required for human survival."[2]

Forty years after founding the Mattachines, Hay told me in a 1990 interview for the *Washington Blade* that he formed the group to "create for ourselves, a gay identity, which at that time didn't exist." His own gay identity was shaped by a lifetime of deep thought, prolific reading and study, a spirit that bridged the gap between contemplation and activism—and by a memorable encounter. When Hay was fourteen, he had a sexual experience with a twenty-year-old who told him of a "silent brotherhood" of gay men that reached around the world. Hay's life's work, and the basis for the Mattachines, was to tap into and, he hoped, unite that brotherhood.

Hay believed that gay men are different from heterosexuals and that those differences go much deeper than mere sexual attraction to other men. He said gay men look at the world differently, are uniquely nonaggressive, noncompetitive, oriented toward sharing and inclined to develop what Hay called "subject-subject" love relationships of equals. What's more, he told me, our calling as gay men "is not only to accept our uniqueness, but to affirm it, make it joyous."

Hay warned against the "spiritual crisis" of what he called gay men's "hetero-imitative" sexual objectification of themselves and one another. In his "A Separate People" essay Hay wrote of the "appalling dichotomy" between the "nurturing sensitivity and concern for each other in a mutuality of sexual intimacy" and "the desolation and alienation from self and from each other that more often takes place as we make sexual objects of ourselves and of each other in pursuit of the traditional and expected behavior in bars and baths."[3]

Hay believed gay consciousness offers the heterosexual majority an alternative that ultimately will save the human race from its aggressiveness and exploitative relationships. He was quick to point out that the salvation depends upon gay people willingly sharing our spiritual gifts with the nongay world. "Our work," he said in our interview, "is not in our community; it's out in the larger world." A gay ghetto wasn't Harry Hay's vision of brotherhood. You might say he was a champion of gay integration—though most assuredly *not* assimilation. Hay cofounded the Radical Faerie movement in 1979 precisely because of what he saw as the mainstream gay community's assimilationist attitude. The Faeries are, as was Hay himself, dedicated to redefining queer consciousness through spirituality.[4] Speaking of the Faeries and looking back to his original goals for the Mattachine Society, Hay told me, "This is what a lot of the stuff I was talking about in 1950 meant."[5]

While Harry Hay devoted himself to raising gay consciousness, Frank Kameny thought the gay movement needed to get more political and radical. Kameny had just finished his research in Tucson for his Harvard doctoral dissertation in astronomy when he was arrested by plainclothes police officers at a San Francisco bus terminal after a stranger approached and groped him. He was relieved he wouldn't have to worry about his employment prospects when he was told his criminal record would be expunged after three years of probation.

After relocating to Washington, D.C., the native New Yorker Kameny taught for a year at Georgetown University, before being hired in July 1957 by the United States Army Map Service. Kameny's superiors questioned him when they learned of his San Francisco arrest, but he refused to provide information regarding his sexual orientation. He was fired soon afterward. In January 1958, he was barred from future employment by the federal government. Neither his Harvard PhD nor his World War II front-line combat veteran status mattered.

But Kameny was not one to slip quietly away and let the matter drop. He filed one of the first lawsuits ever to challenge the federal government's discrimination against gay people. Douglass Shand-Tucci writes in *The Crimson Letter: Harvard, Homosexuality, and the Shaping of American Culture* that Kameny was "the most conventional of men, focused utterly on his work, at Harvard and at Georgetown." Kameny was radicalized by his experience.[6]

In 1961 Kameny and Washington native Jack Nichols organized the Mattachine Society of Washington, D.C., an affiliate of Harry Hay's original in name more than in style. Nichols had been deeply affected at age fifteen when he read Edward Sagarin's 1951 book *The Homosexual in America*. Nichols recounted decades later in a letter to *The Gay Metropolis* author Charles Kaiser that he was most touched by Sagarin's quotation from the prominent African American activist and author W. E. B. Du Bois: "The worst effect of slavery was to make the Negroes doubt themselves and share in the general contempt for black folk."[7] Nichols well understood the harmful effects of self-stigma in gay men's lives.

At first the D.C. group mostly devoted itself to writing letters to people in the federal government. Kameny represented dozens of civil servants trying to save their jobs or obtain security clearances. In 1963, he began his thirty-year campaign for the revocation of D.C.'s sodomy law, which was finally repealed in 1993.

Kameny and Nichols realized that one of the biggest obstacles to gay people's progress in society was the psychiatric profession's classification of homosexuality as a mental illness. In a 1964 speech to the New York Mattachine Society, Kameny said, "The entire homophile movement is going to stand or fall upon the question of whether homosexuality is a sickness, and upon our taking a firm stand on it."[8]

In March 1965, the D.C. group threw down the gauntlet to the psychiatric establishment whose scientifically dubious classification of homosexuality served, as needed, to justify discrimination against gay people. "The Mattachine Society of Washington," read the group's public statement, "takes the position that in the absence of valid evidence to the contrary, homosexuality is not a sickness, disturbance, or other pathology in any sense, but is merely a preference, orientation, or propensity, on par with, and not different in kind from, heterosexuality."[9]

The following month, Kameny, together with other members of the Washington Mattachine Society and members of the lesbian group Daughters of Bilitis, launched the first gay and lesbian protest in front of the White House on April 17, 1965. Ten members picketed against Cuban and U.S. government repression of homosexuals in the first organized protest by gay people demanding equality. On July 4 of that year Kameny and Nichols organized the first annual Fourth of July pickets outside Independence Hall in Philadelphia. Their presence before America's most hallowed building was intended to remind Americans that not all their fellow citizens were granted the equal justice under law promised in the Constitution, written and adopted right there.

Something clicked for Frank Kameny in the summer of 1968 when he heard African American activist Stokely Carmichael on television leading a group of protesters chanting "Black is beautiful!" He knew immediately that gay people could use their own affirmation. "Gay is good" was his answer. When the North American Conference of Homophile Organizations met in Chicago that summer, they adopted "Gay is good" as their official slogan. The group sent questionnaires to all the political candidates that year, asking their views on a "homosexual bill of rights" that would decriminalize sexual acts between consenting adults and remove all legal support for job discrimination against gay people.[10]

Mainstream religious groups at the time were just beginning to stir on the matter of homosexuality. Some of them opened the church door at least a crack to let in the light of new scholarship, science, and social attitudes. In 1964 the Episcopal Diocese of New York became the first mainstream church to support the decriminalization of sexual acts between consenting adults. In contrast, the Catholic Archdiocese responded by fiercely fighting to defend the laws making both adultery *and* homosexuality criminal acts in New York State.

While the mainstream groups struggled to figure out whether and how much they thought God could tolerate homosexuals, some gay men of faith didn't need their fellow believers' approval to know that God loved them, too.

Troy Perry loved church, even as a southern Georgia kid growing up in the 1940s. Sunday mornings he went to his mother's Southern Baptist church. Sunday night he was at the Pentecostal church. He knew from a young age he was going be a clergyman. He started preaching at age thirteen, and was a licensed Baptist preacher by fifteen. People responded to his preaching and he loved it.

"But I knew I was different," Perry told me in early 2016. A psychiatrist told him he was gay because a friend of his abusive stepfather raped him about the time he started preaching. "I was very lonely," said Perry. "I knew I wasn't sick. I went to my pastor at age eighteen and said I had these funny feelings. I didn't know I was homosexual. He told me I just needed to marry a good woman and that would take care of that problem." Perry married the pastor's daughter.

Five years and two children later, the funny feelings had not gone away. In a Santa Ana, California, bookstore, Perry found *The Homosexual in America* and *ONE* magazine, published by One, Inc., an offshoot of Harry Hay's original Mattachine Society in Los Angeles. "The book said I wasn't sick or sinful," said Perry. "It was a normal experience for people, and *ONE* let me know there are other people like me. That changed my life."

It sure did.

Perry was excommunicated from the Church of God of Prophecy, where he was pastor. His bishop "almost had a heart attack" when he found out Perry admitted openly that he was homosexual. His wife found, and read, his life-changing books. She suggested that maybe they could stay together, but he knew better. "It's not fair to you and it's not fair to me," he told her. They separated, she took their two sons to her parents' home—her parents attributed Perry's homosexuality to demon possession—and it would be seventeen years before he saw one of his sons again; Troy Jr. remains estranged.

It took being drafted into the Vietnam War, serving in the military, to yank Perry out of his funk. "The military was like a finishing school," he said, "not only to get me ready as a person of faith, but it gave me confidence in myself." After his two-year service as a cryptographer, Perry said, "Now I'm not afraid of anybody; I'm the butch gay man. But the one part of my life that just ate me alive was my spirituality. That part was so important to me."

When he fell in love with a man for the first time, in 1968, Perry fell hard. So hard that after six months the man told him he was "the most domineering man he'd ever met" and broke it off. Friends told Perry there were "thousands of fish in the sea." He responded, "But I only love *one* fish." He was inconsolable. "I took a razor blade into the bathtub, and cut both wrists," he said. Fortunately his roommate came home, broke down the door, and took Perry to the hospital as he cried uncontrollably. There he had what might be called a *real* conversion experience.

"I really did pray for the first time since I left the church," he told me, "other than telling God what God couldn't do. I said God, here I am, what a mess I've made of myself. I know you don't know me and you won't hear it but I've committed a sin—not the sin of homosexuality, but because I put a human being on a pedestal. I said I hope you will forgive me for that. Well, all at once, as we Christians say, I had the joy of my salvation again."

Suddenly the doctor came in and "talked to me like a Dutch uncle," said Perry. He asked whether he should lock Perry up in the psychiatric ward for seventy-two hours. Perry told him he was going to be okay. "God," said Perry, "spoke to me in a still small voice and said, 'Troy don't tell me what I can and can't do. I love you. I don't have stepsons and daughters.' I knew without a shadow of a doubt that I could be a Christian and could be a gay man. I didn't understand how, but I knew I could be."

It was the same at every church Perry attended: they loved him because he was tall and confident and a great preacher. But as soon as they found out he was gay, they rejected him. "I knelt and prayed and said 'God I can't find any church that will let me go,'" Perry recalled. "I said 'God, I know you called me to preach. You knew me in my mother's womb, so you knew what I was going to be when I grew up. I know my call is to ministry. I'm so hungry to do what you want me to do. If you want me to open a church that is open to everybody, but with a special ministry to the LGBT community, give me a sign to let me know when.'"

"Now" is all he heard.

Perry went to a gay bar owner and asked how to meet the people from the *Advocate*, which was just starting up in Los Angeles. It happened they were due at the bar in an hour. The owner introduced Perry. "I am Rev. Troy Perry, and want to buy an ad," he told them. "With that they shut down. 'Why should we sell you an ad?' They finally said we will give you the first ad if you buy two more. I said fine, I will send you money after taking up the first collection." Perry's roommate went off the deep end when Perry went home and told him. "You're taking an ad in a gay paper with your photo and our home address?" he said. "Nobody's going to come. The police will be there, scooping people up in nets."

Twelve people showed up on October 6, 1968. After six weeks of services in Perry's living room, the new Metropolitan Community Church moved to a women's club, an auditorium, a church, and then a theater that could hold six hundred. The first Christian denomination with a particular ministry to LGBT people dedicated its own building in 1971 with more than a thousand members in attendance. "There was such a hunger in our community," said Perry.

Today MCC has more than three hundred congregations in eighteen countries. It has had buildings torched by arsonists. Eight of its clergy have been murdered. Perry, seventy-five when we spoke, has participated in every major effort to fight antigay discrimination, from Anita Bryant's 1977 "Save the Children" campaign to the campaign for marriage equality in the twenty-first century. He holds honorary doctorates, has participated in White House meetings on LGBT civil rights, hate crimes, and HIV-AIDS. His books *The Lord Is My Shepherd and He Knows I'm Gay* and *Don't Be Afraid Anymore* have comforted and inspired thousands.

Perry has been arrested, spat on, slapped in the face, and had people try to murder him. All because he was a gay man who believes God loves him, too. "My faith gave me resilience," Perry told me, after recalling the struggle he's had in claiming his equal right to that love. But after so many years of struggle and triumph, he added, "We're not going anywhere."[11]

That was *precisely* the sentiment at the Stonewall Inn on Friday night, June 27, 1969. New York police thought it would be just another routine raid of a gay bar. But tonight was different. The young black and Latino kids and drag queens who frequented the Stonewall were in no mood for it. "I was in the back of the bar near the dance floor, where the younger people usually hung out," recalls Philadelphia native Mark Segal, eighteen years old at the time, newly arrived in Manhattan, and a Stonewall regular. As usual, he said, the cops "walked in like they owned the place, cocky, assured that they could do and say whatever they wanted and push people around with impunity. We had no idea why they came in, whether or not they'd been paid, wanted more payoffs, or simply wanted to harass the fags that night."[12]

As the cops emptied the bar, a crowd gathered outside in Sheridan Square. Onlookers jeered and catcalled as a paddywagon hauled away the bartender, the bouncer, and three drag queens. After a lesbian put up a struggle as the officers steered her through the crowd to a patrol car, all hell broke loose.

"Limp wrists were forgotten," the *Village Voice* reported a few days later. "Beer cans and bottles were heaved at the windows and a rain of coins descended on the cops . . . Almost by signal the crowd erupted into cobblestone and bottle heaving . . . From nowhere came an uprooted parking meter—used as a battering ram on the Stonewall door. I heard several cries of 'let's get some gas,' but the blaze of flame which soon appeared in the window of the Stonewall was still a shock."[13] Backups rescued the cops from the flames.

"It was not the biggest riot ever," says Segal, founder and publisher of *Philadelphia Gay News*. "There were probably only a couple hundred participants; anyone with a decent job or family ran away from that bar as fast as they could to avoid being arrested. Those who remained were the drag queens, hustlers, and runaways."[14] Young Puerto Rican transvestites and homeless youths from the ghetto of runaways in the East Village charged against rows of uniformed police officers. "Whoever assumes a swishy queen can't fight should have seen them," says Segal, "makeup dripping and gowns askew, fighting for their home and fiercely proving that no one could take it away from them."[15]

By the next night "Gay Power" was graffitied along Christopher Street. Young gay men, mostly femme according to reports, hung about the streets. Anger and tension hung in the air. Someone threw a bag of wet garbage into the open window of a police car. A concrete block landed on the hood of another patrol car on Waverly Place. Dozens of men immediately surrounded the car, pounding its doors and dancing on its hood. Cops in riot gear swinging their nightsticks broke up a chorus line of gay men. Several dozen queens screamed "Save Our Sister!" as they rushed a group of officers who were clubbing a young man, dragging him to safety.

Trash fires burned, stones and bottles were tossed, and shouts of "Gay Power!" echoed through the Village. When gay countercultural poet-guru Allen Ginsberg arrived on the scene Sunday evening, he commented on the noticeable change along Christopher Street already evident after the Stonewall riots. "You know," said Ginsberg, "the guys there were so beautiful. They've lost that wounded look that fags all had ten years ago."[16]

CHAPTER THIRTEEN

~

Out and Proud

A Community and Movement Emerge

Arnie Kantrowitz was finally unpacking his books and belongings after a hot summer of searching for an affordable apartment in Manhattan. He was twenty-five and about to start teaching English that fall at Staten Island Community College. The fourth-floor walkup on Bleecker Street wasn't his ideal Greenwich Village address, but for $150 a month the L-shaped studio would have to do.

After spending the Labor Day weekend of 1966 moving in, Kantrowitz finally went out for a stroll around his new neighborhood after midnight Monday. He checked out the shop windows, marveled at the heavy pedestrian traffic for the late hour, and then walked down Christopher Street. "Everything changed all at once," he writes in his 1977 memoir *Under the Rainbow: Growing Up Gay*, "as if by some miracle I was glimpsing a black-and-white world suddenly gone Technicolor."

Kantrowitz wondered whether he'd landed in Oz itself. "The street was literally lined with men," he recalls, "chatting in clusters, standing alone in doorways, sitting on stoops, leaning against railings, strolling, everywhere. They took no pains to hide their obvious interest in each other. They seemed to eye each other with cool ease, as if sex were merely a glance away. Dressed sensually in clinging pants, an extra button open on their shirts to reveal their chests, they seemed utterly unabashed, saying what they pleased and acting as they liked."[1]

Kantrowitz practically ran back to his apartment. "[T]heir freedom terrified me," he says. "Even if I didn't look or act like them I didn't want anyone to know I was one of them." He worried about running into other faculty members from the college. But of course the lure of the street was too much to resist. "It didn't take too many days," says Kantrowitz, "before I poked my timorous head outside my turtle shell for another look at the wonders of Christopher Street."

Although he lived so close, Kantrowitz missed the events at the Stonewall Inn in June of 1969. But on March 8, 1970, the police raided The Snake Pit, a bar on 10th Street that the *New York Times* said was "frequented by homosexuals." After the cops forced their way in, grabbed all the money in the register, and arrested 167 patrons, a young Argentine, afraid of losing his visa and being deported, tried to leap out a window of the Charles Street station house to the next rooftop. He fell onto a spiked fence. Firemen had to cut a portion of the wrought iron fence and transport twenty-three-year-old Diego Vinales, still impaled on five spikes, by ambulance to St. Vincent's Hospital.[2] He lived, fortunately, though he sustained massive and lasting injuries.

At a gathering in Sheridan Square to protest this latest raid, Kantrowitz had the experience that finally spiked his own coming out. "I heard the words that changed my life," he says. "Five hundred homosexuals, not timid faggots, but fierce, demanding, beautiful men and women, were disrupting the nighttime with earthquake chants of 'Say it loud: Gay is proud!' No more apologies. No more shame. Gay doesn't just exist," he realized. "It's glad to exist. It's proud. It's not only all right to be a homosexual, it's a good thing! I couldn't believe it. I had to believe it. It was true."[3]

Not long afterward Kantrowitz saw an ad in the *Village Voice* for a meeting of the Gay Activists Alliance. He'd never been much for meetings but thought this one might offer something to explain what was happening to him. Maybe he wouldn't feel strange with these people. "I had to find out if there was such an animal as a healthy, self-respecting homosexual," he says. "Maybe I could even become one if there was." It was when he realized in the GAA meeting that gay people come in every shape, size, and color that Kantrowitz knew he had at last found his people.

His new friends at GAA called him Arnie, not Arnold, and he soon felt right at home. With Jim Owles, the group's president, and fellow member Vito Russo, the three formed a fun and dishy triumvirate and the core of Arnie's gay family. Their shared vision and passion for gay equality was the glue holding this family together. "The gay world was a consuming infatuation," writes Kantrowitz, "and liberation a vision we were reaching for, a vision of a world in which everyone could be honest, a world without pretending, where men could love men and women love women openly."[4]

It was that vision they bore aloft on placards, wore on T-shirts, pinned across their chests on political buttons, and shouted to anyone with ears to hear as men and women of every age, color, and ability marked the first anniversary of the Stonewall uprising.

The Christopher Street Liberation Day parade kicked off from Waverly Place on Sunday morning, June 28, 1970. Arnie Kantrowitz was one of the marshals. He'd come a long way from turning up his jacket collar so work colleagues wouldn't recognize him as one of "them." He was very much one of *us*, and proudly proclaiming it on this first-ever LGBT pride day. Across his own gay liberation lambda T-shirt, Arnie's buttons shouted "Gay Is Good" and "Gay Revolution," and winked "Fellatio."

"Out of the closets and into the streets!" he shouted with the other marchers as they made their way up Sixth Avenue toward Central Park for their planned "Gay-In."

"Curious crowds began to string along the sidewalks," Kantrowitz writes in *Under the Rainbow*, "as we passed up the avenue, flaunting our hearts on our sleeves. There were smatters of giggling, but they were quickly stifled. We were a few too many to offend. The spectators' faces showed amazement, confusion, shock, resignation, unconcern, affirmation. Ours showed two emotions: pride and determination. We were coming out of our closets, however many of us could, but we were coming out together."[5]

As the marchers made their way north, no one had dared to look back lest their number prove to be as few as they feared it would be. "At last we came to the Sheep Meadow," writes Kantrowitz, "our feet hot and tired. I got to the crest of a small knoll before I turned around. There behind us, in a river that seemed endless, poured wave after wave of happy faces. The Gay Nation was coming out into the light! There was hardly a dry eye on that hill. What had begun as a few hardy hundred had swollen all along its route, until we filled half the huge meadow with what the networks and newspapers estimated as five to fifteen thousand people, all gay and proud of it!"[6]

Mark Segal was there that day, too, marching under the Gay Liberation Front's white banner emblazoned with large, entwined same-sex gender symbols. GLF emerged from the rebellious ferment that followed the Stonewall uprising as LGBT subcommunities were coming together for the first time to organize, strategize, and fight back. "Up until that moment," Segal writes in his own 2015 memoir *And Then I Danced: Traveling the Road to LGBT Equality*, "LGBT people had simply accepted oppression and inequality as their lot in life. That all changed."[7]

GLF marked a watershed in the nascent LGBT movement for equality. The group channeled the anger and energy of its mostly young supporters to propel the movement farther than ever before. "Before Stonewall we were polite," writes Segal. "After Stonewall we demanded our equality." GLF sponsored numerous demonstrations, marches, and "zaps" in which protestors would do things like seize a microphone or obstruct an event.

GLF's more militant leanings weren't for every budding gay activist. Its support for the Black Panthers was the last straw for Jim Owles and Marty Robinson, GLF's visionary leader who Segal says was "the one person" who recognized the potential for the Stonewall raid to be the catalyst for a new movement that would bring together all the separate groups and mark "a pivotal point in history."[8] Owles, Robinson, and a few others left GLF and created Gay Activists Alliance in early 1970—when Arnie Kantrowitz saw that ad in the *Village Voice*.

Many of the new generation of activists who thrived on the energy of Stonewall looked at the Mattachine Society's coat-and-tie, blouse-and-skirt politeness as an anachronism, a hangover of an earlier time. Wistful longing for a place "somewhere over the rainbow" was giving way to a new insistence on equality here and now. "We were going to smash that rainbow," says Segal. "We didn't have to go over anything or travel anywhere to get what we wanted."[9]

But it was the Mattachines, the gay men and lesbians who had been chipping away—bit by bit, year by year—at the very bedrock of legal and social homophobia. It would be the Mattachines as well who could claim what is arguably the single greatest accomplishment in the LGBT equality movement: the declassification of homosexuality as a mental illness. Doing so they effectively removed the strongest pillar of legalized homophobia and opened the door to finally become equal citizens and fully vested human beings.

The Washington Mattachines had already made it clear in their 1965 declaration to the psychiatric profession that there would no longer be a market in the homosexual community for their "pseudo-scientific" views of homosexuality. In 1970, the executive committee of the National Association for Mental Health declared that homosexual relations between consenting adults should be decriminalized. The group's San Francisco chapter adopted a resolution asserting, "Homosexuality can no longer be equated only with sickness, but may properly be considered a preference, orientation, or propensity for certain kinds of life styles." Braced by the affirmation, gay activists began to strike with vehement regularity at the American Psychiatric Association.

The late Barbara Gittings, a leading lesbian activist from Philadelphia and close ally of Frank Kameny, relished the zaps of the APA's conventions, beginning in 1970. "A year after Stonewall," Gittings told me in a

1993 interview, "a lot of gay people were raring to go." Off they went to San Francisco, for the APA's annual meeting, where they disrupted a session on behavioral therapy. Gittings recalled telling the psychiatrists, "We want you to talk *with* us, not *about* us."[10]

The doctors who didn't flee the room stayed to listen. As a result, Gittings and Kameny the following year staffed the first gay-positive booth ever to appear at an APA meeting. The exhibit, "Gay, Proud and Healthy· The Homosexual Community Speaks," included photos of happy lesbians and gay men—a novelty for most of the psychiatrists who stopped by the booth. For good measure, and "in the spirit of the times," as Frank Kameny put it, he and others also zapped an exhibition on "aversion therapy," a meeting of antigay psychiatrist Irving Bieber's and the APA's prestigious Convocation of Fellows.

"Psychiatry is the enemy incarnate!" shouted Kameny, seizing the microphone as he and other gay rights activists effectively took over the world's most important gathering of psychiatrists. The Mattachines may have been known for their button-down style of protest, but Frank Kameny was no ordinary Mattachine. He was a man who believed with every fiber of his being that gay *is* good. "Psychiatry has waged a relentless war of extermination against us," he told the assembled doctors. "You may take this as a declaration of war against *you*."[11]

Kameny decried the injury and gave voice to the anger of gay men and lesbians who, for decades, had been subjected to electroshock, lobotomy, "conversion" therapy, and commitment to mental hospitals by psychiatrists who believed they were "sick" and in need of cure. Kameny believed psychiatry's designation of homosexuality as a mental illness was the prop holding up society's disdain of homosexuality. He reasoned that removing it, kicking it out if necessary, would bring the walls of discrimination tumbling down.

The APA's nomenclature and statistics committee met with a group of gay activists, including Bruce Voeller from the newly formed National Gay Task Force (NGTF), who presented the scientific evidence proving homosexuality was not a mental illness. The committee, headed by Robert Spitzer, prepared a background paper on homosexuality for the APA's board. In it they defined the simple standard by which psychiatrists to this day determine mental illness: for a psychiatric condition to be considered a mental illness, it must either cause distress or impair an individual's social functioning. "Clearly," wrote Spitzer, "homosexuality, per se, does not meet the requirements for a psychiatric disorder since . . . many homosexuals are quite satisfied with their sexual orientation and demonstrate no generalized impairment in social effectiveness or functioning." For the record, he noted, "the terms 'normal' and 'abnormal' are not really psychiatric terms."[12]

Two years after Frank Kameny declared war on psychiatry, the American Psychiatric Association's board of trustees voted unanimously in December 1973 to remove homosexuality from the *Diagnostic and Statistical Manual*, the bible of psychiatric disorders. The board acknowledged that "the unscientific inclusion of homosexuality per se in the list of mental disorders has been the ideological mainstay for denying civil rights" to homosexuals. For good measure, they called for the repeal of sodomy laws and for the passage of antidiscrimination measures to protect the rights of gay people.[13] Ronald Bayer, codirector of Columbia University's Center for the History and Ethics of Public Health, pointed out that the APA's diagnostic change "deprived secular society . . . of the ideological justification of its discriminatory practices."[14]

At a time when physicians, including psychiatrists, were held in very high esteem, it was unheard of that the prestigious medical field could possibly include homosexuals. To prove otherwise, former New York City health services director Howard J. Brown, MD came out publicly as a gay man in October 1973. His announcement made the front page of the *New York Times*. He told the paper he decided to come out because times were changing. "You get to a point in your life where you want to leave a legacy," he said. "In a sense this can help free the generation that comes after us from the dreadful agony of secrecy, the constant need to hide."[15]

Brown capitalized on the publicity his coming out generated by helping to found the National Gay Task Force (NGTF) on October 16, 1973, which helped achieve the massive victory with the APA for gay people only two months later. He wrote in his 1976 memoir *Familiar Faces, Hidden Lives*, "The gay activists who converged on Washington on December 15, 1973, were the first group of patients in history to insist that they were not sick and to demand that the label be removed." When the APA voted to depathologize homosexuality, Brown says, "Never in history had so many people been cured in so little time."[16]

Even before the APA's 1973 decision, Richard Pillard, MD had already become the first openly gay psychiatrist in America. Pillard had just turned eighty-two when I interviewed him for this book in October 2015. He recalled his own experience in psychoanalysis as a patient. He was married at the time and had three daughters. After four years of analysis, he realized he was a gay man and needed to find a male partner. He divorced his wife but remained, and remains, close to her and his three daughters. "I concluded I am a gay man," he said, "and this is not a mental disorder."

Pillard said his decision to come out was made somewhat easier by holding a secure job researching psychiatric medications at Boston University, living in a fairly tolerant state, and the beginnings of gay culture around Boston by the early 1970s. Another factor was Howard Brown. "It's amazing to think he was the first medical doctor to become openly gay," said Pillard, noting that it wouldn't attract any attention at all today. But then it appeared on the front page of the *New York Times.* "What an astonishing, momentous thing it was for somebody in his position to be openly gay," said Pillard. "I rejoiced in this and went to New York and met him. He was a charming and intelligent man."

Besides knowing Howard Brown, another inspiration for the newly out Dr. Pillard was an invitation in the spring of 1970 from the Boston University student homophile league. Now he would know other openly gay people right there in his workplace. "Less than a year after Stonewall, the idea of coming out was becoming embedded in our psyches," said Pillard. "I remember telling a colleague I was going to give a talk to the student homophile league, and he said, 'My god, there's a *league* of them?!'"

Pillard said that coming out had immediate rewards. Best of all, he said, there were no more "dark secrets." He thought a moment, then added, "*That* is gay liberation. Freedom from our own fear."[17]

CHAPTER FOURTEEN

~

Love in Action

Showing the World What "Community" Looks Like in the AIDS Epidemic

Not long after the first AIDS cases were reported, in June 1981, New York writer Larry Kramer wrote in the *New York Native*, "This is our disease and we must take care of each other and ourselves."[1] On August 11, Kramer hosted a meeting at his apartment on Fifth Avenue for gay men interested in learning what little was known about the strange diseases that had already killed some of their friends. Five months later, Kramer's living room was again the setting for what would become a historic event. Kramer, together with five other well-known gay men in the city—journalist Nathan Fain, physician Larry Mass, attorney Paul Rapaport, writer Edmund White, and banker Paul Popham, a Vietnam veteran decorated for valor—made plans to form a new organization. They called it, straightforwardly, Gay Men's Health Crisis.

Kelsey Louie, GMHC's CEO, in 2016 looked back at the organization's founding thirty-five years earlier. "August 11, 1981—35 years ago to this day—was a day like no other," he said. "Fear was spreading rapidly since *The New York Times* published the first article about AIDS, titled 'Rare Cancer Seen in 41 Homosexuals,' July 3 of that year. There is no way to put into words how hard and scary it was to be a gay man during that time. So on August 11, 1981, a group of brave men gathered in Larry Kramer's living room, and together they set a course to change history. Choosing hope and strength over fear and helplessness, they passed around a hat and collected $7,000 to fight this rare cancer."[2]

Like so many AIDS organizations that would be formed in the years ahead, GMHC's first service was a hotline—originally nothing more than the answering service of Rodger McFarlane, who would become GMHC's first executive director. At first GMHC was a kind of ad hoc committee of volunteers who contributed time and created services according to their interests and abilities. "We almost allowed anybody to do anything if they seemed responsible and passionate about it," Kramer told me in an interview for *Victory Deferred*, "whether it was doing an epidemiological study, or wanting to start a buddy system, or translating some stuff into Spanish that we would give out in the bars, or designing a brochure, or putting out a newsletter. We didn't have an office; we met in different people's apartments every week."[3] GMHC worked to create a parallel health care and social service system for gay men who couldn't expect compassionate care from "mainstream" providers. As the needs of gay men with AIDS became clear—from home care, to grocery shopping, to writing wills—GMHC found the volunteer resources and money to create the services.

By the end of its first year, GMHC had grown from its original six founders to more than three hundred volunteers. In its second newsletter, GMHC's board catalogued the group's successes: they had raised more than $150,000; distributed twenty-five thousand copies of their first, and one hundred thousand copies of their second, newsletter; produced three hundred thousand brochures (in English, Spanish, Creole, and French—since Haitians in those earliest AIDS years were also believed to be at heightened risk); fielded almost five thousand hotline calls; formed a network of "buddies" to provide practical support for people with AIDS; provided legal and financial advisers; organized community forums; trained medical professionals; and served as a source of AIDS information for the media. All of GMHC's services were provided by volunteers and offered free. Larry Kramer penned the GMHC's board statement that appeared in its second newsletter. "We have never encountered so much love between men as we have felt at GMHC," it said, "and watching this organization grow in response to our community's terrible new needs has been one of the most moving experiences we have ever been privileged to share."[4]

In San Francisco, gay men, lesbians, and their nongay friends, co-workers, and neighbors also were creating programs to serve the city's growing number of people with AIDS, most of them gay men. In July 1981, dermatologist Marcus Conant, a gay man himself, organized a multidisciplinary clinic at the University of California, San Francisco, to serve the alarmingly increased number of gay men with Kaposi's sarcoma lesions—the disfiguring manifestations of untreated HIV infection that affected gay men more than others with the disease. By the following spring, Conant realized he would have no end of Kaposi's sarcoma patients if something wasn't done to prevent them from becoming sick in the first place. "Wait a minute," he said to himself. "It's not enough to sit up here in your ivory tower and diagnose them, you've got to get out there and stop it."[5]

Conant realized he needed political support in the city's politically active gay community to form an organization that would provide information about the new disease. He contacted Cleve Jones, then an aide to city supervisor (and future mayor) Art Agnos, and former right-hand man of assassinated gay city supervisor Harvey Milk. "Marcus said he wanted to start a foundation," Jones told me in an interview for *Victory Deferred*, "and I said I would help him. I had the political knowledge and connections."

The Kaposi's Sarcoma Research and Education Foundation, known today as the San Francisco AIDS Foundation, had little information to give out at first, so little was known about AIDS then. "We rented this one room on Castro Street, and had one phone line," recalled Jones. "That phone started ringing—and it never stopped." Young men began showing up with purple spots on their feet. There were no services available at the time, nowhere for these men to go except the K. S. Foundation. "People would call," said Jones, "and all we could really say was 'we care,' and 'give us your name and number.'"

Like Larry Kramer, Jones recognized that the gay community's response to AIDS had enormous political implications. "It was the beginning of this incredible grassroots movement," he told me. In the foundation's first year, Jones would go down onto Castro Street and wait for someone he knew to walk by. He recalled, "I'd say, 'You! How would you like to serve your people? Come up here and answer my phone, would you?'" Those young gay men were the first class of recruits in the fight against AIDS. Said Jones, "Many of them now hold high administrative positions. Many are dead."[6]

Whitman-Walker Clinic in Washington, D.C., known today as Whitman-Walker Health, sponsored the city's first community AIDS forum on April 4, 1983. "We ran a few ads in the *Blade*," recalled Jim Graham in our interview for *Victory Deferred*. Graham was the clinic's board president at the time and its director from 1984 to 1998 before being elected to the D.C. city council. "We had no idea whether or not people would be interested," he said. By December of that year, the clinic's AIDS Evaluation Unit began to see patients. "There was no pretense of any treatment," said Graham, "and I wouldn't say it was a full diagnosis because there was no test." He added, "We did have the ability to know what was a K. S. lesion."[7]

Like Whitman-Walker, gay health centers across the country that started as STD clinics during the great gay coming-out party of the 1970s—as sexually transmitted infections raged like wildfire among gay men—expanded into providing AIDS services as a natural extension of the work they already were doing in the community. Chicago's Howard Brown Health Center, for example, added AIDS services to its ongoing involvement at the time with the hepatitis B studies of gay men that would soon lead to a vaccine. In other cities, gay health clinics organized AIDS services as freestanding agencies. Boston's AIDS Action Committee, for example, started as a board committee of the Fenway Community Health Center, known today as Fenway Health, and the world's premier LGBT clinical and health research organization.

In Los Angeles, the Gay and Lesbian Community Services Center—today the world's largest and best-funded LGBT organization and known as the Los Angeles LGBT Center—emerged in 1971 from the gay liberation movement that had begun to blossom in LA as early as the 1950s, when pioneering activist Harry Hay formed the Mattachine Society there. The late Eric Rofes, who became the director of the community center in 1985, explained in an interview for *Victory Deferred*, "It was founded by a group of people, including Morris Kite and Don Hill Heffner, who said they were trying to do political organizing among people who had been damaged by societal homophobia. They needed a place to bring people to heal while doing that work."[8]

Although many black gay men dismissed AIDS in the early years as a "white gay thing"—despite the disproportionate impact it was having on black gay men even then—others realized the dividing line based on skin color wasn't quite so black and white. Fortunately there were black gay men who got it and were willing to speak out. One of the most prominent was the Reverend Carl Bean.

In 1975 Bean formed Unity Fellowship in Los Angeles, the first denomination chiefly for gay men and women of color. A decade later, he created the Minority AIDS Project, America's first community-based AIDS service organization run by and primarily for people of color. In the years between Unity's formation and MAP's creation, Gospel singer Bean in 1977 released "I Was Born This Way" with Motown, the most prominent black-owned record label ever. "I'm happy, I'm carefree, and I'm gay," he sang in one of the first disco songs aimed at the gay community.

Bean was openly gay at the time, and in fact never saw himself as closeted. "In the black church," he told me, "the majority of black Gospel music, we were all gay. Everyone knew it; no one thought we were heterosexuals." Motown promoted Bean just like they promoted their other artists. He wouldn't have expected otherwise because, as he said of his growing-up years in 1950s and 1960s Baltimore, "I never rode in the back of the bus in Baltimore. I sat wherever I wished."

Although Bean was a femme boy—"I was a drum major, twirling batons," he said—he felt loved by his community. In the black neighborhood in Baltimore where he grew up, he said "there were drag queens and transgendered people all over the neighborhood." He said it's "just not reality" to believe the black community is as "insanely homophobic" as it's often portrayed. "There were no gangs, there was no fear with my effeminacy, as some called it. I never felt I would be chased or beaten."

One of Bean's teachers, Miss Pearl, "was as white as could be," he said. "She loved me. She wasn't afraid to drive me home." He mentioned her as one of his role models. "There were people really involved in causing change to take place," said Bean. "I think that is a big part of my resiliency. I could always identify those people of good will who had good hearts and were determined to make this society into what it was thought of around the world, as a democracy. Yes the bad stuff was still there, but there was a wealth of good people in America, always has been, trying to get us to live up to what America is supposed to be. *That* is what made Carl Bean."[9]

Bean realized his work needed to include starting an AIDS organization in the black community. "I always knew I had to go home," he told me. In 1985, he formed the Minority AIDS Project as an outreach of his Unity Fellowship Church in South Central Los Angeles—an area that in the early 1990s would symbolize the country's festering racial wounds when riots broke out there after the acquittal of city police accused of beating black motorist Rodney King. "Being black and gay," said Bean, "and having been black and gay in the community, I also knew the only voice that was going to deal with the issue was going to be a black homosexual who had in fact had the experience of being very openly homosexual in the community."

Bean's strongest opponents were other black gay men. As for his idea that MAP would be part of his church's ministry, the others' reaction was "Jesus and gay and black and church? No!" Bean persisted. "I said yes, it will happen, because all of that is alive in *me*, and *I'm* real. I am black, I am Christian, I am gay, and I'm a part of the black church."

Bean is *all* about being true to himself in every setting. "It has never attracted me to be in a Castro or West Hollywood," he told me in our interview for *Victory Deferred*. "I like talking to the old lady in my building in L.A.— she has a nephew who is gay. She's a delight, a wonderful woman. I have a Russian couple who moved over here recently, and we talk. There's gay folk in my building, and there's Asian folk, black folk, Jewish folk, Greek folk. To me, *that's* humanity. Coming from a past of segregation, I don't understand wanting to create segregation. How are we ever going to love, share, bring about these things that we say our country is built on if we're afraid to know each other?"[10]

~

CHAPTER FIFTEEN

Claiming Our Power

AIDS Organizing Proved Our
Ability to Create Change That Benefits All

Larry Kramer tried to kill himself his freshman year at Yale. The most famous hero of gay America's heroic response to the AIDS epidemic was lonely and felt as though he was the only gay student on campus in 1953. Fortunately for gay men and the world, his suicide attempt failed. A quarter-century later, Kramer would likewise survive character assassination by other gay men after his 1978 novel *Faggots* blew the closet door off the world of drugs, promiscuity, and multiple sexually transmitted infections that had come to define "gay liberation" for many gay men in the great coming-out party of the 1970s.

As a pariah within a community of pariahs, Kramer's outsider status gave him the perspective he would need to become the loudest and most visible champion of gay men's fight to awaken the United States to the realities of AIDS. Unfortunately for gay men *and* for America, Kramer also would live into the name he often used for himself—Cassandra, the mythic daughter of the king of Troy, gifted with foresight but fated never to be believed.

"Unless we fight for our lives, we shall die," he wrote in the *New York Native* in March 1983.[1] Before Kramer's article "1,112 and Counting," gay people were doing what they could to care for the sick and mourn their dead with quiet dignity. After the article appeared in gay papers across the country, they grew increasingly unwilling to be quiet about the deaths of gay men and the preternatural silence about the epidemic from elected officials.

A full year before "1,112 and Counting" appeared, San Francisco's gay community already was rousing to action. In March 1982, the Stonewall Democratic Club sponsored the city's first forum on the new disease, calling it "Gay Cancer." Bobbi Campbell, the sixteenth person in San Francisco to be diagnosed with Kaposi's sarcoma and the self-proclaimed "K. S. Poster Boy," came to show the group what the unusual skin cancer looked like. Twelve people showed up.

A hundred thousand people showed up for the National March for Lesbian and Gay Rights on July 14, 1984, as the Democratic National Convention got underway in San Francisco. On the eve of the march, the Sisters of Perpetual Indulgence—Bobbi Campbell was one of the campy gay men dressed as nuns, performing charitable works in the gay community—staged a mock exorcism of a woman dressed as arch-conservative Phyllis Schlafly and ripped off the pants of a Rev. Jerry Falwell look-alike to expose fishnet stockings and a black corset. Both Schlafly and Falwell were in San Francisco at the time, rallying their own antigay forces.[2]

The momentum generated by the July march spiraled into support for an independent gay AIDS activist group in San Francisco. Thirty-one-year-old Paul Boneberg, then president of the Stonewall Democratic Club, was tapped by other gay community leaders to head the new group. Mobilization Against AIDS came into existence in the fall of 1984 with the express goal of organizing street demonstrations, a goal it accomplished by staging monthly protests. Besides its street demos, Mobilization, beginning in 1985, took on the task of organizing the annual AIDS candlelight vigil that the San Francisco People with AIDS Coalition had started in 1983. On the night of March 2, 1983, a dozen gay men with AIDS led the first candlelight march in San Francisco. They smiled bravely at one another and held up a banner that encapsulated their hope and struggle: "Fighting for Our Lives," it said. Gary Walsh, one of the city's first to be diagnosed with AIDS and the one who thought of the idea for the candlelight march, held the banner between Bobbi Campbell and Mark Feldman, an old boyfriend.

The PWA Coalition had asked Paul Boneberg to help them organize the candlelight march in San Francisco, and to get other cities to hold similar marches. Boneberg marveled years afterward at the drive of the men with AIDS who led that first march. "I can't think of another community on earth," he told me in an interview for *Victory Deferred*, "that would think the logical response to being stricken with an unknown disease was to come out, say your name on TV, and organize a march! It directly flows from Harvey Milk, and [his saying] 'Come out, come out! Organize, organize!'"[3]

As the 1980s wore on and tens of thousands of gay men died with still no effective treatment for AIDS, Larry Kramer's nerves were shot. In a March 10, 1987, speech he gave at the New York Lesbian and Gay Community Services Center, today known as the LGBT Center of New York, Kramer laid into the gay community as only Larry Kramer could. "If my speech tonight doesn't scare the shit out of you, we're in real trouble," he told the group. By then, thirty-two thousand AIDS cases had been reported across the country—nearly a third of them in New York. President Reagan still hadn't spoken about AIDS to frightened Americans. "If what you're hearing doesn't rouse you to anger, fury, rage, and action, gay men will have no future here on earth," said Kramer. "How long does it take before you get angry and fight back?" The crux of the speech was Kramer's simple question: "Do we want to start a new organization devoted solely to political action?"[4]

The answer was a resounding "Yes!" Two days later, about three hundred people again showed up at the center where they formed ACT UP, the AIDS Coalition to Unleash Power. The group's first demonstration—a protest on Wall Street against the exorbitant price of just-approved AZT, the most expensive drug ever to that point—introduced what became the group's distinctive brand of street theater. ACT UP took the camp humor and theatricality of the Gay Liberation Front "zaps" to a whole new level.

ACT UP/New York's energy and early successes sparked the formation of ACT UP chapters in cities across the United States and in several other countries as well. In San Francisco, for example, the late activist Hank Wilson told me in our 1995 interview for *Victory Deferred*, "We formed ACT UP here because we liked the name, we got off on the energy of the people in New York, and we loved their graphics."[5] As Larry Kramer told me, "The fact that everybody responded to ACT UP, I think was more just a question of time, and moment, and frustration. It was the right time for it to happen."[6]

ACT UP's brightest moment of media coverage was its October 11, 1988, protest against the Food and Drug Administration. A year to the day after the second March on Washington for Lesbian and Gay Rights, and just after the second showing of the AIDS Memorial Quilt in Washington, D.C., "Seize Control of the FDA" became the most widely publicized of ACT UP's early demonstrations. It was organized by ACT NOW, a network of ACT UP chapters throughout the country that had formed during the 1987 march, primarily to protest the FDA's hidebound procedures for the testing and approval of new drugs.

Activists in T-shirts that said "We Die, They Do Nothing!" plastered the front of the Parklawn Building, the suburban Washington FDA headquarters, with ACT UP graphics and banners that said things like "Time isn't the only thing the FDA is killing" and "The Government has blood on its hands. One AIDS death every half hour." Others provided a nonstop theatrical spectacle for television cameras that ate it up. One group did "die-ins," lying on the ground in front of cardboard tombstones with "epitaphs" such as "R.I.P. Murdered by the FDA." Another group wrapped themselves in red tape. The ten-hour demonstration more or less shut down the FDA and resulted in 176 arrests. On October 24, nearly two weeks after the demonstration, FDA Commissioner Frank Young called for researchers to help speed the process for developing and approving AIDS drugs. For the first time in history a group of "patients" and their advocates had succeeded in forcing the FDA to budge.

Peter Staley was a twenty-four-year-old bond trader on Wall Street in 1985 when his doctor diagnosed him with the "pre-AIDS" stage of HIV infection known at the time as AIDS-Related Complex. He thought he only had a bad cold. He went to a support group for gay men with AIDS in August 1986. Looking back, he told me, "Nineteen of those twenty guys were like 'Woe is me, I'm tainted meat. I can't have sex again and have very little time to live.'" That fatalism didn't fly with Staley. "I was like, 'I'm not coming back to this meeting!' I was having none of it," he said. "I just wasn't ready to bring that self-loathing into it."

After he was handed a flyer on the way to work, Staley decided to check out what became the organizing meeting of ACT UP. Although he was closeted at first, he chaired ACT UP's fundraising operations before coming out at work and going on disability leave. When he took part in ACT UP's first-anniversary demonstration on Wall Street on March 24, 1988, he was interviewed by a local TV station that broadcast his image with the caption "Peter Staley, AIDS victim."

Next to Larry Kramer, there is probably no one who is less a "victim" than Peter Staley.

Like other white, gay, urban men in the 1970s, Staley said, "We were mostly privileged gay white guys in the city and those gay ghettoes and the closet allowed us to have a sense of privilege and a life that a lot of us were enjoying." But "it was a shock to most of us," he added, "when we discovered how much we were hated, that our government was going to do nothing as we began to die en masse. The nice and protected lives we built were being yanked out from under us. I think there was a collective indignation. I think we were shocked."

ACT UP provided Staley's introduction to gay history, and he was impressed by what he learned. "I was a closet case on Wall Street when I became an activist," he said, "so I knew little of our history. I barely knew about Stonewall when I became HIV-positive." Someone in ACT UP suggested he check out *The Times of Harvey Milk*, winner of the 1984 Oscar for best documentary.

"I had absolutely no idea," said Staley, "there was this politically active community that was thriving in San Francisco at the time that was so huge and strong it could win against a ballot initiative [the 1978 Briggs initiative that would have banned gay men and lesbians from teaching in California public schools] and spark the White Night Riots." In the biggest uprising since Stonewall, the gay community in San Francisco erupted in fury on the night of May 21, 1979, after Harvey Milk's fellow supervisor and killer Dan White received a lenient sentence because his addiction to junk food allegedly impaired his judgment.[7] Knowing what he learned about the gay community in San Francisco "absolutely informed everything I did after that," said Staley. "I found history *hugely* motivating."[8]

Other gay men who didn't identify with the privileged white gay men radicalized by AIDS drew from other sources of identity and experience in responding to the frightening politics of AIDS. ACT UP's logo "Silence = Death," the most iconic image of the AIDS epidemic, was created by a consciousness-raising collective of artists pulled together in 1985 by Brooklyn, New York, artist Avram Finkelstein. "It was no accident that three of the six members of the collective were Jewish," Finkelstein told me in an interview. These men knew from the Jewish community and their own family histories how fear of those branded as "different" can escalate to official condemnation, round-ups, and even concentration camps.

When William F. Buckley Jr. in 1986 called for gay men to be tattooed on their buttocks to "warn" prospective sex partners they might have AIDS, the group struggled for six months to figure out what an appropriate poster response would be about. Finkelstein said they wanted something iconic. They considered the rainbow flag, the lambda symbol, and the pink triangle gay men were forced to wear in Hitler's concentration camps during the Holocaust. "We rejected the pink triangle," Finkelstein told me, "because we were Jewish, and even though William F. Buckley was talking about tattooing people, which definitely relates to the history of the camps, we weren't sure that was the right symbol because it would telegraph other things—and one of them was the intonation of victimhood."

But they kept coming back to the pink triangle. When they inverted it, they knew they found what they wanted. The phrase "Silence = Death" "happened literally in ten minutes," said Finkelstein. "I had seen some phrases in the news: 'The silence is deafening.' I asked the collective, 'What about gay silence is deafening'? Someone else said 'silence equals death.' Someone else said 'equals should be an equal sign.' We all jumped up and screamed."[9]

The inverted pink triangle became the perfect symbol for gay men who were likewise overturning old ideas about homosexuals and what it means to be an American. Who else but proud, openly gay men would have the nerve—in the face of a highly stigmatized and deadly epidemic—to reject society's stigma and insist on discussing the actual facts of an exploding, deadly epidemic?

It took enormous courage and audacity to push back against the mountain of shame our fellow Americans expected us to bear silently as the price of being what they considered abominations. But we had likewise rejected the stigma that psychiatry had forced on us for decades, labeling our "different" sexual orientation a mental illness. "I definitely think there was something about that moment," said Peter Staley, "and that community definitely supported everybody's shedding of shame and instilled a feeling of indignation and pride."[10]

Never was that indignation and pride expressed as simply and powerfully as it was in the Denver Principles and the People with AIDS (PWA) self-empowerment movement the principles spawned. A group of gay men with AIDS from New York and San Francisco met during the Second National AIDS Forum, held in Denver in 1983 in conjunction with the annual lesbian and gay health conference, and created a document that would literally shape the world's response to AIDS.

Bobbi Campbell—San Francisco "K. S. Poster Boy," Sister of Perpetual Indulgence, and nurse—took charge of the room as a dozen people with AIDS met together in a hospitality suite during the conference to talk about how they might organize themselves. They made plans for a coalition of political groups in all the cities with large AIDS populations, proposing that the local groups join one another in forming a national group. Campbell also conveyed the wish of his fellow San Franciscan, Mark Feldman, who succumbed to AIDS just before the conference, that terms like *patient* and *victim* should be rejected because they were disempowering. It took a bit of convincing, but the New York contingent joined the group from California to insist that those with the disease be known simply as "people with AIDS" or "PWAs."

The PWAs who met in Denver realized they shared the same frustration with not being listened to by their health care providers—or even, too often, by those who were providing services to them in the new AIDS organizations that had mostly been started by gay people. They drafted a manifesto known as the "Denver Principles," a series of rights and recommendations for health care providers, AIDS service organizations, and people with AIDS themselves. The Denver Principles became the charter of the movement for PWA self-empowerment. Among them was the recommendation that people with AIDS "be involved at every level of AIDS service organizations," and that they retain the right "to full explanations of all medical procedures and risks, to choose or refuse their treatment modalities, to refuse to participate in research without jeopardizing their treatment, and to make informed decisions about their lives."

These gay men with AIDS were not a passive lot. As they put it in the preamble of the Denver Principles, "We condemn attempts to label us as 'victims,' a term that implies defeat, and we are only occasionally 'patients,' a term that implies passivity, helplessness, and dependence upon the care of others. We are 'People with AIDS.'"[11]

POZ magazine founder and Body Counts author Sean Strub was already a legendary direct-mail fundraiser in New York for LGBT organizations when he joined, and raised big bucks for, ACT UP/New York. He said in an interview for this book in Milford, Pennsylvania—where he was mayor at the time—that the creation of the Denver Principles "was not only the first time a group of PWAs got together to strategize politically, but the first time in the history of humanity that a group of people with a disease gathered together to have a political voice in decisions that would affect their lives."

Then again, it was radical for homosexuals considered mentally ill to challenge the psychiatric profession—and win. That victory had propelled the gay equality movement from arguing to be accepted, to claiming our right to exist. In too many quarters, as the fear and bigotry unleashed by AIDS amply demonstrated, it was a radical act simply to say gay men's humanity was equal to that of heterosexuals.

Strub pointed out that when New York musician and longtime AIDS activist and survivor Michael Callen interviewed PWAs for his 1990 book Surviving AIDS, he found that long-term survivors had three things in common: they could define a purpose for their lives, a reason they wanted to survive. They believed that survival was possible. And when asked what they had done to treat their HIV infection, the length of their list said everything. "Those who were living long had longer lists," said Strub. "They were the seekers, the ones going out and seeking things that might potentially be helpful to them." He added what he considers a fourth factor. "I think maybe the piece Michael didn't have in there that became enormously important in ACT UP—and I think feeds one's resilience—is being part of a community."[12]

Peter Staley agrees. For him, as for thousands of gay men, finding so many others who rejected victimhood changed—and probably saved—his life. Staley believes the supportive, mutually affirming, socially and politically engaged community he found in ACT UP still exists. "Even though a lot of people say they have less sense of community these days," he said, "one thing that never died down was the indignation. I think whatever got lit in 1987 has stayed pretty bright on the indignation front. As a people now, we will not be denied. And that is history. We know that if we are indignant and angry and push all the political levers that we know we have, that we've used in the past and used successfully, we can push back."[13]

The light was dimming and the temperature dropping in San Francisco on an early September afternoon in 2015 as I sat with Paul Boneberg for an interview in the front window of illy Caffè. A couple blocks down Market Street was Castro Street, still the symbolic heart of San Francisco's gay community and the namesake of the city's neighborhood hardest hit by AIDS. Literally thousands of gay men died there. Now sixty-three, it's been years since Boneberg was the first director of Mobilization Against AIDS, the granddad of AIDS protest groups. We spoke about the leading role the gay community has played in San Francisco's response to the HIV-AIDS epidemic since the beginning, the model it created of low-cost, community-based care and support services for homebound people with life-challenging illness, and the personal and community empowerment that were both strengthened as a result.

"One of the things I'm most proud of," said Boneberg, "is San Francisco's trying to embrace the wholeness of its own diversity. I'm proud of the community's response, and my role in it." He said he hopes "no other queer community" has to face a massive disaster like AIDS and the flood of homophobia it engendered. As in every catastrophe humans have faced throughout history, there were only two options for gay men in San Francisco when the viral cluster bomb erupted in the community: fight or flight. "AIDS made us choose," said Boneberg. "Most chose to stay and fight." In his characteristically understated manner, Boneberg added, "It is my experience that our community is heroic."[14]

AIDS gave gay men new words to use in defining "gay" that better suit a people who were tested by the fire of terrible illness, death, and stigma—and survived. Four words that come to mind are: *heroic, brave, courageous,* and *proud.* Larry Kramer made it clear in his landmark 1985 play *The Normal Heart* that the AIDS epidemic gave gay men a new, powerful identity to claim for ourselves. Kramer's alter-ego Ned Weeks says, simply, "That's how I want to be defined: as one of the men who fought the war."

Kramer put it a little differently in our 1995 interview for *Victory Deferred.* We talked in the living room of his Fifth Avenue apartment, the setting for some of gay America's most historic moments, including the world's first AIDS fundraiser in 1981 and, in 1982, the formation of GMHC, the world's first AIDS service organization. Reflecting in particular on ACT UP, Kramer said, "Singlehandedly, we changed the image of gay people from limp-wristed fairies to guerrilla warriors."[15]

On a sweltering late July afternoon in 2015, the air conditioner in his history-filled living room blasting at full tilt, I reminded Kramer of the quotation I had borrowed from *Faggots* as the epigraph for the opening chapter of *Victory Deferred*. In it the Krameresque protagonist Fred Lemmish marks his fortieth birthday saying, "It's the beginning of the summer of our lives." What, I asked Lemmish's creator, would he say if a forty-year-old Fred Lemmish walked in and a now eighty-year-old Larry Kramer met him. "What would you tell a younger version of yourself?" I asked. "I tried to kill myself my freshman year at Yale," said Kramer. "The younger Fred Lemmish almost wasn't around to be anything but the younger Fred Lemmish. I don't think so much about that. Somewhere along the line I was able to work out that I love being gay, that it was the most important thing in my life."[16]

~

CHAPTER SIXTEEN

Love (and America) Won

Our Successful Push for Marriage Equality Moved America Closer to Fulfilling Its Promise

"Mr. Marriage," as Evan Wolfson would come to be known, moved to New York to work with Lambda Legal, shortly after graduating from Harvard Law School in 1983. Outside his new job with the nation's oldest and largest LGBT legal organization, the twenty-six-year-old Wolfson didn't know any gay people in the city at the time, so he decided to march in his first gay pride parade with the group from Yale. He had graduated from Yale in 1978 with a bachelor's degree in history, a subject that is still his passion even as he himself has helped to make history.

One of the people in the Yale group was history professor John Boswell. Wolfson told me in an interview that reading Boswell's 1980 book *Christianity, Social Tolerance, and Homosexuality* was one of the major life experiences that led him to write his third-year law school paper, titled "Samesex Marriage and Morality: The Human Rights Vision of the Constitution."[1] "As somebody who loves history," said Wolfson, "being able to read of my story, which I was now able to claim as *my* story, through this dimension of history already meant a lot to me. It really gave me an insight that inspired me. The insight was that it had been different how gay people had been treated and exalted over different periods of time. That made me think that if it had once been different, it could be different again." When he met Boswell in the parade, Wolfson said, "We immediately clicked and talked all the way down Fifth Avenue about same-sex marriage."[2]

For the next thirty-two years Evan Wolfson would *keep* talking about same-sex marriage. The man described as the "architect" of the marriage-equality movement believed that by claiming for ourselves the vocabulary of marriage—love, commitment, connectedness, freedom—gay people could transform America's understanding of us, and make clear why exclusion and discrimination are wrong.

As the gay community staggered under the impact of AIDS in the 1980s, and activists debated what the equality movement's priorities should be, few agreed that marriage should be a top priority. Some resisted marriage altogether, arguing it was little more than a patriarchal hangover. Others had strategic concerns, doubtful their fellow Americans would ever allow same-sex couples to wed. Not only that, but they feared the fight for marriage equality could set back the movement for LGBT equality itself.

As it turned out, AIDS propelled the marriage equality movement—just as it did the broader LGBT equality movement. "AIDS was a wake-up call," said Wolfson. It woke up gay people to our vulnerability in being excluded from legal protections for our relationships. AIDS also made activists realize they needed to exchange gay people's traditional "leave us alone" posture toward government for a "let us share and participate from within" approach.

Wolfson said AIDS also woke up nongay people. "Americans got to see this very different vision of who gay people were," he told me, "and that helped set the stage for changing hearts. I think AIDS played an enormous role in paving the way to change hearts and minds and understanding in the non-gay world so we could change the law *and* change our place in society."[3]

Many of the hearts and minds that needed changing belonged to gay men and lesbians themselves. One of the corrosive effects of self-stigma among gay men is the common belief that gay relationships can't last, or that sex is the only way gay men are connected to one another. Others were opposed to "surrendering the noble outlaw position," as Wolfson put it. But he said that a lot of the resistance to making marriage equality a priority "was due to being taught we couldn't have it, were not worthy of it, that our love was not as serious, enduring, didn't need the same kind of support and protection that a 'real' deep procreative marriage nurtures. People had a lot of doubt about it and a lot of coping strategies for coping with not having it. They were not only told they couldn't have it by hostile anti-gay people, but by fellow gay people."[4]

After President Bill Clinton signed the 1996 Defense of Marriage Act (DOMA) into law, denying any federal recognition of same-sex marriages, Wolfson, as Lambda Legal's marriage project director, organized national LGBT groups to meet and plan for how to achieve the freedom to marry.

He was nicknamed "Mr. Marriage" and "The Paul Revere of Marriage" as he traveled the country telling people that the freedom to marry is coming.

A $2.5 million challenge grant from the Evelyn and Walter Haas Jr. Fund provided the fuel Wolfson needed to launch Freedom to Marry in 2003. The campaign to win marriage-equality nationwide would work to build momentum aimed at eventually pushing either the Supreme Court or Congress to act.[5] As gay and lesbian attorneys filed lawsuits and waged court battles, Freedom to Marry encouraged local LGBT advocates around the country to organize their efforts around marriage in their own communities and states.

When Massachusetts led the way on same-sex marriage in 2004, many other states doubled down to deny gay people the freedom to marry. The Republican Party's longtime strategy of using social issues to frighten Americans into supporting them used fear of same-sex marriage to turn out conservative voters in 2004. Thirteen states voted to amend their constitutions to outlaw same-sex marriage. President George W. Bush, supporting an amendment of the U.S. Constitution to ban same-sex couples from marrying, won election to a second term.

Just before Election Day, Wolfson admonished legal professionals gathered in Minneapolis for the National LGBT Bar Association's annual Lavender Law Conference to dig in for a longer battle. In a speech called "The Scary Work of Winning," he told the group that even with the losses expected in the election, the number-one lesson was that "wins trump losses." He said that even the movement's one victory, in Massachusetts, "gives fair-minded Americans the opportunity to see and absorb the reality of families helped and no one hurt when the exclusion of same-sex couples from marriage ends."[6]

In 2008, the California Supreme Court declared it unconstitutional to deny same-sex couples the right to marry. Thousands of couples took advantage of their right and legally wed. But on November 4, 2008, voters overruled their own Supreme Court and supported Proposition 8, another antigay state constitutional amendment, by a slim 52 percent to 48 percent margin. Suddenly thousands of legal marriages were declared illegal. "Prop. 8" came into immediate effect the day after the elections. Demonstrations and protests in California and across the country followed—as did numerous lawsuits challenging the proposition's validity and effect on formerly legal same-sex marriages.

Meanwhile on the other coast, Connecticut's Supreme Court on November 12, 2008, struck down the state's civil union law and declared that same-sex couples had a constitutional right to marriage.[7] Nicknamed the "Constitution State" because its 1639 Fundamental Orders is widely viewed as the first constitution in what became the United States, my own home state now helped lead the way on marriage equality.

"Prop. 8" became a rallying cry for activists. Even nongay people were shocked to see an entire class of Americans stripped of a fundamental human right they took for granted. Now bigger guns got involved. Tim Gill, the openly gay Quark software founder, launched the Gill Action Fund to build a team of political strategists and help focus LGBT funders to invest in state-level LGBT rights campaigns. As the ACLU, GLAAD, Lambda Legal, and the National Center for Lesbian Rights mounted court challenges in various states, Freedom to Marry kept up its effort to enlist allies among labor unions, religious groups, African American and Latino civil rights organizations, and the business world.

Although state courts upheld Proposition 8, federal courts ruled it unconstitutional. On August 4, 2010, U.S. District Chief Judge Vaughn R. Walker, a gay man, said the state's constitutional amendment violated the federal constitutional rights of gay men and lesbians to marry the partners of their choice. Walker pointed out that singling out gay people to deny their right to marry created an "irrational classification on the basis of sexual orientation." He added, "Plaintiffs seek to have the state recognize their committed relationships, and plaintiffs' relationships are consistent with the core of the history, tradition and practice of marriage in the United States."[8]

Antigay Prop. 8 supporters naturally appealed Walker's decision. But a Ninth Circuit Court of Appeals panel asked the California Supreme Court to rule whether Prop. 8 proponents had the right to appeal (called "standing") if the state itself didn't appeal. The court ruled that they did. Prop. 8 remained in place for a while longer while appeals continued to the U.S. Supreme Court.

Besides organizing in the states, the marriage equality movement's "Roadmap to Victory" strategy included challenging the federal Defense of Marriage Act. Between 2010 and 2014, Freedom to Marry's budget ballooned to more than $13 million. The group set its sights on New York, knowing a victory in the third-largest state would reverberate across the country. Just before midnight on June 24, 2011, the New York Senate approved the freedom to marry.

After analyzing more than eighty-five sets of research data from state marriage campaigns in 2010, Freedom to Marry realized they needed to change their messaging. When voters were asked in one Oregon poll, "Why do couples like me get married?" 74 percent responded "for love and commitment." When the same voters were asked "Why do same-sex couples get married," 42 percent responded "for rights and benefits." Only 37 percent responded "love and commitment." Twenty-two percent didn't answer the question, presumably because they had no idea why same-sex couples would want to marry.

The group realized they needed to emphasize love and commitment, and make clear gay people didn't want to redefine marriage; they wanted to participate in the institution. Freedom to Marry shifted its messaging toward helping voters understand why same-sex couples want to marry—and why the Golden Rule, treating others as you would like to be treated, applied to the issue.[9]

In February 2011 the Obama administration announced that the U.S. government would no longer defend DOMA because it had determined the law violated the 14th Amendment of the Constitution. Although presidential candidate Barack Obama had supported civil unions but not same-sex marriage, President Obama still opposed same-sex marriage while supporting the repeal of DOMA. Freedom to Marry enlisted the support of senior members of the Obama administration as well as celebrities and leaders to pressure the president, particularly after he indicated his openness to "evolving" on the subject.

Vice President Joe Biden stunned many with his comments on NBC's *Meet the Press* on Sunday, May 6, 2012. When asked about President Obama's "evolving" views on marriage equality, Biden said, "I am absolutely comfortable with the fact that men marrying men, women marrying women, and heterosexual men and women marrying one another, are entitled to the exact same rights, all the civil rights, all the civil liberties." He also made clear that it was the president, not vice president, who made policy decisions. For Biden, the debate boiled down to a simple question of "Who do you love?" and "Will you be loyal to the person you love?" He explained, "That's what people are finding out is what all marriages, at their root, are about, whether they're marriages of lesbians or gay men or heterosexuals."

The vice president framed the issue in personal terms. He recalled meeting a gay couple's children at a fundraiser in Los Angeles two weeks earlier. During a question-and-answer session at the fundraiser, Biden said a gay man asked him, "How do you feel about us?" In response, Biden asked the owner of the house, "What did I do when I walked in?" The man said, "You walked right to my children. They were seven and five, giving you flowers." To which Biden recalled responding, "I wish every American could see the look of love those kids had in their eyes for you guys. And they wouldn't have any doubt about what this is about."[10]

Everyone expected Biden's comments would intensify pressure on Obama to evolve into a supporter of marriage equality. In fact, only three days later, on May 9, 2012, the president's evolution was obviously complete when he sat down to an interview in the White House Cabinet Room with openly lesbian *Good Morning America* journalist Robin Roberts. "At a certain point," he said, "I've just concluded that for me personally it is important for me to go ahead and affirm that I think same-sex couples should be able to get married." Obama said he had changed his views partly because of gay friends who had prodded him, and conversations with his wife and daughters. Echoing Freedom to Marry's messaging, he added that the Golden Rule also factored into his "evolution."

Obama's then-presumed Republican opponent in 2012, Mitt Romney, immediately opposed the president's announcement. No one knew what political impact Obama's change of heart might have on his reelection campaign underway. It wouldn't change any laws, but it could certainly drive the conversation forward. Public support for same-sex marriage was growing, and same-sex couples were featured in popular television shows. Vice President Biden had credited *Will and Grace* with changing many hearts and minds about gay people. But there was opposition by white working-class voters, who didn't strongly support Obama anyway, and by many African Americans who did.

Openly gay U.S. Representative Barney Frank, Democrat of Massachusetts, didn't worry about the politics. "This country is moving," Frank told the *New York Times*, "and what's interesting is every time somebody does something that's supportive of our rights, it turns out to be (a) popular and (b) not very controversial." He said many Americans already assumed Obama supported same-sex marriage anyway. "Politically, it's kind of a non-event," he said.[11]

In a kind of legal two-fer—with twice the victory for gay and lesbian people as well—the U.S. Supreme Court on June 26, 2013, ruled in *Hollingsworth v. Perry* that those who had appealed Judge Walker's decision had no standing. It dismissed the appeal and ruled that the California's Ninth Circuit had erred in allowing it. This left Walker's original federal district court ruling against Proposition 8 as the final outcome. Same-sex marriages in California resumed almost immediately afterward.[12] On the same day the Supreme Court ruled that Section 3 of DOMA, "Definition of Marriage," created "a deprivation of the liberty of the person protected by the Fifth Amendment." Section 3 stated that the federal government would recognize the word *marriage* as applying *only* to a legal union between one man and woman as husband and wife, and the word *spouse* as a person of the opposite sex who is a husband or a wife.[13]

New Yorkers Edie Windsor and Thea Spyer first met in a West Village restaurant in 1963. In 1965 they began dating after reconnecting in the Hamptons, and got engaged in 1967. They were legally married in Canada in 2007—forty-four years after they met. New York governor David Paterson in 2008 had ordered state agencies to recognize same-sex marriages performed in other jurisdictions. But the real impact of DOMA became clear after Spyer died in 2009. Because the federal government under DOMA didn't recognize even same-sex marriages that were legal in a state or another country, Windsor was forced to pay $363,053 in federal estate taxes on the estate Spyer left entirely to her—a massive bill no heterosexual widow had ever received. Edie Windsor wanted a refund.

By the time her lawsuit made its way through the courts up to the Supreme Court, Windsor got more than she ever dreamed. In *United States v. Windsor*, the court held that the U.S. government's interpretation of "marriage" and "spouse" as applying only to opposite-sex couples violated the Fifth Amendment's due process clause, which says to the federal government that no one shall be "deprived of life, liberty or property without due process of law." The Court held that the Constitution prevented the federal government from treating legal heterosexual marriages differently from legal same-sex marriages, and that such differentiation "demean[ed] the couple, whose moral and sexual choices the Constitution protects."[14]

Thousands of supporters in the brilliant June sunshine outside the Supreme Court building waved American flags and rainbow flags, cheered, and wept joyful tears. When Edie Windsor came out to the front steps, the crowd chanted her name. She put it plainly: "I wanted to tell you what marriage meant to me. Marriage is different. It's a huge difference. It's a magic word—for anyone who doesn't understand why we want it and why we need it, it is magic."[15]

Roberta Kaplan, one of Edie Windsor's attorneys, said in a speech to one of the country's largest synagogues, where many members in 2016 voted for Donald Trump, "We always believed that we would win our case if we could convince the judges that the marriage that Edie had with Thea, despite all the bigotry and homophobia, was really no different than their own. We succeeded."[16]

President Obama hailed the DOMA ruling as "a victory for American democracy."[17] In a formal statement the day after the ruling, Obama said, "We are a people who declared that we are all created equal—and the love we commit to one another must be equal as well. . . . The laws of our land are catching up to the fundamental truth that millions of Americans hold in our hearts: when all Americans are treated as equal, no matter who they are or whom they love, we are all more free."[18]

"More free," absolutely. But still not quite equal. The *Windsor* decision set the federal government in action to equalize benefits for same-sex couples legally married in their own states. But now there were so many different "classes" of marriage in the country—different-sex couples who could marry in any state, remain legally married wherever they went, and have their marriages recognized by the federal government; married same-sex couples whose marriage might be recognized by their state and now the federal government, but perhaps not by the state next to theirs; and married same-sex couples whose marriage was recognized by the federal government but not by their own state.[19] Same-sex couples legally married in one state could drive across the state line into a state that banned same-sex marriage and find themselves legally single again.

Clearly this patchwork quilt was coming apart at the seams. Growing public support and political progress, boosted by the *Windsor* decision, gave rise to legal challenges in every remaining state with a marriage ban. By the fall of 2014, there were already five same-sex marriage cases seeking U.S. Supreme Court review. The court denied review, which meant the five states where federal judges had struck down marriage bans (Indiana, Oklahoma, Utah, Virginia, and Wisconsin) now had to abide by those judges' decisions. In one week alone, sixteen states were forced to recognize same-sex marriage.[20]

Finally on January 16, 2015, marriage equality supporters learned that the Supreme Court would consolidate cases coming out of four states and review the Sixth Circuit Court of Appeals ruling that had upheld marriage discrimination in Kentucky, Michigan, Ohio, and Tennessee. Thousands of friend-of-the-court briefs were filed in *Obergefell v. Hodges*, from a cross-section of Americans including faith leaders, mayors, medical and public health figures, and leading American businesses, including forty of the Fortune 100. Freedom to Marry aired TV ads in Washington, D.C., and in key states with the simple messages "America is ready" and "It's time."[21]

The Supreme Court agreed on June 26, 2015—exactly two years to the day after it overturned DOMA, and twelve years after its six to three decision in *Lawrence v. Texas* overturning sodomy laws nationwide and affirming that consensual intimate sexual contact was part of the liberty protected under the Fourteenth Amendment. "No union is more profound than marriage," said the Court's majority opinion, "for it embodies the highest ideals of love, fidelity, devotion, sacrifice, and family." The Court acknowledged that the men and women who brought the cases bundled together into *Obergefell* were simply asking for "equal dignity in the eyes of the law." At long last, the Court said, "The Constitution grants them that right."[22]

"I always believed we would win," Evan Wolfson wrote in a *New York Times* op-ed piece just after the Court ruling, "but I didn't expect to cry."[23]

I asked Wolfson what kept his hope alive for the three decades between the time he wrote his 1983 law school paper on same-sex marriage and the triumph at the Supreme Court. "I believed it was a fight worth fighting and that we could win," he said. "It was not only around winning marriage, but about what would improve the situation for *all* gay people. It would become an engine that would help change non-gay people's understanding of who gay people are, and it would change things on all fronts. I believed we could change people's hearts and minds, and that there was a pathway."

Wolfson said there are three necessary ingredients for any movement to succeed—"or any of us to succeed in life": hope, clarity, and tenacity. He explained, "Hope you can win; believe in it. Clarity about your strategy and what you need to do. Tenacity in spite of challenges and obstacles." He said he possesses these qualities himself and they are evidence of his own resilience. "I do have hope and clarity as to where I want to go and what to do to bring people along," he explained. "I have tenacity. I worked to win the freedom to marry for thirty-two years. We had severe, painful blows and disappointments, and many people pronounced us dead and said it wasn't worth fighting for and dangerous. I really believed that we could win, trusted that other people would rise to fairness, and that we could make the case to them in the legal environment, but also in the personal contacts and conversations. That is what kept me going."

That and a good man. One of the ironies of Wolfson's advocacy for marriage equality was that he was, as he puts it, "whinily single" for the first nearly two decades. Wolfson married his husband, Cheng He, on October 15, 2011, after being together as a couple for a decade before they wed. "I knew all this intellectually, but wasn't experiencing it personally," said Wolfson. When I asked how his marriage contributes to his resilience, Wolfson said of his husband, "He is good, smart, funny, caring, and keeps me in my place but also gives me tremendous support. That is a wonderful thing to have in my life."

What would Wolfson tell a young gay boy about the historic events he has shaped and witnessed? "You are part of a community," he said he'd tell the boy, "that has offered the most resonant, inspiring movement in decades. You are part of the community that has helped America move to become a more perfect union, that has offered the most inspiring example of belief in what America stands for at its best."

But what happens when heroic action isn't required on a daily basis—as it was in the dark early AIDS years, as it was in more subtle ways in the decades and centuries of secrecy and subversion before Stonewall, as it was in the lives of millions of gay men who did their best to live with dignity and pride when the entire social order insisted they were criminal, sick, second class, and even less than human? "There is still plenty of need for heroism and activism," said Wolfson. "It's never done. There is always going to be something else to do. Even though we won the freedom to marry, and that was an enormous, historic triumph, we're not done with even the primary list of things we need to achieve as a movement."[24]

There is always going to be the need to live heroically, to tell your story as one of survival and triumph rather than defeat and surrender. There will continue to be the need to tell our story, the story of gay men, as one in which we are the heroes and not the victims. Claiming our community's history as a part of our own story is the best way to live powerfully and with a sense of belonging to a long line of heroic men (and women) worthy of celebration—and emulation.

PART III

A HOME IN THE WORLD

~

Overview:
Part III

It is easier to build strong children than to repair broken men.

—Frederick Douglass, 1855

Most boys, gay and nongay, don't have the good fortune to be brought up to love themselves exactly as they are. From our youngest age we are told that "real boys" don't cry or feel this or do that, that to be worthy of love and esteem we must be true to a constricted idea of what a boy, or a man, is supposed to be, do, think, say, and feel. For a boy who is different in some way, criticism, put-downs, and even outright rejection are among the common ways families show their discomfort with his truth. If they are religious or hold antigay cultural values, they frequently try tipping the scale by claiming God is on *their* side.

What a marvel, then, to see a young gay man in his early twenties after being raised by a loving mom and dad, within a faith community—strong, confident, happily coupled, and pursuing his dreams and the life he dreamt of in New York City. It's equally marvelous to chat with a young straight guy, just graduated from college, about how having two gay dads has benefitted him in the dating marketplace. In a class of resilience all their own are the gay youth who aren't fortunate to grow up in stable and supportive homes. You know you are beholding something mighty in the human spirit, something important, when you hear the stories of homeless and other at-risk LGBT youth who have managed to defy the worst odds to come out intact on the other side of their troubled growing-up years, ready to embrace their future.

Finding "our place" where we can enjoy the community's embrace at a level that supports our resilience is all of our challenge. "Doing" friendship, building community, is where we find LGBT America at our most creative and resourceful as we create specialty bars, clubs, and circles for those with shared tastes or concerns. One of the most special is the drag house and ball scene. There largely working-class and poor young gay men, many of them African American and Latino, find a safe place where they can be true to their deepest selves, where they *matter*. Many others bring their own hunger for connection to places like the Los Angeles LGBT Center and community centers like it across the country. Even more of us—more than half, according to a big Pew Research Center study—find the connectedness we need, and the strength it gives us, in our faith.

We gay men nurture our resilience by routinely creating communities for ourselves, drawing from the collective economic, emotional, professional, and spiritual resources they provide. Our friends and networks of friends are the foundations and pillars of our communities, as is the nuclear family—at least its ideal—for the heterosexual world in which most of us are reared. Peter M. Nardi, professor of sociology at Claremont College, writes in Gay Men's Friendships: Invincible Communities, "Gay men's friendships may someday become the cornerstone of a new structure of social and personal relationships that has the power to transform everyone's lives and to create a new invincible community and culture of dignity and equality."[1] Of course the strengthening agent of *all* our communities is the mysterious bond of friendship between gay men, best defined by the heroic actions it regularly inspires—the powerful force Walt Whitman called "the manly love of comrades."

CHAPTER SEVENTEEN

~

How to Raise a Gay Son

Straight Parents Become Staunch Allies After Their Son Comes Out to Them at Fifteen

After he finished bawling, Sean Duggan posted photos on Facebook of his mom and dad's new tattoos. "My parents have been super-supportive all the way," he told me in an interview for this book at the LGBT Community Center in New York City, just a few days before I was to interview his parents back home in Connecticut. "I had one boyfriend through the first half of college," he said. "It ended explosively, and they were there to pick up the pieces. I have been with my current boyfriend since then. They wanted to meet him and be supportive in any way they can. There is nothing about me being gay that they have never been supportive of, which has always made me feel good."[1]

Tim and Kathy Duggan have stood by their son since he came out to them his junior year of high school. Not only that, but they took on Sean's coming out as an opportunity to learn and grow themselves. By the time we sat down for an interview in their backyard in Norwich, Connecticut, in August 2015, they had been active in the southeastern Connecticut chapter of PFLAG for seven years. The group had even sent Kathy to their national conference in Washington. They had "come out" as the parents of a gay son to all their family and friends. Kathy had even served as a coadvisor for the Gay-Straight Alliance (GSA) at Norwich Free Academy—her, the two Duggan boys', and my own high school.

But a tattoo? This was another magnitude of "outness," a deeply personal yet very public testimonial of their commitment. Sure enough, there they were: on Kathy's right forearm is tattooed the word *Equality*; on Tim's, the Human Rights Campaign's "=" logo.

I first met Kathy and Tim at a PFLAG meeting in Norwich, the Duggans' and my own hometown. I interviewed them for an article I wrote about gay teens' risk for suicide after a rash of gay teens killed themselves in 2010. The article ran on the front page of the *Norwich Bulletin*, the daily newspaper. The couple has lived here their whole lives, and they have extended family in the area, too. A large color photo of Sean sitting between his parents on the sofa in their living room accompanied the story.

Kathy and Tim didn't expect to have a gay son. "As the mother of two sons," said Kathy as we shared dinner in their home for that earlier interview in 2010, "I never expected to have a son-in-law, or to see my son holding hands with another boy." A petite, attractive, and vivacious woman, Kathy is being uncharacteristically understated. What she's not saying is Sean's coming out was the shock of her life.

During dinner I was quickly aware of the affection and comfortable interactions between the parents and both of their sons. Sean was then a college freshman, and Brian was a high school senior and football player. It also became clear pretty fast that Tim and Kathy's love of their sons, one gay and one straight, is far stronger than their regard for "what others think." Their independent mindedness may not be unusual in Norwich. After all, the eastern Connecticut city still prides itself on playing an important role in the American Revolution beyond "merely" being the hometown of both Benedict Arnold and Samuel Huntington, a signer of the Declaration of Independence. Nevertheless, being a straight married couple of gay activists is still *highly* unusual in Norwich.

Not too long after Sean came out to them, Tim and Kathy started attending meetings of the local PFLAG chapter. The southeastern Connecticut PFLAG group meets monthly for a potluck dinner and discussion in the basement of the white clapboard Noank Baptist Church, in the charming little coastal village twenty miles south of Norwich. Barbara Althen, the now-retired former GSA faculty advisor at nearby Ledyard High School and longtime president of the PFLAG chapter, told me, "Noank Baptist Church took on PFLAG as part of its opening and affirming position." She recalled Tim and Kathy's initial arrival at PFLAG—"a lot of Catholic baggage, a lot of crying"—but made abundantly clear that they had "elevated" themselves, risen above any reservations they might have had to model for their sons the acceptance and unconditional love they wanted them to know in their family.[2]

Since 1972, PFLAG has been helping parents like the Duggans, and others with significant LGBT people in their lives, to adjust to the reality of their loved one's "difference." When Jeanne Manford marched with her son Morty Manford in the 1970 Christopher Street Liberation Day March in New York, the first LGBT Pride march, so many gay men and lesbians asked Jeanne to speak with their parents that she decided to start a support group. The first group of twenty people met at the Metropolitan-Duane Methodist Church (known today as the Church in the Village) in Greenwich Village. PFLAG today has four hundred chapters in all fifty states, the District of Columbia, and Puerto Rico, in cities, towns, and even rural areas like much of eastern Connecticut. Formerly known as "Parents, Family, and Friends of Lesbians and Gays," the group in 2014 formally changed its name to PFLAG.[3] Whatever its official title, the PFLAG group *always* gets the loudest applause in Pride parades.

Like so many parents of gay kids who make their way to PFLAG, the Duggans had to learn to put aside their own expectations and hopes to discover their son as he knows himself to be. They wanted to show their love for Sean in every way possible because, as Tim put it, "We're a family that loves and supports our children."

They had no idea at its beginning where their journey as the parents of a gay son would take them. "We went to PFLAG as the 'walking wounded,'" said Kathy. "We needed support, and I needed to look into another mother's eyes and cry. I had to give up the idea of Sean walking down the aisle of St. Patrick's Cathedral with his bride." For his part, Tim said, "It's comforting to sit in that room with other parents with gay children, because you don't have to explain to them." Kathy said, "The most interesting thing about PFLAG is that at some point you realize you have gone from needing help to providing it."

Although there was a Gay-Straight Alliance (GSA) at Norwich Free Academy (NFA) when Sean was a student there, he didn't participate in it after he came out at fifteen. "They were people who didn't fit in anywhere else, with black fingernails, wearing rainbows," he told me in our first interview, when he was nineteen. "I had all the support I needed. I almost went to one meeting and looked in the door and thought, 'None of these people are like me.'"

GSAs are so important for *so many* kids precisely because they feel they are the only one like themselves. Findings from the GLSEN 2015 National School Climate Survey show that even in largely "blue" Connecticut, schools are not safe places for most LGBTQ high school students. They report being victimized in some way—from name calling, to pushing, to physical assault. Yet only half report the incidents to school staff. Of the incidents reported, only one in three of the students who reported an incident said it resulted in effective staff intervention. In a state that has had legal same-sex marriage since 2008, one in five Connecticut LGBTQ high school students were persecuted—and disciplined—for public affection in their schools that doesn't result in similar action for non-LGBTQ students.[4] Clearly it will take time for society to understand that LGBTQ youth have crushes and rushes, and like to hug their friends and love objects—just like young people everywhere. Until then, GSAs provide a safe space for LGBTQ youth to explore for themselves what it means to be gay, or maybe not gay but just "different."

Sean was fortunate. "If I hadn't been getting all the love from my family," he said, "I think I would have reached out to GSA." He did, however, participate in the GSA all four of his undergraduate years at Eastern Connecticut State University. But even then it wasn't a matter of finding support but making friends and sharing the experience of being in college.

Chuck Lynch, the GSA faculty advisor while Sean was at Norwich Free Academy, told me in an interview for my 2010 *Norwich Bulletin* article, "What's really nice about the GSA is it creates a community where the kids can be themselves, and be safe and secure. It doesn't solve all their problems. It's not going to change their parents' point of view, but it can change how they react to it and deal with it." Lynch pointed out that although young people today face many different challenges from what he and I faced growing up, some difficult experiences are very much the same. "When the kids casually mention an alcoholic parent or something like that," he said, "I think what it was like when I was their age growing up with an abusive alcoholic father, and I think about how much work it's taken to get from there to here—the therapy, Al-Anon, self-help books. I thought, 'Wow! It's tough being a gay kid, even today.'"[5]

Each year, the NFA group sponsors "Ally Week," which spotlights friends and other supporters of LGBT youth. There is also the annual "Day of Silence," when students nationwide take a vow of silence to bring attention to antigay rhetoric, bullying, and harassment in their schools. For Connecticut GSAs, the most popular event is the annual True Colors conference at the University of Connecticut. Sponsored by Hartford-based True Colors, Inc., the conference brings together about two thousand young people and educators from across the state for workshops, entertainment, and, probably most importantly of all, the chance for sexual minority youth to meet others like themselves and know they aren't alone.

The year before we met, Tim, Kathy, and Sean went together to the True Colors conference. Kathy and Tim have shared what Sean calls their "hearts and rainbows" story with Sean's college GSA. Kathy calls Sean a "PFLAG success story." She and Tim credit Sean's gayness for expanding their family's "pretty amazing capacity to love," as Kathy described it. "We've had incredible experiences being part of the gay community," she said. She mentioned the media interviews and even meeting Ellen DeGeneres's mother, Betty, at the PFLAG conference in Washington. Most importantly, though, Kathy said, "Sean's being gay prepared us to be even more welcoming in our family."

In fact, after Sean left for New York, Tim and Kathy became involved in the life of a young black man named Tuzar. Tim knew him from the NFA football program he's been involved with since Brian was on the team. Tuzar was about to age out of the foster care system and had nowhere to go. "He is basically an adopted brother now," said Sean. "He lives at the house and goes to college now. That speaks to who my parents are: They heard about this kid in need, didn't know him, just knew he was on the team, that he was a good kid and struggled in school but just needed a good foundation, so they reached out to him." When I asked Kathy for a family photo, the newest member was in it, too.

"If Sean indicated he's lucky to have us, we're doubly lucky," Kathy told me, knowing I had just seen Sean in New York. "There's nothing he could do that would make me prouder. He's successfully supporting himself, and in a successful relationship, in the toughest city in the world."[6]

Sean had always pictured himself living in the Big Apple since going there in kindergarten to see *The Lion King*. "We walked out into Times Square," he told me, "I looked up and said I am going to live here some day. I didn't know how or why I was going to get here." He *did* know, however, he wasn't going to be satisfied living in Norwich his whole life. But unlike so many gay men of my own age (fifty-eight as I write this in 2017) and older, Sean never felt he *needed* to leave Norwich to live as an openly gay man in the big city. "It was about not wanting to live in a small town," he explained, "not moving to the city to 'be gay' because I could be that at home. I didn't have the need to get here for that reason; it's just where I saw my life going."

Working for an upscale photo studio on the Upper East Side at the time of our interview, and living in Harlem with the same boyfriend he'd been with since college, I asked Sean whether he plans to get married. The Supreme Court had issued its same-sex marriage decision not long before our interview, which means he can get married anywhere in the United States and know his marriage is legal in every state of the union. "Absolutely, at some point in the future," he said. "It was never a question for me that I was going to get married. It would just be to a guy." He added that there will probably be two children, too—one adopted and the other "through some biological route"—because he himself appreciated having a sibling when he was growing up.

More than anything, Sean looks forward to recreating the kind of loving family he grew up in. "When I was growing up," he said, "I didn't know that every family didn't have two parents who loved each other. I told my parents, 'I want to have what you guys have and what you've made, this solid family. You've got kids and you raised them, and everyone loves each other and gets along.'"[7]

~

CHAPTER EIGHTEEN

Husbands and Dads

Pioneering Massachusetts Couple Finds Resilience in Marriage and Fatherhood

The road to marriage and parenthood wasn't a given, nor was it easy, for the first gay male couple in Suffolk County, Massachusetts, to coadopt a child that wasn't either partner's biological offspring.

Joe Levine and I first met in Boston, in 1984, when we both lived in "boys' town," the just-beginning-to-gentrify South End, and Joe was a biology professor at Boston College. Looking back he told me he "internalized the party line" that becoming a father just wasn't an option for gay men when he came out in the 1970s. The native New Yorker said he made "occasional forays" into the Manhattan gay party scene with friends, while attending Tufts and for a few years after graduation. He recalled the powerful "tribal" feeling of dancing in one famously exclusive New York nightclub full of "A-list" men. "I remember specifically one night when I was really into it," he said. "This spectacular room was filled with God knows how many hundreds of good-looking, successful New York men, dancing shirtless to music spun by an incredible DJ, having a fabulous time, and, by doing so, basically saying 'Fuck you!' to straight society. That was the kind of defiance that I got strength from." By the time he finished his PhD in biology at Harvard, he had settled down . . . somewhat.

Steve Cadwell got strength from growing up in a big Yankee family on a Vermont farm—one of six boys. "Some of what gave me resilience," he told me, "was having a place that I could come back to and draw from. There was this solid sense that I came from somewhere." But Steve knew from his earliest years that he was a sissy boy. He had a gentle spirit and loved pretty things. He went through tremendous anguish and heartache trying to be true to what he felt inside against the social pressures to conform. Then of course in his growing-up years of the 1950s and 1960s there was the shame and stigma of being officially classified as mentally ill for being homosexual. At one point in his early twenties he was committed to the state mental hospital to be "treated" for homosexuality after all the stress drove him to a nervous breakdown.

As it turned out, the only thing wrong with Steve was he had internalized the messages that said the gentle, loving person he knew himself to be was sick. "I had a lot of privileges," he told me, "white, male, middle class, WASP. And even with all of those, I internalized a lot of the self-hate of homophobia." Although he enjoyed his moments as a "disco queen" in the 1970s, Steve knew that coming out for him would have more to do with what he did by day than with boogying at night. He knew the field of social work was one of the first to be open to gay culture and pride, which appealed to him. He also knew he wanted a career that melded his work and personal identities, "where I could be all of who I am and there wasn't going to be a closet." Earning a PhD in Smith College's prestigious social work program set him on his way to becoming one of Boston's leading psychotherapists for gay men and others in the LGBT community.

On top of his career choices, Steve always wanted to be a parent, too. For him it was about wanting to live in a more relational way, through parenting, something he also does in his work as a therapist. He'd seen it modeled by his mother, who had always accepted his difference and even gave him a doll when he was a boy. His father provided well for his large family, but like so many men of his World War II generation he was emotionally detached. Joe's father, on the other hand, was eager, interesting, and engaged, according to Steve. "Some of my attraction to Joe was his warm and loving dad," he joked.

Like so many gay and straight men alike who grow up with distant fathers, Steve thought he was somehow responsible for his father's distance. But as he came to better understand men like his dad, he realized he wasn't the reason for the man's lack of warmth. He realized his father was healing from his own trauma. "All my brothers were having some version of this trouble in finding him," he said. But as their dad moved through his elder years, Steve said he became "more accessible and connecting as we were struggling to find him."

Joe recalled a summer afternoon when he and Steve, and Steve's entire clan, were sharing a cousin's cottage in Boothbay Harbor, Maine. "I suddenly realized that all six boys were glued to this picnic table and John was talking," he said. "It turned out it was the first time in quite a while that he was willing to talk about his wartime experiences to the boys." Steve said his father was able to "come out" and share much more emotion. "He just had anger before. Then it was the softest love. He would weep when we would get together. He was very expressive in appreciating us."

By the time Joe and Steve met, in 1986, Steve had worked through most of his family issues and was completely "integrated" into his family as an openly gay man. Joe's full integration with his own family was unfolding in fits and starts, but didn't fully happen until after he met Steve. When they had their *first* commitment ceremony, in the fall of 1986, Joe's mother wouldn't let him invite her best friend because she hadn't yet "come out" about having a gay son. "It was after meeting Steve," said Joe, "and realizing what a wonderful man he is," that Joe's parents' fears were finally put to rest. "At first their fear was that gay men don't have relationships and they die alone," he said. "Six months after the ceremony, a package arrived, and it was a wedding gift from Mom's best friend."

In 2003, Steve and Joe had a legal civil union in Vermont. Now their love was legally binding, at least in Vermont. They held the "big hoopla" in a Vermont hotel close to where Steve grew up, and where his family often celebrated Thanksgiving. Lots of family. Lots of friends. Joe's mom *and* her best friend; his dad, sadly, had died by then. They even had a party planner who dubbed herself "dominatrix of ceremonies." Then in 2004, the couple "eloped," as they put it, and got married legally in their own state of Massachusetts after it made same-sex marriage legal that year.

"I always wanted to get married," said Steve. "I fantasized this as a child. I didn't get the male role in that; I probably fantasized more about being the bride than the groom in my early fantasies." He believes this kind of fantasizing actually helps build gay kids' resilience. "It builds the capacity to believe we can play any role we want, in spite of what others say," he told me. Many people would respond to Steve's declaration that he was gay by saying "But you'd be such a good father!" Steve finally reached a point where he rejected the lies and hurtful labels—"child molesters," for example—ignorant people impose on gay men. He finally understood that he didn't have to grieve the loss of being a father just because he was gay. He could be gay *and* a parent! He sought out role models of men who had chosen parenthood, and wanted more and more to be a parent himself. That's how he was able to believe with conviction that not only would he *make* a good parent but also there was no reason he should *not* be a parent.

For his part, Joe said he probably would never have become a parent if he hadn't paired up with Steve. "Steve hadn't put the option of being a parent out of the picture the way I had," he said. Steve helped Joe to think differently about parenting. Rather than assuming that being gay preemptively disqualified him from being a father, he began to think "just because I'm gay doesn't mean I can't become a parent."

Steve and Joe had been living in the racially and economically integrated Dorchester section of Boston for seven years by the time they adopted. It cost them tens of thousands of dollars in legal fees, and a great deal of stress, before Steve finally traveled to Guatemala to bring back their newborn son. He would be called Isaac, and would be raised in a love-filled home, thousands of miles, and worlds, away from his birthplace, by *two* devoted dads.

As fixtures of the neighborhood, Steve and Joe felt accepted before and after Steve became Isaac's Daddy and Joe became his Abba. Joe said, "We had been there long enough for people to get to know us as a couple, not as single men who were out tomcatting around all the time. We had a fabulous garden and were active in the neighborhood. So people *knew* us." On a political note, he added, "That's when I realized one of the reasons the radical right is so vehemently against gay adoption. Having a child *normalized* us, and integrated us into 'normal' straight society in a way that could never have happened as gay men without a kid. We were at PTA meetings. We were picking up kids at day care. We were at soccer games, bringing water, car-pooling, and doing what all the other parents were doing."

Steve said that belonging to the gay "tribe" had given him the confidence to determine for himself what he wanted. When Isaac reached school age, they entered him in the lottery for magnet schools in Boston . . . and lost. They also wanted a safer neighborhood in which to raise their son. "We *loved* our neighborhood," Joe recalled, "and in fact, some people we knew couldn't believe we were so upset about leaving a place they would never have even considered living in." They then decided to relocate to Concord, twenty miles northwest of Boston. "We went through our own 'suburba-phobia' about how people would see us," he said. "We were sort of pioneers out here in Concord. In Dorchester, there were some gay couples with kids. We could have gone to Jamaica Plain and been surrounded. But we chose Concord, partly for the excellent school system, but also because we liked it out here. This town is far beyond 'liberal' into progressive. We knew we wouldn't be pre-judged the way we would have been back then in certain other Boston burbs."

Their decision to choose Concord echoed their thinking about parenthood itself: "Why *shouldn't* we be able to choose where we want to live?" as Steve put it. They formed their own local network with other parents they met. "There was less of the identifying as a 'gay family' per se," said Steve, "and more as just another family. Our friends locally, at least at first, were the parents of Isaac's buddies from school and soccer."

That is certainly how Isaac remembers growing up. He was twenty-two and had just graduated from Eckerd College, in Florida, when we ran into each other in the Church Street Marketplace in downtown Burlington, Vermont, in early August 2016. I was there to do an interview for this book. I had forgotten that Joe and Steve told me Isaac moved to Burlington after his graduation until I heard my name in the busy marketplace.

Over an exceptional Italian dinner at Pascolo Ristorante, I asked Isaac whether anyone had harassed him for having two dads. "I was never bullied," he said. "Concord was so accepting." In a really interesting twist, he said that after high school, where everyone knew he had two dads, he discovered that having two dads gave him a competitive advantage with girls because of its uniqueness. "Girls in college didn't know I had two dads," he explained, "so I'd meet them at a party and they'd say 'so tell me about yourself,' and I'd say I have two gay dads. They love it. They think it's so cool. It's such a great ice-breaker." After telling another friend in Florida that he had two gay dads, the guy said, "Really? You're so normal."

How was it for Isaac to grow up with so many men, gay and straight, all rooting for him? I mentioned that a section of this book was going to focus on the importance of reliable, consistent male mentors. "It's nice. I like it," he said. "I get the gay side from Steve and Joe's gay male friends. Then I have the straight uncles who want to play hockey and are into sports. So it's the best of all worlds."

I reminded Isaac that one of the right-wing smears against gay people is that we try to recruit and convert children into homosexuals. "You are proof that two loving gay men were not out to corrupt a kid," I said. He laughed and recalled a time when he was a boy. His parents bought him a leotard and took him to dance class. "I hated it," said Isaac. "The leotard became part of a Superman outfit. That's when Steve said they knew they were raising a straight child."[1]

I asked Steve and Joe how marriage and being co-dads, parents, has strengthened their resilience as individuals and as a couple. "The resilience we have had as individuals and as a couple," said Joe, "is because our first ceremony, in Dorchester, offered an intentional venue for telling people that we know it's not going to be a bed of roses, there will be rough spots, and we are asking for your help when those tough spots come—whether in the relationship, or in parenting, or parenting and society. Knowing we have that backup from family and friends is a significant part of resilience."[2]

Besides being a therapist, Steve in 2014 created a one-man show that he has since performed from coast to coast. *Wild and Precious* traces his life journey from sissy farm boy, through the wild and crazy 1960s, the early gay rights movement and disco era of the 1970s, the devastation of AIDS in the 1980s, and his biggest role ever as an out and proud gay man married and raising a son of his own with his legally wed husband, Joe. The show's final, triumphant image is a great blue heron taking flight, rising slowly, majestically, off the water. It ends with Steve draped in the rainbow flag. His takeaway message: Inner peace comes of accepting our own differences, and resilience comes from integrating all our parts.

"It's right here, *under* this rainbow of our smiles, affirming, loving, accepting—not the hate and pushing away," Steve said in a 2014 interview we did for the *Huffington Post* after he performed the show at Fenway Health in Boston. He said he never quite understood the appeal of holding onto the "over the rainbow, never reachable pathos" of Judy Garland, and the gay men who hung onto the old hope of "maybe someday" being equal and free. "That's why in my piece I weave it in as this aching sense of 'will we ever'—but then coming to the other side of the rainbow of our pride and power, and we have it right here," he said, patting his heart. "Dare to be different," he says at the end of *Wild and Precious*. "Make a difference. Be the difference. Be wild! Stay precious! We're only as free as our least are free."[3]

CHAPTER NINETEEN

~

Becoming Their Story's Hero

Helping At-Risk Gay Youth Find Strength in Their Resilience

"I want to be a surgeon."

It's a clear, confident statement thousands of young men and women make all the time in looking ahead at their lives. But for Sami Medina, self-destructive behavior was the more familiar norm. "The angry Goth kid," as the twenty-six-year-old described his teenage self, acted out the belief he couldn't seem to shake growing up, that all the bad things he experienced were his fault: his distant single mother, the psychiatric hospital admissions between ages seven and seventeen, the rape by a cousin at age five. "Growing up in a world full of therapists, people talking behind your back," he said, "makes it difficult to trust." He added, "The only person I did trust was my best friend, who recently died."

Sami's mom blamed her emotional distance from him on her own difficult childhood. She was only seventeen when he was born. At fifteen Sami realized it wasn't good for him to live with his mom. So he lived in a residential program for kids who couldn't fit in with their families. He lived with friends for a year, then lived with an aunt. Around age thirteen, Sami's therapist wanted him to have a mentor. Hartford, Connecticut–based True Colors, Inc.—the sexual minority youth support and advocacy organization that sponsors the annual True Colors youth conference at the University of Connecticut—matched Sami with Eddie, a black gay man in his late forties at the time, and his husband. Sami calls them Pop and Poppy. "They've been a great resource for me," he said. Sami came to realize his "Goth phase" was aimed at keeping people away. Cutting made him feel "alive in the moment."

Then it was smoking cigarettes. "If it's not one thing, it's another," he said. "I'm used to things always changing. What I want more than anything is stability."

I met Sami for our interview at Eastern Connecticut State University, where he was a sophomore earning his room and board as a resident assistant. "Things are working out for me," he said. The tears spring from his eyes, slip below the rim of his glasses, streak down his cheeks. But they are tears of defiance, not defeat, as he talks about his late friend. "If I have to be alone," he said, "I'll do it."[1]

Fortunately, Sami doesn't have to handle it alone. Kamora Herrington is the mentoring program coordinator for True Colors who matched up Sami with his "gay dads." She told me the kids she works with tend to be queer and in "the system," the foster care system. She said it's common in her job to hear from these youth "how entitled they are," that "the world owes them something." Sami was different, though. "Sam understood that he lived in this really unfair world and he had to make it work," she said.

"I believe wholeheartedly in mentoring," said Herrington. She noted that one of the "biggest benefits" she has seen in mentoring relationships between adult gay men and younger men, fifteen to eighteen or so, "is taking 'gay' off the table" for young gay men who arrive "over-the-top gay." She recalled twenty-six-year-old Mick's experience. "He came to us covered in rainbows, with a lisp. He was a virgin but he gave the impression that he was a slut. He had it all envisioned: he was going to be a Broadway star, live in a penthouse, and be driven around in a limousine."

Herrington said that few young gay people have the opportunity to see stable, mature gay men and lesbians, or functional same-sex relationships. "In our community, no matter what we say about marriage, we don't often see what a working relationship looks like," she said. So True Colors matched Mick with Joe, who had wanted to be an actor when he was younger but now did something else as his full-time job. "Mick is now a very grounded human being," said Herrington. "He does dinner theater. He would like to work for Disney; that is his dream. But he has reevaluated his dreams and is now realistic. He lives in Orlando."[2]

Like Sami and Mick before True Colors helped them find mentors, too many young gay men don't have a responsible older gay male role model. They find out on their own, sink or swim, how to navigate the world as a *gay* man, and the gay world as a *young* man—each with its own risks and rewards, privileges and perils.

Most American males grow up with what psychologist William Pollack calls the "Boy Code," the messages instilled in a million ways from our youngest age telling us that "real" boys must keep a stiff upper lip, not show their feelings, act tough, and be cool. Pollack writes in his book *Real Boys: Rescuing Our Sons from the Myths of Boyhood*, that "perhaps the most traumatizing and dangerous injunction thrust on boys and men is the literal gender straitjacket that prohibits boys from expressing feelings or urges seen (mistakenly) as 'feminine'—dependence, warmth, empathy."[3]

So many gay men learn we are "different" from other boys by having the fact pointed out and ridiculed by bullies during our young, most impressionable, years. Our young peers become pint-size enforcers of the Boy Code—using shame and even violence to enforce conformity to the absurd notion that every male is heterosexual and expresses his maleness only within a limited, permitted range of emotions and behaviors.

As every gay man knows who has been insulted or assaulted for his actual or perceived sexual orientation, there are steep penalties for violating the Boy Code as there are for anyone who is "different" from the presumed (typically white, heterosexual, middle-class) standard. The 2015 GLSEN National School Climate Survey—a biannual online survey of 10,528 students between ages thirteen to twenty-one and grades six through twelve, in all fifty U.S. states and the District of Columbia—found that even though things have gotten somewhat better, American LGBT students still face extraordinary levels of abuse and discrimination in the nation's public schools. The survey, covering 3,095 unique school districts, found that 98.1 percent of the student respondents reported hearing the word *gay* used in a negative way; 57.6 percent felt unsafe at school because of their sexual orientation; 31.8 percent missed at least a day of school in the last month because they felt unsafe; 71.5 percent avoided school functions and extracurricular activities because they felt unsafe; 27 percent were physically harassed (pushed or shoved); 13 percent were physically assaulted; and 48.6 percent reported being electronically harassed. Respondents who reported higher levels of harassment also reported lower self-esteem, lower grades, and were twice as likely not to pursue postsecondary education. Perhaps the survey's most disturbing findings of all were these: Of those who reported being harassed or assaulted, 57.6 percent of them chose not to report the incident, mainly because they didn't expect anything would be done about it. Of those who did report what happened, 63.5 percent said nothing was done about it.[4]

How does a gay kid survive the trauma he suffers for being different in a culture that still condemns his difference as something bad or "less-than" and wants to mold him into the same shape it tries to mold every boy? Robert Pollack says the most important thing a family can do to support their gay son is to keep loving him, "to convey to him, as soon as he shares his feelings, that he is still loved through and through, that his sexual orientation will not in any way diminish how much he is admired and respected. These are the things a boy needs most to hear."[5]

But what of a boy whose family actually rejects him? Forces him out of the house? In 1979 Dr. Emery Hetrick, a psychiatrist, and his life partner and coeducator on gay and lesbian issues Dr. Damien Martin, a professor at New York University, were moved by the story of a fifteen-year-old boy who was beaten and thrown out of his emergency shelter because he was gay. They gathered a group of concerned adults and created what they called the Institute for the Protection of Lesbian and Gay Youth (IPLGY) to assist young people who needed support. The organization was renamed Hetrick-Martin Institute in 1988 to honor its founders.

Today HMI is the nation's oldest and largest LGBTQ youth services organization, annually serving more than two thousand young people between ages thirteen and twenty-four, from thirty-eight states across the country. It supports them with programming focused on arts and culture, health and wellness, counseling, education, and job readiness. In its main New York City location at 2 Astor Place in Manhattan, Hetrick-Martin also serves more than eleven thousand hot meals a year; 81 percent of HMI youth members (as they are called) cite the need for food as their main reason for coming to HMI. The institute founded and hosts the Harvey Milk High School, a four-year, fully accredited transfer public high school operated by the New York City Department of Education. The most vulnerable youth can find acceptance here, and learn without the threat of physical violence and emotional harm they likely experienced at their former schools.

Thomas Krever, Hetrick-Martin's CEO, told me in an interview at his office that every young person coming to HMI starts with a mental health intake. The way HMI frames the young people's stories to engage their resiliency distinguishes its approach to marginalized, traumatized, vulnerable youth. Krever called it a "positive youth development" model. Instead of a "deficit" model in which trauma is the touchstone ("the 'woe is me' poverty factor," as he put it), the PYD approach builds on the young person's resilience. "It's about believing in a young person's strength, even when they don't believe in it yet," said Krever. "There would be a very different feel in this conversation," he said of our interview, "if we were talking about a deficit model rather than strength. And [the young people] feel that and pick up on that. Young people vote with their feet. Which organization would you go to—one that says 'It's okay, honey, you'll be okay,' or the one that says 'That's okay. You're gonna do it anyway. You got through the doors, let's start with that.'"

It comes down to choosing either a victim mentality or the opportunity to own something, said Krever. "The very nature of PYD is the opposite of victimization; it says these things happen, but *despite* them you're going to succeed because you're *here* when you could have chosen *not* to be here." That choice alone offers much to work with. Said Krever, "It already means the young people are coming to us with a modicum of what I say is a level of *heroic* resilience."[6]

Since its beginning with six beds in a church basement, the Ali Forney Center has grown to become the largest agency in the country dedicated to LGBTQ homeless youth. Carl Siciliano founded AFC in 2002, to protect LGBTQ youths from the harms of homelessness and empower them with the tools they need to live independently. The organization's namesake, Ali Forney, was a gender nonconforming teen who fled home at thirteen, bounced around the foster care system, was beaten, and ended up living on the streets. Before he was murdered in 1997, Ali was dedicated to helping other young people and advocated for the safety of homeless LGBTQ youth. The Manhattan-based agency today serves nearly fourteen hundred youth each year through ten housing sites and a multipurpose drop-in center. President Obama in 2012 named Siciliano a White House "Champion of Change," noting the widespread recognition of the Ali Forney Center's high-quality and innovative programming.

Siciliano told me in an interview at his office that he's thought about resilience throughout his career of youth work. He said that when young people come to AFC, "they're often in desperate situations." First things first: stabilize them, help them get IDs, access medical benefits, and find housing. AFC offers two types of housing, emergency and transitional, which can last up to two years. "Everything we're doing is about building resilience," said Siciliano.

In his decade of work with homeless adults before starting the Ali Forney Center, Siciliano encountered many people who had lost hope. Something he likes about working with the youth is "they haven't given up on themselves." But that doesn't mean the young people are *easy* on themselves—or one another. "Something I see very strongly when kids come to us is self-hatred projected out to each other," said Siciliano. It shows when they "throw shade" at others, publicly trash talking and disrespecting them. "We don't encourage shade, or threats," he said. "We really try to build and support resilience." He said the key to building resilience in the young people who come to Ali Forney—or any youth, really—is "having an adult show you that you are precious and loved."[7]

Of the estimated 1.6 million American adolescents who will experience homelessness this year, LGBT youth account for an astonishing 40 percent.[8]

Yet research is limited on these young people's equally astonishing resilience—or on the resilience of LGBT youth in general who are victimized because of their sexual orientation or gender expression.

One Chicago study of 425 lesbian, gay, and bisexual youth between the ages of sixteen and twenty-four found that 94 percent had experienced some form of victimization perceived to be a result of their sexual orientation. Gay and bisexual males reported higher levels, and black gay youth had the highest levels of victimization of all. Importantly, only one-third of the sample reported clinical levels of psychological distress. The researchers suggest the youth who didn't experience distress had resources in their lives "that make them resilient against these ubiquitous negative experiences." Both peer and family support were found to help promote resilience—which the researchers define as "a process encompassing positive adaptation within the context of significant adversity." Family support was particularly important for younger LGB people, though less so as they aged. Peer support, on the other hand, continued to be the single most important source of protection against the impact of homophobic victimization, regardless of age. The researchers recommend supporting GSAs and lesbian, gay, and bisexual youth centers as settings where sexual minority youth can socialize and form friendships with other "different" youth like themselves. The Internet, too, can be useful for forging friendships and romantic relationships that provide support and can even become offline relationships, too.[9]

An even more fundamental way to support the resilience of LGBTQ youth is by supporting their families before disapproval of homosexuality spins out of control into homelessness and the many pernicious effects it has on youth. San Francisco State University professor Caitlin Ryan and her colleagues reported in a 2009 *Pediatrics* article on their groundbreaking survey of 224 white and Latino lesbian, gay, and bisexual young adults, aged twenty-one to twenty-five, that LGB young adults with high levels of family rejection during adolescence were at high risk for harm, injury, or even death. Compared to their peers from families that reported no or low levels of rejection, young people from rejecting families were 8.4 times more likely to report attempting suicide, 5.9 times more likely to report high levels of depression, 3.4 times more likely to use illegal drugs, and 3.4 times more likely to report having engaged in unprotected sexual intercourse.[10]

Caitlin Ryan happens to be a native of my own hometown of Norwich, Connecticut. She is also a leading expert on the role of families in shaping their LGBT children's health and well-being. Coauthor with noted lesbian pediatrician Donna Futterman of the landmark 1998 book *Lesbian and Gay Youth: Care and Counseling*, Ryan is an internationally noted clinical social worker with nearly forty years of research and practice experience focused on LGBT health and mental health. In 2002 Ryan launched the Family Acceptance Project, based at San Francisco State University. The project has developed print and video educational materials, and conducted hundreds of workshops, to help families in the United States and a number of other countries from all kinds of ethnic, racial, religious, and socioeconomic backgrounds. The concepts developed from the project's work provided the basis for an "official" practitioner's resource guide called *A Practitioner's Resource Guide: Helping Families to Support Their LGBT Children*, which Ryan herself authored for the Substance Abuse and Mental Health Services Administration (SAMHSA), part of the U.S. Department of Health and Human Services.[11]

Ryan told me in a 2013 interview for *The Atlantic* that the Family Acceptance Project has found their respectful approach to the families they work with to be met in kind. "Meeting families where they are," she said, "we build on family strengths to show them what we've learned from our research, and help them understand that some of the ways they have treated their children have been putting them at risk."[12] For example, many parents believe they are helping their gay child by discouraging him from expressing what they consider inappropriate behavior for a boy. "Parents," says a project brochure, "think they are helping their children survive in a world they feel will never accept them by trying to prevent them from learning about or from being gay. But adolescents feel as if their parents don't love them, are ashamed of them, or even hate them."[13]

Ryan said it's important to realize that gay, lesbian, and bisexual youth are coming out at younger ages. "When most people think of gay youth," she said, "they think of sixteen-, eighteen-, or twenty-year-olds—not twelve years old. That is the reality of what we're dealing with now." She said there is a misconception among many parents, clergy, and health care providers "that someone needs to be an adult to know they're gay." They don't understand that sexual orientation is about more than sex. "If they think it's only about sex," said Ryan, "they wouldn't know that on average, whether someone is gay or straight, they become aware of their first crush at an average age of ten."[14]

Despite the ever-earlier coming out of so many youth, Ryan said the focus on serving young LGBT youth has been the same: peer support and, to some extent, from individual providers, but not through the family. "Family has always been seen as an adversary," she said, "so there have not been services for families, certainly not for families that speak a language other than English, or who are socially conservative, to provide accurate information for them about what sexual orientation means."

By the time of our interview for this book in late 2016, Ryan had already trained more than thirty thousand health educators, clergy, families, and LGBT youth programs. At one of the oldest and largest national LGBT programs, she said of the activists in her audience, "their eyes were like saucers" as she overturned everything they were doing. Ryan said the activists had assumed, erroneously, that the youth wouldn't want to talk about their families because it was too painful. In fact, helping them talk about their families is an important step in helping them heal.

Traditionally, in dealing with troubled LGBT youth, families "were seen as the enemy, not as a resource," said Ryan.[15] The assumption was the families didn't love their children, maybe even wanted to hurt them. But she said the reality is exactly opposite in many instances. "We found they *did* love them," she said. They even attributed their extreme actions—such as kicking the gay kid out of the house—to care and concern, not wanting to *hurt* the gay family member. They themselves didn't perceive their words or behavior as hurtful. Often the parents mistakenly believe their child will "choose" not to be gay if they show him what it will cost him in lost family support.

A lot of the project's work involves storytelling, said Ryan, helping families to reframe their story of having a gay child, as well as the story the gay child tells himself about his family. It aims to move the needle from a discussion about morality to well-being, helping families understand that sexual orientation is about emotions and relationships, not only sex. It gives parents the opportunity to share their hopes and dreams for their child. The Family Acceptance Project's educational materials and workshops help them to reframe how they think, and suggest strategies to build the skills they need to support their gay child in a healthy way. Ryan said parents often begin to change the dynamic simply by listening to their child. "*That* is accepting behavior," she said.

The benefits of accepting behavior can be as tremendously positive as the effects of rejection can be harmful. "It's a health hazard to remove young people from their families," said Ryan. "Research shows that when children are removed from home for reasons of abuse or neglect, and placed in custodial care, their health risks skyrocket." By contrast, the project has found that increased family support reduces substance abuse, HIV risk behaviors, and suicidality. "This is exciting," said Ryan. "This is a low-cost, low-tech approach that has benefits for the family. It not only strengthens children, but it also strengthens families."[16]

It also helps ensure that the story a gay kid tells himself *about* himself can be one of acceptance, belonging, and connectedness. It can give him the courage he needs to say something like Sami Medina's "I want to be a surgeon." No matter the directions his heart and interests take him—even if he unfortunately finds himself homeless because of family rejection, as reports from Hetrick-Martin Institute and the Ali Forney Center illustrate—the loving support of consistent, reliable adults in his life will help guarantee that today's young gay boy grows into tomorrow's confident, healthy gay man, the hero of his own story.

~

CHAPTER TWENTY

Invincible City of Friends

From Drag Houses to Community Centers, LGBT Americans Take Our Communities Seriously

D.C.'s Capital Pride Festival went on as planned on Sunday, June 12, 2016. But the more somber mood of that day's festival was a marked contrast to the hilarity of the Capital Pride Parade the day before. Overnight the mood had darkened after a man brutally transformed the popular Orlando, Florida, LGBT nightclub Pulse into the scene of America's worst-ever mass shooting. Forty-nine men and women were gunned down as they enjoyed a Saturday night at the club, among their friends, in their community, in the place where they felt safe.[1]

President Obama put it well when he addressed the nation that afternoon. Unlike most Republicans that day, who either chose to ignore the tragedy or to blame the LGBT community for "causing" it by simply existing, the president said, "This is an especially heartbreaking day for all our friends—our fellow Americans—who are lesbian, gay, bisexual or transgender. The shooter targeted a nightclub where people came together to be with friends, to dance and to sing, and to live. The place where they attacked is more than a nightclub—it is a place of solidarity and empowerment where people have come together to raise awareness, to speak their minds, and to advocate for their civil rights."[2]

Signs and slogans declared support for the LGBT community at Pride events and candlelight vigils around the country and across the world. Iconic buildings, including the Eiffel Tower and the Sydney Harbor Bridge, were lit up in rainbow colors. In San Francisco, thousands gathered in the Castro district for a vigil at Harvey Milk Plaza. In New York, the Empire State Building dimmed its lights in respect for the victims while thousands packed into

Sheridan Square outside the Stonewall Inn to publicly share their grief and solidarity. Only a year before, the crowds were there at the newly designated national monument, the site of the 1969 riots that launched the modern LGBT equality movement, to celebrate the Supreme Court's decision legalizing same-sex marriage.

Reporting on the tragedy from Orlando, *Washington Blade* editor Kevin Naff in a touching and thoughtful column called "A Tribute to Gay Bars" wrote, "Where outsiders see only a bar or club, we see a community center or the place where we formed our closest friendships or met our significant others. Our bars and clubs have played a heroic role in supporting the community, serving as gathering places in times of triumph and tragedy and helping to raise countless dollars to fund our causes, to fight HIV, to aid our own. When the government turned its back, the first dollars to fight AIDS came from the bar and club scene."[3]

I was in Washington during the week after the attack to do interviews for this book. One of them was with a short black man with an outsized persona and equally big commitment to the LGBT community far out of proportion to his physical stature. I knew enough of his story from an earlier phone interview to know it's one of courage, resilience, and survival. It's also about finding one's talents and true home.

Donnell Robinson is better known around D.C., and far beyond, as Ella Fitzgerald, D.C.'s premier drag queen. For thirty-six years, Ella has hosted the weekend drag shows at Ziegfeld's, the city's leading venue for top-quality drag entertainment. A 2001 *Washington Post* profile described Ella as "the doyenne of Washington drag queens, zipping around on the stage like a fire engine with the siren blaring."[4]

The siren isn't blaring today. But the crush of people in line ahead of us for Sunday brunch at Freddie's Beach Bar & Restaurant in Arlington, Virginia, parts when Freddie himself, an old friend, escorts Donnell/Ella—his friends call him "Donnella"—and his interviewer to what is arguably the best table in the house, front and center, as if it had been awaiting his arrival.

Star power has its privileges, and Robinson knows how to wield it to advantage—whether to procure a prime table in a restaurant, inspire Pride Day crowds as a marshal (once again), or lead a roomful of people wanting to party on a Saturday night in a solemn 2:00 a.m. tribute to the forty-nine Orlando shooting victims. "At two, we came out on stage and had forty-nine candles," said Robinson describing the vigil at Ziegfeld's only hours earlier. "It was six queens and me. They played Christina Aguilera's brand-new song 'Change,'"[5] dedicated to the Orlando victims, released only three days earlier. "Everybody is playing it around the world," he said.

Robinson has been thinking a lot about the horrors in Florida. "They showed a clip on TMZ," he told me, "where the queen had just walked off stage at Pulse, had just done a performance. They were throwing money up on stage. All her friends and fans who had been around her, tipping her, gone. That really hit me hard. I thought about it all day yesterday and Friday. Just imagine what that little queen is thinking and how she's feeling because that could have been her." Speaking as Ella Fitzgerald, mother of the drag house at Ziegfeld's, Robinson said, "I told the queens last night, we're very blessed because it could have been one of us out of town working at that club." He explained that "a lot of our queens travel" and perform all over the place. Ella herself sticks mainly to D.C., her "own little universe."

Robinson's universe has certainly expanded far beyond the farm he grew up on in western Virginia. "I was feminine as a little boy," he told me. After his parents divorced, he stayed with his mom for a year and a half until she remarried. She took his sister and brother, while Robinson stayed with his grandparents. He was in eighth grade when his grandmother told him, "If you're not going to help your grandfather outside, you're going to stay in the house and be my assistant. You're going to cook, clean, hang drapes, iron, and at night you can play in my apron."

That's when the drag started. Robinson was already the class clown when comedian Flip Wilson created his "Geraldine Jones" character, the sassy black church lady always claiming "the devil made me do it." A girl who was the same size gave him her red dress. The school librarian had the same wig as Geraldine, so Robinson bought it from her. "I don't know how I knew, but I brought it home and used pink sponge rollers to flip it, like Geraldine's," he said. Robinson won the eighth-grade talent show as Geraldine Jones. He reprised the role four years later, during his senior year of high school. He missed a lot of school his junior and senior year of high school, not only because of chores on the farm but also because school officials told him he and his drag were "too much." He didn't have mentors in or outside of school, and didn't do so well in some classes, though he was an A student in dramatic arts. "I hid the fact that I was gay until I was fifteen or sixteen," he told the *Washington Post*. "Drag was my escape, I guess."[6]

After high school, his grandparents knew life would be tough for a 5´2˝ black femme boy in farm country. "My grandfather gave me a couple grand and I moved to Arlington, and started doing drag," Robinson told me. When he revived his Geraldine Jones act in the 1975 Halloween party comedy category at the D.C. gay nightclub Pier 9, he won. "They put me to work the next week," he recalled. "I've been blessed. Forty-one years later I'm telling this story." He is also marking thirty-two years since taking a friend's advice and going to beauty school to become the talented and successful hair stylist he is, earning the funds it takes to support a fancy for feather boas and sequined dresses.

In his career as D.C.'s most famous drag queen—hosting Ziegfeld's weekly "Ladies of Illusion" drag shows since they started July 4, 1980, and a Washington institution for nearly as long—Donnell Robinson has been through it all, including the worst years of the AIDS epidemic. His first friend to die was Joe, better known as Marlo Thomas, who introduced him to the Academy of Washington, the city's oldest continually operating LGBT organization and most prestigious drag organization until changing times and budget shortfalls forced it to disband in 2015.[7] "It got to the point that I could not cry anymore," said Robinson. "It seemed like we were in a daze, just waiting for the next person to die. It seemed there was a funeral a week. Just in our drag community it seemed like there was."

Changing times have come to Ziegfeld's as well, including its 2006 eviction from 1325 Half Street Southeast and 2009 relocation to 1825 Half Street Southwest. The old site was part of an entire block of gay community businesses razed to make way for the new Nationals Park baseball stadium. Robinson said drag itself has also changed. "It's all about a pageant," he said. "Everybody wants a crown." When he was starting out, there weren't so many transsexuals doing drag. He has never wanted to transition. "I love my drag," he said. "But I am still a man even if I'm a drag queen. I like my penis." He learned from the best, including legendary female and male vocal impersonator Jimmy James. "Because of Jimmy James, I started using the microphone and singing," said Robinson. "In high school I was in a cappella choir, so I thought I can do that. I was a baritone. I learned a lot from Jimmy James back then. He was one of my mentors on the show side."

At sixty-one, Robinson often finds himself mentoring younger men. "I've encouraged a lot of my kids, as I call them," he said. He cites his own example to show them how to prepare for the long haul, how to navigate their own aging with no serious financial or medical worries other than the usual aches and pains. As for himself and "Ella Fitzgerald D.C.'s Premier Drag Queen," he's happy doing his drag show only on Saturday nights. "My body's worn out, and they wonder why I hurt after all those years of running around in heels," he said. Now he wants to find a manager and maybe make a movie of his life. At night, he said, "I look at my drag and wigs, pray, and I go to sleep."[8]

Donnell Robinson, and Ella Fitzgerald, *earned* his/her status in the Washington, D.C., community. Hair stylist extraordinaire. D.C.'s Premier Drag Queen. Adoring fans, gay and straight. His place in the community—a fixture in every Pride parade, riding atop a convertible, waving regally to the crowds—didn't come only from entertaining the troupes as a chunky little black drag queen with big hair and a bigger mouth (ask Ella's fans!). It was hard work and much love poured out in the community, over many years. The community loves Ella because Ella has given so much love to the community.

Few young and aspiring drag stars ever attain Ella's status and serenity. The 1990 documentary *Paris Is Burning* made clear that most of the young poor and working-class black and Latino femme guys in the drag ball community never get the opportunity. Their dreams of luxe lives, white weddings, and wealthy husbands come second to basic survival in a hostile, sometimes brutal, world. In an early scene, we hear a young man's voiceover recounting his father's warning about his interest in drag and the ball community: "I remember my dad said you have three strikes against you in this world. Every black man has two, they're black and male. But you are black and gay, and if you're going to do this full fucking time, you're going to have to be stronger than you ever imagined." A later voiceover puts the theme of black drag queens' resilience in the bigger context of the black community in general: "We as a people for the past four hundred years are the greatest example of behavior modification in the history of civilization. We have had everything taken away from us, and yet we have all learned how to survive."[9]

Like other LGBT community institutions, the balls and houses serve to support their members' ability to survive, and even thrive, in a hostile world. The fact that their participants are largely young gay men of color and limited financial resources testifies to a powerful resilience worthy of further attention. In fact, a survey of 263 ball and other community event attendees in Los Angeles found that participation in balls and drag houses offers support and a positive identity. The respondents—83 percent Black/African American and 7 percent Latino, 66 percent identifying as gay or some other same-sex sexual identity, and averaging nearly twenty-four years old—commonly reported experiences of rejection, racism, and homophobia. When asked what brought or attracted them to the ball community, they typically described feelings of acceptance and lack of judgment—opposite what they had felt from family, friends, and their communities based on their sexual identities.

When participants who actually won a ball were asked to describe how they felt after winning, they reported feeling validated, important, and recognized for their efforts. The researchers noted, "The idea of being recognized for their efforts in front of their 'family' and friends led one respondent to report that he had become 'more accepting I guess of myself.'" They suggest participants' sense of pride and validation "may serve to address experiences of internalized homophobia," noting that survey data indicate 30 percent of male respondents agreed with the statement "sometimes dislike myself for being sexually attracted to men," 50 percent reported sometimes wishing they were not sexually attracted to men, 22 percent reported feeling conflicted about having sex with men, and a third (34 percent) reported sometimes feeling guilty about having sex with men.

It "may be a sign of resiliency," say the researchers, for the young men in the study who seek refuge in a subculture, like the houses and balls, where they can become a part of a group or family whose membership reflects their own interests and beliefs. The house and ball communities offer "a safe space and an alternative to the discrimination and potential social marginalization" that young African American men who have sex with men face. In particular, the idea of shamelessness, or pride in oneself—a core value of the community—"can potentially counter the effects of homophobia, both external and internal, as well as depression and other mental health conditions." The researchers recommend that service providers and others working with young African American and Latino gay men encourage them to be "shameless" and express their true selves. They liken this shamelessness with regard to sexuality to ethnic pride, which has been identified as a protective factor among adolescents for risk behaviors such as substance abuse and sexual risk.[10]

Offering the kind of safe space and "shamelessness" the ball community offers its members, LGBT community centers have played an enormous role in supporting the resilience of both individuals and the community itself. The premise of the first gay and lesbian community centers in the country, in Los Angeles and in Albany, New York, was as simple as it was revolutionary: lesbian and gay people deserve to live open, fulfilling, and honest lives free of discrimination and bigotry, with access to culturally competent social services, as equal partners in the cultural and civic life of the community.

In the 1980s, the centers were at the forefront of HIV caregiving, education, prevention, and advocacy. In the 1990s, the community center "movement" spread to smaller cities and towns. In 1994, the directors of the centers in Dallas, Denver, Los Angeles, Minneapolis, and New York launched the National Association of LGBT Community Centers to mark the twenty-fifth anniversary of the Stonewall Rebellion. By 2000, nearly half the country's one hundred LGBT community centers were the only staffed nonprofit LGBT organization in their area—the first entry point for people seeking information, coming out, accessing services, or organizing for political change. By the time the association changed its name to CenterLink in 2008, it had three full-time employees. The group produces an annual summit meeting for LGBT community center executive directors and board leaders, and each year provides technical assistance and support to more than five hundred individuals and centers around the country.[11]

Before becoming CenterLink's executive director, Terry Stone directed the Northwest AIDS Foundation in Seattle. He recalled in an interview how the foundation, like so many HIV-AIDS organizations in cities and towns across America, "acted as a sort of community center, where people came to volunteer, where gay and lesbian people came because it was a chance to be active. It was the place where the big galas took place." His experience of working at the grassroots level on HIV-AIDS taught Stone the value of community centers as focal points, purposeful communities in themselves, able to leverage the LGBT community's assets to the benefit of all. It also taught him lessons he applies in his own life. "I learned resilience," he said. "It happens at community centers all the time. It's not always roses, and you sometimes have to take two steps back so you can take two or three steps forward. It's in our ability to recover from the difficult things we're faced with. From the AIDS epidemic we learned resilience. One of the key things to our health is our ability to bounce back and continue to move forward."

Stone, about to turn sixty-five when we spoke, said his experience with AIDS seems to have had unexpected, even positive, effects as life has moved along. "I think it prepared us for part of our later lives," he said. "I lost a daughter six years ago. She was thirty-six years old and died of a pulmonary embolism. People have asked what I've learned from the experience. I realized that I saw so many of my friends die at an early age. This was much more personal, but it still helped me find balance in grieving, celebrating, and moving on. My mom is getting older. I'm seeing changes in her and figuring out what my role as a caregiver will be when I'm with her. I think I learned from my earlier experiences with AIDS, the courage and the heroic nature of what I saw around me."[12]

Lorri L. Jean, the longtime CEO of the Los Angeles LGBT Center, was one of the founders of CenterLink. She regularly ranks high on lists of the most influential gay and lesbian people in America, including being listed twice on *OUT* magazine's list of the most powerful gay and lesbian people in the nation. In 2014 *Los Angeles* magazine named her as one of the ten most inspiring women in Los Angeles. She holds a law degree from Georgetown University, and has been legally married to her wife, attorney Gina M. Calvelli, since 2008. Jean has helmed the world's largest organization providing programs and services to LGBT people in two extended stints, first from 1993 to 1999, and then again from 2003 still to this writing in early 2017.

She has grown the organization's revenue budget dramatically from $8 million when she first took over running the organization in 1993 to $97 million last year; built the first $10 million endowment for an LGBT organization in the country; and is leading a $40 million capital campaign for what will become the Anita May Rosenstein Campus, scheduled to open in early 2019.

Jean is in an exceptional position to have observed the trajectory of gay men's and other sexual minorities' health over the years, from when an HIV diagnosis was still a virtual death sentence to a time when many more are living with HIV than dying from AIDS. She told me in a telephone interview that when she first arrived at the center, "the vast majority of the work we were doing was healing the wounds of homophobia and transphobia that our clients arrived with." But even then there was a new, bigger vision for the center. "We had a dream of another kind of service and program," she said, "where we weren't just trying to fix people and heal their wounds, but trying to celebrate our wellness as individuals and as a community."

In the 1970s, said Jean, "when there was so much oppression and little freedom, everyone came to the center, from the moguls on down." That changed over the years, so the donors didn't come to the centers anymore. One reason was that gay men who used to get their HIV testing and care through the center could now just see their private physicians. In 1998 the center opened The Village at Ed Gould Plaza, a multipurpose office-theater-meeting-exhibit building, to help bring the community together again. "We didn't use the word *resilience*," said Jean, "But it's what we were thinking that kind of place would be."

The new campus promises to "be the most iconic thing in our community," said Jean. The striking glass and steel building pictured on the center's website is nearly as impressive as the entire campus's role. The website says, "The revolutionary new campus will include up to one hundred units of affordable housing for seniors, one hundred beds for homeless youth (double the number we currently have), new senior and youth centers, up to thirty-five units of permanent supportive housing for young people, a commercial kitchen to feed homeless youth and seniors, ground floor retail space, and three hundred fifty subterranean parking spaces for residents and visitors to The Village."[13] Said Jean, "The $118 million project, more than a city block long, is not only going to bring together our most vulnerable, youth and seniors, but is going to have them right across the street from where we've been celebrating our wellness, creating a multigenerational place of safety and celebration. People are so excited about it!"

It's hard to wrap one's mind around what the Los Angeles LGBT Center represents for our community, for the city of Los Angeles, and literally for the world. It demonstrates so boldly and publicly what LGBT people are capable of doing—and how well we take care of our own people. Imagine the millions of individual acts of courage, resilience, and strength that occur on any given day at the center. Imagine, if you can, the coordination, energy, and talent it takes to provide the services that are the center's heartbeat: health services alone include primary, HIV, and transgender medical services; mental health and addiction recovery services; a pharmacy; and clinical research. Social services and housing serve youth, transgendered men and women, seniors, and provide legal services, discussion and support groups, too. There is Triangle Square, a 104-unit affordable housing apartment building for seniors. Then there are the theaters, galleries, and meeting spaces. And befitting a leading institution like the center, there are leadership and advocacy services as well, including training social service providers, caregivers for seniors, government agencies, and law enforcement officials to help them better serve the diverse LGBT community.

"For all the progress we've made," said Lorri Jean, "the vast majority of our clients are coming to us because they need to be *more* resilient. They come to us because they have suffered in a homophobic and transphobic society, and they need help. We help build their resiliency one person at a time." At the same time, she added, "We're trying to build it in bigger groups and the movement. It not only makes a difference in individual people who can then make the whole movement stronger, but we have legions now of people who have survived whatever they were dealing with—who were resilient enough, with a little bit of help, to make it through whatever they were dealing with."[14]

LGBT subcommunities, like the drag and ball community, and our brick-and-mortar community centers like the Los Angeles LGBT Center, are both the bulwarks of our resistance against homophobia and living examples of how we are continuing to make our "over the rainbow" dreams come true here and now. "I dream'd in a dream I saw a city invincible to the attacks of the whole rest of the earth," wrote the renowned nineteenth-century gay American poet Walt Whitman. "I dream'd that was the new city of Friends. Nothing was greater there than the quality of robust love, it led the rest—it was seen every hour in the actions of the men of that city, and in all their looks and words."

Whether it's in the drag house and ball scene, in the gay men's STD clinic, or at the Los Angeles LGBT Center, gay men and all our friends in our many LGBT communities show one another daily and in a myriad of ways "the quality of robust love" in actions, looks, and words. We embody Whitman's dream, living in freedom and working together to fulfill the promise of this nation that America's most influential poet loved with his whole homosexual heart.

~

CHAPTER TWENTY-ONE

God Loves Us, Too

The Inside Truth About Religion and Homosexuality

The young black and Latino guys at the Magic Johnson Clinic at Carl Bean House in Los Angeles aren't likely to be thinking about the *name* of the AIDS Healthcare Foundation clinic. Sure, everyone knows Magic Johnson's story about coming out as HIV-positive in 1991 and leaving his brilliant basketball career. But a black preacher-slash-gospel-slash-disco-singer taking buses and subways around Los Angeles in the 1980s, ministering to black gay men dying from AIDS, won't likely come to mind as they await their STD testing or results. The story of Carl Bean House is lived every day. So is the story of Carl Bean himself, and it's a story of profound faith.

"I really believe resilience for me, faith for me, has far more to do with practical experience," said Reverend Bean in our interview for this book. "Seeing the practical experience of the faith idiom lived out. That is what makes me resilient. I don't think you just get that from hearing Bible verses. We had to see people *live* their faith experiences."

Bean lived *his* faith by forming the Unity Fellowship in South Central LA, the first Christian denomination for LGBT people of color, and its Minority AIDS Project, the nation's first HIV-AIDS service organization run by and for people of color. "Unfortunately the institution became more important than the practicality of living [faith] day-to-day," said Bean. "When they say 'the church' today, they aren't talking about people who ascribe to living a certain way in the world, they're talking about the institution. So we see protecting the institution while children are being molested—rather than challenging people according to what they *do*."[1]

Bean is one among the multitudes of gay men and other sexual minority people of faith whose religious beliefs and spiritual values shape and drive their lives. Their lived faith challenges the erroneous view that "all" LGBT people are antireligion, or that all religion is antigay.

The false dichotomy between "religion" and "gay" owes significantly to the news media's overreliance on conservative evangelical antigay commentators, as a 2012 GLAAD report on religious voices in mainstream media stories about LGBT equality makes clear. Antigay religious conservatives have shaped a public perception of "all" of us as unanimously antireligion—and all religion as unanimously antigay. It's simply not the case, even within the LGBT community. There is a widespread perception that where it comes to religion and homosexuality, they are best left separate. But that is not the reality for a substantial number of us.

GLAAD's three-year study of mainstream news coverage about the intersection of religion and LGBT-related issues showed the media overwhelmingly quoted or interviewed sources from evangelical Christian and Roman Catholic organizations to speak about LGBT people's lives. Although evangelicals account for 26 percent of the U.S. population, evangelical organizations comprised 50 percent of all religious organizations cited by the media. Not only that, but evangelicals accounted for almost 40 percent of all the negative comments about LGBT issues made by religiously identified spokespeople. Those speaking on behalf of the Roman Catholic hierarchy contributed another 12 percent. Most pro-LGBT sources were presented without any religious affiliation—reinforcing the erroneous impression of a fierce wall of fire between "religion" and "gay."[2]

That wall is far less fierce than many in the LGBT community itself might suspect. In fact, a 2015 Pew Research Center report, called *America's Changing Religious Landscape*, found that an impressive 59 percent of lesbian, gay, and bisexual Americans (the study didn't assess transgendered individuals) consider themselves "people of faith"—the largest percentage (48 percent) of whom are Christian. Another 11 percent identify with faiths other than Christianity, particularly Judaism, Islam, and Buddhism.

It's especially interesting to note that Pew's survey of more than thirty-five thousand Americans found that the percentage of adults over age eighteen who describe themselves as Christians dropped nearly eight percentage points in the seven years since its previous survey, from 78.4 percent in 2007, to 70.6 percent in 2014. Over that time, the percentage of religiously unaffiliated Americans—describing themselves as atheist, agnostic, or "nothing in particular"—jumped more than six points, from 16.1 percent to 22.8 percent.[3]

So what's going on? When Americans are moving away from religion, how is it so many LGBT people consider themselves people of faith, or at least affiliated with a faith community? The numbers make clear the inaccuracy of claiming that "all" gay people reject religious faith—or that "all" religious faiths reject gay people.

Fortunately for those gay men inclined toward one of the "organized" religions, or simply a spiritual approach to life, change is as visible as the rainbow flag outside a local "welcoming" congregation. "The change may be due to the fact that the rising tide of LGBT acceptance is allowing more people in conservative communities to come out who wouldn't have a generation ago," said Matthew Vines, author of *God and the Gay Christian*, in an interview with the *Advocate* about the Pew study. "Especially for LGBT people who greatly value marriage, family, and community, the legalization of marriage equality makes a major difference in their ability to be able to envision a future for themselves that makes coming out worth the cost. As they continue to come out in higher numbers in the years to come, they will likely cause the number of religiously affiliated LGBT Americans to rise, and they will also help to build a bridge for other LGBT people to re-engage with faith if they wish to do so."[4]

Of course *many* wish to do so, as the Pew study suggests. Rev. Troy Perry, founder of the Metropolitan Community Churches (MCC), for decades has ministered to the spiritual wounds of LGBT people and their oppressors. He has seen, and helped exorcise, a lot of religious pain. He doesn't make light of the pain, nor does he recommend throwing away your own spirituality because a particular denomination disapproves of your sexuality—even if that denomination is the one you grew up in. "Being a spiritual person doesn't mean you have to join a church," he said in our interview for this book. For Perry it all comes down to three things: hope, healing, and heaven. "I always want to give people hope, not throw the baby out with the bathwater," he said. "No matter what you've been taught you can still be spiritual. You can still find your spirituality. Work it out for yourself. You don't have to listen to anybody else."

We all need healing, said Perry, "because there's still oppression sickness in our community." He explained, "We're not like other minority groups. An African American family has other African Americans. Other families are taught their stories; our kids have to be taught and re-taught over and over again, because they never hear the story, that we have a history, that we have made a difference."

Which brings us to heaven. "You can have heaven right here, right now," said Perry. "We don't have to wait till we die. I believe in the hereafter, but I believe we can have some of it here, now."[5]

James Melville ("Mel") White flashed into public awareness like a bolt from the heavens in 1994, when the former ghostwriter for the Revs. Jerry Falwell, Pat Robertson, and Billy Graham came out as a gay man. He had already been installed on Pride Sunday, June 27, 1993, as Dean of the Cathedral of Hope Metropolitan Community Church in Dallas—the largest LGBT-oriented congregation anywhere, serving approximately ten thousand congregants in the Dallas area. At his installation, Reverend White proclaimed, "I am gay. I am proud. And God loves me without reservation."

White's bestselling 1994 book *Stranger at the Gate: To Be Gay and Christian in America* was a revelation for many Americans, including many gay Americans. It exposed the fact that we truly *are* everywhere—even, in Mel White's case, in the good graces of America's best-known evangelicals and outspoken homophobes. Until he chose honesty, that is.

Publication of his memoir inspired public soul-searching on both sides of the alleged gay-religion wall. It also launched the next phase of White's diverse career. After three decades that had included teaching communication and preaching at the evangelical Fuller Theological Seminary in California, and producing dozens of documentaries and other media projects, White and his partner, now husband, Gary Nixon, formed Soul Force, Inc. The group is dedicated to teaching Mahatma Gandhi and Martin Luther King Jr.'s principles of nonviolence and organizing people of faith to do justice and confront religious leaders whose antigay rhetoric White believes "leads to the suffering and death of God's lesbian and gay children."

Little more than a month after he was appointed national "minister of justice," an unsalaried position for the United Fellowship of Metropolitan Community Churches, White was arrested February 15, 1995, for "trespassing" at Pat Robertson's CBN Broadcast Center. National news media followed the story of his arrest, twenty-two-day prison fast, and what White called the "little victory" that followed. After his fast, Robertson visited White in jail and then went on the air to say clearly that he "abhorred the growing violence against gay and lesbian people." White later said, "Pat Robertson is not our enemy. He is a victim of misinformation, like we all have been. In the spirit of Jesus, Gandhi, and Martin Luther King, Jr., we must go on believing that Pat and the others can change."[6]

I asked Mel White in an interview for this book how he survived the slander and attempted character assassination that followed his coming out—coming as it was from the evangelical world, the right wing, that had been his world all his life. First of all, he said the term *evangelical* itself is problematic because of its close associations with homophobia. Even the word *Christian* is suspect. "Basically the term *Christian* is no longer germane, helpful, or even safe to use," said White. "We can use it in closed circles, behind closed doors. But we don't want to admit it in public because the definition has gone terribly awry."

That doesn't mean White has rejected his Christian faith. When he and his son Mike White appeared in two episodes of CBS's show *The Amazing Race*, White answered the question about whether he is a Christian, saying, "No I am not a Christian as it is popularly defined. I am a mediocre follower of a first-century Jewish carpenter." In fact, he attributes his own resilience to a "very personal relationship with Jesus." He explains that his understanding of Jesus was formed when he was just a boy. "Jesus was always nonjudgmental, a friend, a mentor, a buddy," he said. "My relationship with Jesus was not about sin. That was at ten or eleven years old at the altar, but after that it was Jesus and me all the way."

That relationship has drawn richly from White's imagination, and he's the first to say so. When he was at the Cathedral of Hope, living in an area outside Dallas the locals avoided because of its KKK history, White said, "The long country roads gave me a chance to take long walks. I always pictured Jesus walking with me, talking with me. No matter how sophisticated we may be, it comes back to that. I'm a little embarrassed to say this, but I talk to Jesus every day." For good measure, he said he also sometimes would walk with Gandhi, too. "When reading deeply in Gandhi, I would talk with the guy. I would say the same thing of Martin Luther King, Jr. and Gandhi, they walk with me."

One time imagination became real, when White was in jail for his trespassing violation at Pat Robertson's studios. "I was fasting twenty-one days," White told me, "and I was a basket case. I would just pray and cry. I was in solitary confinement and for a white boy with privilege and entitlements, well, I would just cry. My cell would fill up with all these people. In that room were all the people I admire and they were all looking at me, quizzically, like, 'What is wrong with you?' It was as if they were saying, 'Are you kidding? This is what you wanted—the chance to make your point in a dramatic way.'"

As real as the figures seemed, White said he is "okay thinking it was just my imagination" because in fact his imagination "did wonderful things for me." At that point in our conversation, White choked up a bit talking about how his vision had given him strength to carry on in the face of near-constant public condemnation from the evangelical community he had been such a deep part of. "Jesus is the one person I know about who is absolutely accepting, especially of the outcasts," he said. "Jesus was an outcast. God came to earth as an outcast, and could have come as a king. That story has always held me close. I feel like a leper some time. Well, Jesus met with a lot of lepers." Somehow, added White, "with all my right-wing propensities, the church's craziness, they gave me that Jesus. That was the church's gift to me with all their sickness. If you want to talk about resilience, that's all I've got for you, that Jesus pulled me through—and it was my imagination, my understanding, my vision, of Jesus that did it."[7]

Anyone who thinks Mel White's faith is only in his head is advised to visit his website (melwhite.org), where the notion of anything otherworldly is dispelled at once. You learn quickly the reverend's faith is deeply rooted in an understanding of social justice that goes back to, well, Jesus. He can't abide injustice, precisely like the first-century Jewish carpenter himself. White's book *Holy Terror: Lies the Christian Right Tells to Deny Gay Equality* (originally published in hardcover as *Religion Gone Bad*) goes inside the fundamentalist leaders' "holy war" against sexual minorities. In an email message White said, "The book clearly illustrates from an LGBTQ perspective a twenty-five-year history of the religious right in their rush to control the U.S. government that ultimately succeeded with the election of Donald Trump."[8]

Prominently featured on the website at the time of this writing in early 2017 is a link to *How to Resist Extremism!: A Pocket Guide to the Practice of Relentless Nonviolent Resistance*. The image on the cover is titled, "Learning how to protest is learning how to live." The guide is a bible of how-to information for Americans committed to fighting injustice in all its manifestations in our country, including LGBTQ rights—but also in such other areas as women's rights, immigration, voting rights, the environment, prison reform, seniors, gun reform, and health care reform.[9]

This list of progressive priorities pulls together the political vision of equality and social justice long championed by the LGBT movement, the moral tenets of White's and millions of others' personal understanding of faith, a vision of a society that embraces its diversity, and a further fulfillment of the American founders' own vision of a "more perfect union." You might say it's the real "homosexual agenda"—the moral force behind the political movement, the power behind many of the community's leading figures, and the source of tremendous comfort and inspiration during the darkest of times.

When Sharon Kleinbaum in 1992 became the first rabbi for Congregation Beit Simchat Torah in Manhattan, the nation's largest LGBT-focused Jewish congregation was staggering under the impact of AIDS on its gay male members. "I was thirty-three years old and I was burying my age cohort," Kleinbaum told me in a May 2016 interview at the CBST's impressive new sanctuary and office space on Thirtieth Street, dedicated only weeks earlier. "We lost at least forty percent of the male members of CBST," she said.

Kleinbaum recalled ministering to a Jewish man who was closeted, married to a woman, and developed AIDS. He was convinced God was punishing him as he was dying. "I spent a lot of time with people from that kind of background, trying to convince them to believe in a different kind of God," said Kleinbaum. She believes that CBST, and progressive faith communities like it, play an important role in helping people "not give up on religion but to transform it, to become a different kind of religion."

The religion she practices takes doing justice seriously, as another of Kleinbaum's early recollections with CBST shows. "When I came here, I had to fight with Jewish funeral homes to bury anyone [who died from AIDS] with dignity," she said. "They were burying them in plastic body bags, which is against Jewish law and custom." Another AIDS memory: "We would sometimes do separate funerals where the community that actually knew the person could speak about them in the fullness of their lives, and not pretend it was cancer."

Still another remembered experience that brought the light of faith into a very dark place: "I did a wedding, before it was legal, for a congregant who was dying from AIDS," said Kleinbaum. "He couldn't get out of bed and his partner sat next to him on his hospital bed. A deli platter was brought into the hospital room. He died a few days later. The dignity and love and sense of humanity in that hospital room was spectacular. It was so inspiring, such a hopeful feeling of being powerful, not victims."[10]

When CBST dedicated its new home on April 3, 2016, now–Senior Rabbi Kleinbaum wrote in the official dedication program, "Our commitment to spiritual seeking is matched by our commitment to social justice, and we act on our commitments. The world needs spiritual renewal and it cries out for racial and economic justice. At CBST, we take both prayer and activism seriously. Our home is expansive, inclusive, and notable."[11]

That is precisely the argument Imam Daayiee Abdullah makes about Islam. Believed to be the only openly gay imam in the Americas, the Georgetown law degree–holding, Detroit-born, and Southern Baptist–bred son of a postman and a school teacher came out at age fifteen and discovered Islam at age thirty-three, while he was studying in China. His first Quran was in Mandarin. He converted, and went on to study the religion in Egypt, Jordan, and Syria.

"Islam adapts to culture," Abdullah said in an interview over coffee in Washington, D.C., where he lives and serves as the spiritual leader of the Light of Reform Mosque, a congregation of mostly LGBT Muslims. Abdullah's experience of coming to Islam by way of China was fortuitous because China already had a long history of gay emperors and military leaders.

"When Islam came in, it didn't affect their Muslimhood," said Abdullah, unlike the harsh fundamentalist Saudi Arabia–style Wahabi (think Sharia law). Abdullah said the fundamentalists "get mad because they know I know that translations are slanted" to support their antigay prejudice.

I knew Abdullah would be busy the week of our interview in light of the Orlando shooting the previous weekend. In fact his phone buzzed with calls from people wanting his time. He said the shooter Omar Mateen's goal was to turn groups against one another. He wanted to divide the community by its differences. Instead his heinous act had the opposite effect. Said Abdullah, "Queer, Moslem, black, Asian, Disney—all communities—are working together in coalition. This is why the response was so quick."

A 2013 Aljazeera America profile of Abdullah focused mainly on the positive aspects of his faith and work. But it still included the kind of obligatory antigay comments so many in the media feel obliged to include, as the GLAAD study showed, in this case from conservative Muslims rather than fundamentalist Christians. Some local imams have refused to greet him, and others across the country have complained his work performing same-sex marriages—fifty as of the article's publication—is not "legitimate" and he should "control his urges."[12]

LGBT people of faith, regardless of their particular affiliation or religious labels, consistently affirm pluralism, community, and a shared commitment to doing justice and showing mercy—precisely the values organized religions espouse even if they are not always practiced. They largely ascribe to the rituals and traditions of their faith, including the Christian, Jewish, and Muslim groups seen here. But unlike more traditional approaches to religious faith, there is genuine room for the singular experience of the individual believer. Each person truly is regarded as a unique and welcomed expression of God and the "human rainbow." As Imam Abdullah puts it, "There is room for dialogue and discussion, but too often religious organizations take the position of *authority*. Well, the authority is the *text* and then you read it through *your* experience."[13]

This open-hearted view of faith, and the essential role of personal experience in shaping it, clashed head on with the traditional top-down approach when V. Gene Robinson on November 2, 2003, was consecrated as the Episcopal bishop of New Hampshire. The first openly gay bishop in any major Christian denomination that claims its bishops descend from Jesus's apostles became a lightning rod for every homophobic attack imaginable.

The Episcopal Church, the U.S. portion of the global Anglican Communion, has only 1.8 million members in the United States. But it has had an outsized role in American public life since it was the leading denomination in the thirteen original colonies. It has been the denomination of more American presidents than any other. Likewise Robinson's consecration in New Hampshire has had an outsized role in forcing the Episcopal Church, and the global Anglican Communion, to choose sides. Either it had to stand fast for its understanding of Christian faith and justice by supporting LGBT people or bend to the condemnations from conservative bishops in the United States and the developing world. The church made its choice: in January 2016, the Anglican Communion voted to suspend the Episcopal Church from voting and decision making for three years because of the American church's support for same-sex marriage.[14]

Even before the Episcopal bishops could consider Robinson after his election in New Hampshire back in 2003, charges of sexual misconduct were filed against him, one for harassment and another for allegedly being linked to a porn website. "I was locked away in my hotel room while this was being investigated," Robinson told me in an interview for this book. "A priest from my diocese brought me a small calligraphed framed piece. 'Sometimes God calms the storm, but sometimes God lets the storm rage and calms his child,' it said."

Unbeknownst to the priest, another priest had already sent Robinson an aerial photo of a hurricane in the Atlantic. Among the swirling clouds, and right in the center, was a clear blue sky. "Being at the center of the storm while the storm raged around me became the mantra by which I survived," said Robinson. He later persuaded his editor to title his 2007 memoir *Eye of the Storm: Swept to the Center by God* because, said Robinson, "I wanted to indicate that I didn't believe I brought myself to that calm eye of the storm, but only God could do that."

Robinson told me he didn't see himself as courageous in leading the way or abiding the bullying he endured—the death threats, twenty-four-hour bodyguards, "all that stuff," as he put it. "I just thought of it as doing the next right thing, putting one foot in front of the other and knowing I could always change course." In fact, he said, he was so calm that he took an hour's nap before the consecration. "That is how palpably close God felt and how calm I felt despite the storm raging around me. That is what sustained me during that time." What a time it was, with news headlines across the world about the controversy over a gay man who claimed the equal right to God's love. One "Christian" newspaper called Robinson's consecration "A Day of Infamy." There was much worse, too.

But the highly public character crucifixion of the most divisive figure in Anglican church history since Jesus wasn't Vicky Gene Robinson's first experience of suffering—or profound resilience.

Born to poor sharecropping tobacco farmers in Kentucky, he began life on earth with a massive birth injury. The pediatrician told him when he was about thirteen that he'd had to "mash" the newborn's misshapen head back into a roundish shape so his twenty-year-old mother wouldn't be terrified looking in his coffin. He wasn't expected to live, so his parents combined the girl's name they had picked, after his paternal grandfather Victor, and Gene from his mother's name Imogene. "There was a time I was quite bent on changing it," said Robinson of his name. "I hated it." But like growing into one's features with age and development, he said, "I never quite got all the paperwork to change my name. Every time I sign my name 'V. Gene' I remember my history." So did his mom. "Mother had always said she thought God had saved me for something," said Robinson. "She gave me a card on the night of the consecration that says, 'Now I guess we know what it was.'"

Nineteen bishops, led by Robert Duncan, the Episcopal bishop of Pittsburgh, warned in a statement of a possible schism between the Episcopal Church and the Anglican Communion over Robinson's consecration. Archbishop of Canterbury Rowan Williams said he expected it "will inevitably have a significant impact on the Anglican Communion throughout the world and it is too early to say what the result of that will be." While Peter Akinola, archbishop of Nigeria, led the anti-Robinson bishops in Africa, Desmond Tutu, the archbishop *emeritus* of Cape Town known for his generous, embracing understanding of God's love, stated that he did not see what "all the fuss" was about, saying the election would not roil the Church of the Province of Southern Africa.[15]

"If you are absolutely certain of God's love, then everything else turns out to be very small potatoes," said Robinson, looking back from retirement. "Keeping that in mind, everything got put into perspective for me. So it didn't matter that the archbishop of Kenya said that I was unconsecrated, or that Satan entered the church, or that the archbishop of Nigeria said gay people are lower than dogs. I'm a child of God and nothing can take that away." If you believe that, he added, "It will all roll off you like water off a duck's back."

I wondered how Robinson would convey this kind of faith and resilience to younger gay men. "Obviously I come at this from the world of institutional religion," he said. "Everybody comes to church looking for God, and what we give them is 'church.' I tell LGBT audiences all the time: Don't ever confuse the church and God. The church often gets it wrong and God never does. If you tell people to believe in the church, you spend most of your time talking about religion when in fact the thing that will stand people in good stead is a relationship with God. If you're talking about candles, liturgy, architecture, politics, you're not equipping people either for a satisfying life or accomplishing anything good."

Robinson said he'd recently been thinking about the religious hymns he grew up with, like "Blessed Assurance." He didn't care for them back then. "I used to run screaming away from them," he said. "They represented everything I hated: old-time religion, where people didn't have a brain." He has reconsidered. "I think those hymns got it right," he explained. "So the effect of blessed assurance is the ability to withstand almost anything because if you are certain of God's love for you, there is almost nothing you can't do."[16]

PART IV

AT HOME IN OURSELVES

~

Overview: Part IV

The strongest oak tree of the forest is not the one that is protected from the storm and hidden from the sun. It's the one that stands in the open where it is compelled to struggle for its existence against the winds and rains and the scorching sun.

—Napoleon Hill (1883–1970)

Most gay men, like everyone else, spend a lot of our time at work. Being comfortable in our workplaces is paramount for our happiness and ability to function at our best. Since the Stonewall riots and the political awakening they sparked, being "out" has been viewed as an indicator of a gay man's self-acceptance and healthy functioning. But the fact is we're not all out in the same way or to the same degree. There are those who are comfortable discussing their off-work activities with co-workers, and others who prefer to maintain boundaries between their work and personal lives. We each choose for ourselves how we will balance the two within our own understanding of what integrity and integration require of us. Some gay men have had to make their choices in the glare of the media spotlight; most of us simply decide in the privacy of our own minds who we will be and how we will conduct ourselves while at work.

One of the most important choices for gay men is in how we balance our gay identity with all the other aspects of ourselves that contribute to making us the men we know ourselves to be. We have much to learn from men I call "doubly different, twice as strong," those who, by birth or circumstance, are not only gay but are different from the white, heterosexual "mainstream" in another way too. They may be black, Latino, Asian—or living with a physical disability. Whatever it happens to be, these men are adept at looking beyond the gay community alone for their cues about survival and resilience. Drawing, as needed, from their various identities, they show the rest of us how to balance all of ours.

In the decades since gay men were expected to accept the stigmatizing diagnosis of a mental illness merely for not being heterosexual, scientists' understanding of what makes us tick has expanded tremendously. So have the interventions they create to help us avoid HIV or to live with the virus if we're infected, and to see inside our own behavior. The exciting new trend in medical and mental health care known as "trauma-informed care" promises to be a powerful antidote for exactly the kinds of traumas that disproportionately afflict gay men—including, most particularly, childhood sexual abuse. Root out the shame and self-blame, and genuine healing becomes possible. Support gay men in feeling good about themselves, help them feel hopeful about their future, and, lo and behold, they want to protect themselves and their partners because that is what healthy men do.

Another powerful thing they do is take the ax to tired old stereotypes among gay men of how "older" guys look, think, or behave. For each one of us, the challenge is to affirm ourselves across *all* the seasons of our lives. It can become harder to do when the man in the mirror looking back at us isn't the cute young thing our minds want us to believe still exists, all evidence to the contrary. Adjusting our expectations of aging bodies and faces, and accepting ourselves at every age, are both liberating—and the keys to aging well.

Good health at any age is strengthened by claiming for ourselves the power of gay men's proud history of resisting our external and internal oppressors, politically organizing our efforts to disrupt the status quo that made us society's whipping boys, and deconstructing the closeted state within society and in our own lives. As we reject the shame we have been expected to bear—for being "different" from others' expectations, for having HIV, for the myriad of other reasons people persecute others who are not themselves—we grow in psychological stature. We become better able to resist the temptation to see ourselves as anyone's victims when we no longer victimize ourselves.

At the end of the day, each and every day, each of us has a choice to make—regardless of our sexual orientation, skin color, ancestry, or zip code: How do we tell *our* life's stories to *ourselves*? Are they tales of overcoming adversities, scaling our economic, psychological, or other hurdles, and pushing onward toward the life we want? Or are they tales of woe about life's unfairness and our bad luck? Choosing to be the hero of our story and a proud heir of gay men's heroic legacy of courage and resilience powerfully supports our health and helps us build a strong community.

~

CHAPTER TWENTY-TWO

Integration

The Power of Authenticity in Our Work Lives

Rich Rasi knew from the time he was in first grade at Our Lady of Lourdes School in Utica, New York, that he wanted to become a Catholic priest. When he was only three, Rasi had a religious experience of a loving, healing, and accepting God. Not only did he feel compelled to express his faith in loving service to others, but he felt a strong sense of having himself received love, healing, and acceptance. This is the God he believed was calling him to become a priest.

Even when the institutional church—by then his employer—in the early 1980s tried to convince him to reject his homosexual orientation, Rasi knew his own vision of God was true to his personal experience, and would have to prevail in his life if he was ever going to find peace. Although Rasi and I were close friends at the time, it was only years later that I learned the details of his struggle when he wrote about it in a collection of essays he coedited, called *Out in the Workplace: The Pleasures and Perils of Coming Out on the Job.* His own personal piece was titled "Dis-Integration."[1]

After being ordained as a priest on May 18, 1975, Rasi said, "My workplace was my life. I ate, slept, prayed, and worked all in the same basic environment." Although he was surrounded by, and worked with, people he came to love, Rasi was lonely for the gay man within him who could be himself only in his visits to gay bars and among longtime gay friends. "These friends," he said, "helped me keep the secret of my priesthood well-hidden in gay circles and the secret of my gayness almost totally hidden in vocational circles."

Not long after we met, in the fall of 1980, Rasi put his new doctorate to use as a staff psychologist at Boston College, a Catholic college run by Jesuits. There he became a fully licensed psychologist. He also began to attend services sponsored by Dignity, the LGBT Catholic community. After a while, he offered to celebrate Mass for the group. "Some of my gay priest friends went crazy," said Rasi. "After all, there had been recognized spies from the cardinal's office seen in the congregation. What if the word got back? I could be defrocked!"

Rasi knew he could lose his job—actually both his jobs, as a Catholic priest and as a Catholic college psychologist—just for addressing the group. "But," he said, "I was so very tired of living with the constant threats of doom I had experienced all my life." He decided it was time to come out, at least to a small gathering of students. "The heavens did not cease to exist," he said afterward, "the walls did not come tumbling down, and no one left the room screaming."

Instead, he left the room feeling good about what he had done. He felt scared, too, because he "knew it was another step out of the workplace closet." Over the next four years, those steps got more frequent and bolder. He started talking about the needs of gay and lesbian students at staff meetings with other counselors in his department at Boston College. He even admitted to being gay himself, at least to a few people with whom he felt safe.

Then one day he was called to a meeting with the counseling services director. The man spoke about a former counselor, also a priest, who had started to advocate for gay and lesbian students years before Rasi arrived at the college. Although he couldn't explain exactly how, the director said this man had "caused a lot of trouble" for the department. The bottom line: Rasi was told he could no longer talk about gay and lesbian issues publicly at the college—nor in meetings of the counseling staff.

But it was too late. Rasi had already become known on campus as the "gay counselor," and students were seeking him out for that reason. Being silent wasn't an option he considered seriously because, as he put it, it would be "deeply regressive" on a personal level. This is when he realized the gap between his personal and professional lives was starting to close. He knew there was no going back. The way forward was uncertain at best.

The next year, Boston College decided not to renew Rasi's contract. The counseling services director and his supervisors claimed he was not displaying professional conduct and that his clinical skills needed improvement—though they couldn't specify how or why. Rasi was outraged that all they kept saying to him was, "You just don't get it," as if there was something wrong with him that he was willfully ignoring.

Rasi decided to resign his position at the college rather than be fired. He felt an enormous sense of relief. Then a most amazing thing happened when he decided to put himself in a place where he could do his job as a self-accepting and out gay man: he found his real life's calling as an openly gay therapist. Today, Rasi Associates—a team of twelve, including a psychiatrist, psychologists, and clinical social workers—carry on Rich Rasi's dream of making the therapy practice "a place where gay men, lesbians, and other individuals seeking to integrate spirituality and psychology could find a place to go," as their website (rasiassociates.com) puts it. Rich lived to see his dream come true before his death in 2002. The women and men he worked with continue to honor his legacy and carry on his vision. "He was our friend, our colleague, our mentor," says their website. "He is our inspiration now."

Rasi Associates's owner and president Lourdes Rodríguez-Nogués, EdD, Rasi's *Out in the Workplace* coeditor and a close friend of his, told me in an interview in the group's Boston office, "The disaster at Boston College showed Rich that what he could not do was compromise his principles that were central to who he was as a human. If you believed God was a loving God, then you, Rich, had to stand up."

She recalled learning of Rasi's experience of having polio as a little boy in the early 1950s, when the doctor said he'd never walk again. "Not my boy!" his mother said. She rubbed his legs with holy oil, and prayed. Rasi had no hint of polio as an adult. "He experienced that as a miracle," said Rodríguez-Nogués. "That formed him and was part of his 'anything is possible' attitude."

Rasi used holy oil from his Melkite Catholic tradition in the healing services he led for Dignity—not as a magical potion, but to symbolize his profound belief in healing. "Everyone has a chance for healing," said Rodríguez-Nogués, "and if you step up to the plate you will not only be a better person but you will touch more lives." She points to Rasi's experience of coming out, leaving his job to be true to himself, and the healing that flowed from him to so many people because of his integrity.

"If your personal life is lived with integrity, you bring that to your work," said Rodríguez-Nogués. "If you can maintain integration, so that your personal and professional lives are connected, then there is integration. Integration is being who you are, and learning how to *be* in the world. If you can do that, you will be healthier, saner, and you will have better mental health."[2]

Reaching this place of integration, where we are as comfortable being gay in our workplace as we are in our personal life, is not only good for us, it's also good for those we work for—as Brian McNaught explains so well in his book *Gay Issues in the Workplace.* McNaught, one of America's foremost corporate diversity trainers, writes, "Employers who want a cohesive, productive work force ideally want gay, lesbian, and bisexual employees who are as comfortable with themselves and with their work world as possible."[3]

Those employees are valuable, too. Yet, said McNaught in an interview for this book, too often gay men undervalue ourselves as employees in the workplace. "I don't think we've paid enough attention to what we bring to the table," he said. When he asks gay and lesbian employees in a business setting about all the things that negatively impact their lives because they are gay or lesbian, "they can come up with dozens."

But they're mostly quiet when McNaught next asks them what positive ways their company benefits because of their unique skills as gay men and lesbians. "My message for some time has been it's time for a change in the way we look at ourselves, being victims," said McNaught. "Getting sympathy for our plight is understandable. But it's time to move forward, not be victims, and say, 'Look, I bring a lot to the table.'"

McNaught offered as an example an openly gay man whose company wanted to send him to Saudi Arabia, but knew that a common problem for American men working in the Middle East is that instead of seeing themselves as guests, and on par with their Middle Eastern colleagues, the Americans would instead come across as patronizing, with the attitude that the American way is the best way. "The American executive wanted to be sure that the openly gay man understood and was prepared for the challenge," said McNaught. "The gay employee explained with confidence that since childhood, he has had to blend into a crowd, not drawing attention to himself. He said he was very skilled in reading a room, and quickly assessing who was the one he needed to avoid, and who were the ones that posed no threat. Not asserting himself with a patronizing attitude would be easy for him. He had this unique talent."[4]

Besides our talent for blending in, another common quality of gay people—our high level of empathy—is an extremely valuable quality in the corporate world, according to Todd Sears, founder of OUT Leadership in New York City. The global consulting firm advises major corporations on how to benefit from engaging with the estimated $3 trillion LGBT market and "the hugely significant international LGBT+ talent pool," as the group's website (outleadership.com) puts it. "We know that LGBT+ inclusion positively impacts business results, and that including LGBT+ people at the most senior levels of executive leadership is powerfully beneficial for business bottom lines; we help our advisory clients achieve greater Return on Equality™."

In an interview for this book, Sears said, "Whenever I speak to groups of young LGBT leaders, I always tell them they are incredibly lucky to be gay. Because they're gay, they number one have a very different sense of the world. They are more empathetic leaders. This allows you to understand others' struggles, understand yourself more. That is a huge opportunity not everyone goes through. They also have access to a very exclusive and important club of people who are very engaged and successful, and 95 percent are eager to help others in the community."

Sears recalled a panel of CEOs at one meeting who spoke about how their experience as parents of gay sons had made them more empathetic. The idea that equality in the workplace offers value seems to be catching on. "When you look at how this was an idea I had five years ago," said Sears, "and now we have a global organization with sixty-six companies, a hundred fifteen CEOs who weren't just willing to sign something or give me a quote, but to host and be on the record to say this matters to them." As an example of the impact of mattering to the big boss, Sears said, "To have the CEO of the largest bank in Asia—with three hundred thousand employees—say so in front of the media in Asia, is pretty exciting."

For gay employees, Sears said, "Anyone who feels valued as part of a team is going to be more productive. It's not some simple linear equation." He said gay men in particular tend to suffer from what he called the "best little boy in the world syndrome," tending toward being overachievers to compensate for not feeling quite equal or feeling they need to hide their gayness. "Especially on Wall Street, and in corporate America," said Sears, "gay men had in some cases the ability or opportunity to hide. In some places they channeled their identity into work. In some places they had to remain hidden on the way up."

For his money, Sears said that "covering"—not the closet—should be the main point of discussion where it comes to the workplace. "Even though you are out," he said, "you may not be out to all your colleagues. You may not be out about your boyfriend." He cites the late British Prime Minister Margaret Thatcher as someone who had to "cover" her lower-class accent when she went into politics. "Covering is a universal experience," said Sears, "whether gay, straight, whatever." He said that 40 percent of gay people in the workplace are closeted, but 80 percent are "covering" in some way. For gay men, Sears said that covering "is a feeling that I need to actively hide an aspect of my identity for reasons in my environment—homophobia, no support, discrimination." Sharing, on the other hand, means "I can uncover that I have a boyfriend, but I choose not to." He added, "There are people who don't want to talk about their sex life, whether they are straight or gay."

Of course sharing, the degree to which we choose to reveal our personal lives in the workplace, is up to each of us. But overall, we gay folk have a lot going for us in the work world—certainly in its upper levels. Said Sears, "These corporations and leaders understand the loyalty and talent in the community. There is definitely research showing that from a workplace perspective LGBT folks—gay men and lesbians in particular—are as or more engaged than straight peers, have more education than straight peers, and have more drive to succeed."

Not only do we offer the loyalty and talent they want, but Sears said companies recognize the value of our unique experiences of growing up "different" and needing to survive and thrive in spite of the obstacles cast in our way. "That is very much what companies are looking at," said Sears, "how resilience translates into employee health, into productivity, into the bottom line."[5]

For Stephen Snyder-Hill, it took a near-death experience in Iraq to shock him awake to the high price he had paid to stay closeted in his job as a U.S. Army soldier.

Snyder-Hill felt like a sitting duck as artillery rained around the armored vehicle he was driving during one of the battles of Desert Storm—the first of his two wars. As he waited for the final explosion that would likely kill him, he happened to look at a picture inside his driver's hatch of his brother and his girlfriend. "All those years of hiding who I was, being scared of it, and not admitting or understanding it stopped right then," he writes in *Soldier of Change: From the Closet to the Forefront of the Gay Rights Movement.* "My whole life had been fake. And if I were to die, I would never have been honest with myself, never let myself love another person. I was so scared, and I felt like I was going to die alone. I promised myself, in those couple of seconds until the next artillery shell came in, that if I made it back, I was going to finally start living my life for myself."[6]

Recalling that day in 1991, Snyder-Hill told me in an interview for this book, "I promised myself that if I ever got out of that, I would never deny myself love again."

After his tour of duty, Snyder-Hill returned to his native Ohio, went back to college, and tried to understand himself as he came out. The activist spirit first stirred in him after he came upon a photo he'd taken years earlier at the Dachau concentration camp in Germany. He wanted an image that would speak to him, so he snapped a picture of a uniform with wooden shoes. When he came upon the photo in a shoebox, he couldn't believe what he saw on it: a pink triangle. The man who had worn that uniform also wore the symbol the Nazis used to identify gay men in the camps, an easy way to target them for particularly harsh treatment. "I was instantly connected," said Snyder-Hill. "That somebody who wore that uniform and died could have been me."[7]

In May 2010 Steve Hill met Josh Snyder, who would become his best friend, life partner, and now legally wed husband. "I had to train Josh to be a military spouse under Don't Ask, Don't Tell," said Steve. "We would be sleeping at night and it would be twelve o'clock, my soldier friends would call and say we're going to come over and play video games. We would rush like a fire drill, and go downstairs, take all the pictures off the wall. Then I would be sitting there and my friends would call again and say we're drunk, we're not going to come over tonight. So I was sitting in my own foyer, in my own home, my private sanctuary, my safe space, and I looked down at all these pictures in my hands. I just looked at him and said, 'I am so sorry.' He just said, 'You know, I am going to just go sleep at my house tonight.'"[8]

If that wasn't hard enough, Steve got deployed again. Twenty years after his first war, he was going back to Iraq. He told Josh that if he would wait for him, he'd marry him. Josh said he would wait, no matter what. Some of the couple's hardest moments were when they had to hide their relationship. Like the time Josh got to visit Steve at the airport in Seattle, just before Steve's deployment. Steve recalled, "The wives were all exchanging information, saying this is going to be hard but we'll get through it. And Josh and I were hiding under an escalator, crying together, to say goodbye. It was so hard."[9]

While he was deployed in Iraq, Steve often thought about the irony of being a gay soldier. "I'm thinking, I'm fighting for everybody else's freedom and it's something I don't have. I'm fighting for freedom that I don't own myself."

While he was home on leave from Iraq halfway through his deployment, Steve and Josh decided to get married. With a five-day waiver in hand, they drove from Ohio to Washington, D.C., and got married on Tuesday, May 3, 2011—at the grave of Leonard P. Matlovich, in Congressional Cemetery.

Technical Sargeant Matlovich (1943–1988), a Vietnam War veteran and recipient of the Purple Heart and Bronze Star, was the first gay service member to intentionally out himself to fight the military's ban on gay service members. When Matlovich's picture ran on the September 8, 1975, cover of *Time* magazine, he became the first openly gay person to appear on the cover of a U.S. newsmagazine. Matlovich's headstone does not bear his name but does feature two pink triangles with the inscriptions, "Never Forget" and "Never Again." Most famously, the stone reads, "When I was in the military, they gave me a medal for killing two men and a discharge for loving one."[10]

"What better way to honor this man who fought for freedom and rights that he couldn't have?" said Snyder-Hill. "When he died, he couldn't be married, it wasn't legal. You couldn't be in the military and be gay. So it was a profound thing for us." So profound, in fact, that Steve and Josh bought the plot next to Matlovich's grave—originally intended for Frank Kameny—and will be buried next to him when their time comes.

Talk of repealing the Don't Ask, Don't Tell policy surfaced while Steve was back in Iraq, now wearing a titanium wedding ring. "I wasn't taking it off for anybody," he said. "I knew I'd have to dodge questions." He considered the implications of DADT's repeal. "I thought it would be amazing if, for the first time, I didn't have to worry about losing my retirement if somebody saw a picture on my computer of Josh."

As the presidential campaign moved along in 2011, Steve recalled that some of the Republican candidates said they wanted to reinstate DADT, which was repealed in 2010. "Josh and I kept saying somebody needs to speak up," he said. So they decided to record a video and sent it to the moderators of an upcoming primary debate. Although they originally intended to keep it anonymous, the video question was selected for the September 22 debate in Orlando, moderated by Fox News anchors Chris Wallace, Bret Baier, and Megyn Kelly. The 2010 repeal of the Don't Ask, Don't Tell Policy had just gone into effect two days earlier.

"In 2010," said Snyder-Hill (just Hill at the time) in the video projected into the Orange County Convention Center, his gray Army T-shirt straining from his muscular arms, the very image of an American soldier, "when I was deployed to Iraq, I had to lie about who I was because I am a gay soldier and I didn't want to lose my job. My question is, under one of your presidencies, do you intend to circumvent the progress that has been made by gay and lesbian soldiers in the military?"[11]

"For merely asking this question, Captain Hill was met by scattered boos from the crowd, boos that grew into a chorus," writes human rights activist and former *Star Trek* actor George Takei, in his foreword for *Soldier of Change*. "It was appalling and outrageous. Apparently, the mere acknowledgement by a soldier that he was gay was enough to rile the crowd."[12]

Even more appalling were the candidates' responses to Snyder-Hill's question. Former Sen. Rick Santorum's comment was typical. He vowed to roll back DADT because, he said, "Any type of sexual activity has absolutely no place in the military." Santorum's idea was that homosexuals and heterosexuals alike should "keep it to themselves." Requiring the military to recognize the full equality of its gay members would be granting a "special privilege," according to Santorum.

"The boos aren't what killed me," said Snyder-Hill. "What killed me was Senator Santorum's response to the boos. In one second, on national TV, he reduced my entire twenty-six-year honorable career, highly decorated, to just sex."[13]

Snyder-Hill's story exploded in the news media. Republican denigration of gay people was nothing new. But an American audience booing a soldier deployed on active duty in a war zone certainly was. "Rick Santorum said he wants us to be like everybody else, to 'keep it to yourself,'" said Snyder-Hill in our interview. "If any straight person had to live the way we lived, they would be going crazy if they couldn't come to work and talk about their wife or the movie they went to, and had to make up fake pronouns, and watch what they're saying We're bombarded with people *not* keeping things to themselves."[14]

Besides writing *Soldier of Change*, both Steve and Josh Snyder-Hill have shared their story in guest appearances in the media and at universities and Pride events across the country. Steve told me he had asked himself what exactly led him to this "remarkable, courageous thing to put yourself out there?" Looking back over his life, he said it was "going through the army and lying, having to hide who I was, the resiliency that built up over the years that led to this volcano on the twenty-second."[15] Both Steve and Josh realize the importance of their story for many others, and of what Steve calls "human moments" in changing people's hearts and minds. "For years," said Steve, "people would talk about soldiers who were gay as 'them'; they never had a face. Now it was indisputable. Now it was Steve Hill, so you couldn't say it was somebody who never served, somebody without a face. It was a real human being, with a name, who is over there fighting for you."[16]

Of course, not all fighters are "over there"—or soldiers. One of our most famous nonsoldier fighters, very much on the inside, is Barney Frank. The personal journey of the now-retired congressman from Massachusetts, the first member of Congress to come out voluntarily, is a fascinating story of how one gay man moved from living a kind of schizoid existence, separating his private identity as a gay man from his highly public work life, to a place of complete integration. As in so many of our stories, the moral of this one lies in the greatly increased personal happiness, professional success, and even improved health that followed Frank's coming out.

Like so many gay men, Frank's strong empathy for others' challenges strongly motivated his work—in his case, inside the world of politics rather than in today's corporate world where OUT Leadership founder Todd Sears said it's so highly valued. In his 2015 memoir *Frank: A Life in Politics from the Great Society to Same-Sex Marriage*, Frank writes, "I chose a political career—even when I assumed it meant forgoing a satisfactory personal life—because nothing was more important to me than doing all I could to reduce the suffering inflicted on vulnerable people by unfair social arrangements."[17]

Frank rode in a car in Boston's second annual Pride parade in 1972, after he was elected to the Massachusetts House of Representatives. "It was my first step into the world of gay politics," he writes in his memoir.[18] Back then he thought he could publicly support gay equality while keeping his own sexuality private. In an interview for this book he called this his "hermetic seal" phase. The next phase, said Frank, "was being a public advocate for gay people though being closeted." He explained, "The way public organizations worked in the seventies is that you could be supportive without outing yourself. The Human Rights Campaign wasn't the 'Gay Rights Campaign,' information came in brown wrappers. It was a way to give people who were being victimized by the prejudice, but who couldn't fight openly, a way to fight."

After six or seven years, Frank realized it wasn't going so well. "I was emotionally suffering from not having a private life," he said. He knew he couldn't be open and have a political career, at least not the career he wanted. "I had to choose between a much better political career and being out. I had being out on hold." He figured if he gave up his political aspirations, his political experience would make him an effective advocate. "That is what I planned to do," he said, "and then I unexpectedly got a chance to run for Congress because the Pope ordered the congressman from the district next to mine, a priest, not to run for Congress." Frank was elected to the U.S. House of Representatives in 1980 with 52 percent of the vote, and was re-elected by wide margins until he retired, three months shy of seventy-three, at the end of his sixteenth term in January 2013.

The third phase of Frank's journey was in Washington. "Away from home," he said, "there is a little more cover for what's going on. I had an active social life with both gay and non-gay contacts, but with no public expression of sexuality, gay or straight." But that wore thin after a few years, too. "In fact, it just became impossible to be a fairly prominent public figure and keep my private life secret," said Frank.

Finally, in 1987, Frank knew the time had arrived for him to come out. "I decided I couldn't live anymore with those self-imposed constraints on me," he said. "So, I became the first member of Congress to come out voluntarily." He was determined to live as a gay member of Congress with no more constraints than a straight person would have. "That worked very well," he said.

Until, that is, the closet exacted one more toll. His name was Stephen Gobie. While Frank was still publicly closeted in 1985, he hired Gobie, a hustler, for sex. They became friends and Frank let Gobie live in his house, paid him from personal funds to be an aide, housekeeper, and driver, and even paid for his attorney and court-ordered psychiatrist. Frank evicted Gobie in 1987 after Frank's landlord reported that Gobie had brought females to Frank's home. Gobie figured he had a scandal-made-for-TV-movie on his hands and tried to sell the salacious story to various media outlets before giving it, free, to the right-wing *Washington Times*.[19]

"The normal way to hurt me would have been to out me," said Frank. "But I had already done that myself. So, he claimed I facilitated his prostitution career. He had used my parking privilege and I fixed some parking tickets for him."[20] Identified by the *New York Times* as "one of two acknowledged homosexuals in the House [the other was the late Rep. Gerry Studds, D-Mass.]," Frank asked the House Ethics Committee to investigate his relationship with Gobie "to ensure the public record is clear."[21] The committee found no evidence Frank had even known of Gobie's activities. But the House still voted 408–18 to reprimand Frank for his relatively minor offenses. In one of the bolder acts of political hypocrisy on Capitol Hill, Republican Rep. Larry Craig led attempts to censure and expel Frank. Years later the congressman would be arrested in 2007 for propositioning an undercover cop in a Minneapolis-St. Paul airport bathroom. Frank publicly called Craig a "hypocrite" for so moralistically condemning something Frank had done while in the closet from inside Craig's own toilet stall–size closet.[22]

From the time of his 1987 coming out, after taking "a little bit of a haircut with the hustler," as he puts it, Frank has lived completely openly. Even the scandal, and the reprimand, didn't create impediments afterward and Frank is widely considered the most prominent gay politician in the United States. From 1987 on, Frank said, "The boundary issue disappeared." Also in 1987, he had read a biography of Adam Clayton Powell Jr., the legendary African American congressman from Harlem. "He refused to accept segregation, and insisted on being treated fairly," said Frank. "His rule was he would not accept anything less than anyone else."

Two decades after his coming out, Frank's public image was ratcheted up considerably after he became chair of the House Financial Services Committee in 2007—and one of the most visible elected officials in America during the years of the Great Recession, the housing market collapse, and banking industry bailouts. The Dodd-Frank Act, which he cosponsored with Connecticut senator Christopher Dodd, became the largest financial industry reform since the Great Depression.

Fortunately for Frank, he had Jim Ready by his side during this highly stressful time. The two met in the summer of 2005, when Frank traveled to Maine to attend a fundraiser for the group working to prevent the repeal of the state's LGBT antidiscrimination law. Ready was then still with his partner of thirteen years, Robert Palmer, whom Frank had known since he was a Massachusetts state legislator and Palmer was a leading advisor to Gov. Mike Dukakis on prison issues and a senior executive at Polaroid. Palmer was seriously ill at the time, and had given his blessing to Ready to pursue a possible relationship with Frank after Palmer's death. "In an extraordinary example of love at its most generous," Frank writes in *Frank*, "he began to think of Jim's future after his own death and mentioned me as a potential partner. With that in mind, he insisted—as Jim later told me—that they attend the Ogunquit fundraiser at which I spoke."[23] Palmer died on January 4, 2007.

After Ready settled Palmer's estate and spent time healing, he and Frank started dating. "By that summer, I was deeply in love," writes Frank, "experiencing at sixty-seven more profound feelings than ever before."[24] The couple married on July 7, 2012. "The hero of this part of the story was my husband," Frank told me in our interview. "Here's this guy who followed politics, had his own job, and suddenly he finds himself on *60 Minutes* and in the public spotlight." He said Ready was somewhat unhappy when their engagement leaked before they had told all their family members. "On the other hand," said Frank, "Rachel Maddow said that night that 'the best thing in the world today' was our engagement announcement, because I was the first member of Congress to be in a same-sex marriage." From that time forward, he added, "Everything has been fine and we have been under no more stress than any heterosexual couple."[25]

Being out as a gay man, and married to a supportive husband, has been extremely good for Frank's health—and his career. "I eat to deal with stress and have a tendency to gain weight," he told me. "When I first decided I could live as a gay man even without going out publicly, I began to exercise and lose weight. I think if I had remained closeted I would not have been in as good physical condition."

Then there were the benefits for his work in the House. Although his gay and lesbian friends were "obviously delighted" when he came out, Frank said his straight friends "tried to dissuade" him. "My friends in the House who were the best advocates for gay rights wanted me not to come out, to live my life. They said that if you come out, you will be marginalized." Frank told them he realized what they said could happen, but he didn't want to live his life in the closet anymore. He said that when he finally came out "there was not as much of a negative as people were afraid of." Not only that, but Frank said, "I had my liberal colleagues saying to me, 'We're glad you did that because you're better at your job.' I was happier. I had a lot more emotional energy for the job—and the job takes a lot of that."

Maybe the surest sign that Frank was a man changed by love and coming out was what others said about him when he wasn't present. "Later," he told me, "when I was chair of the committee during the midst of the financial crisis, Jim repeated that he was frequently told they were glad he was here because Barney was easier to deal with."[26]

The first time Michael Guest heard about gay people, it wasn't with the word *gay* but *homosexual* when his father was preaching from the pulpit, or *fag* from other kids. He hadn't internalized that he was gay, and wouldn't until long after leaving home. "I didn't have role models," Guest told me in an interview for this book.[27] "I didn't relate to those guys on television newscasts, wearing hot pants and feather boas and dancing in the street. That's all I really knew. And I was very much focused on academics and what I wanted to do in life, what I wanted as a career."

That career was diplomacy. It wasn't easy for Guest's parents to see him pursue the diplomatic career he dreamed of. They had expected him to carry on the family "business" and become a Southern Baptist preacher in South Carolina, like his father, grandfather, and uncle. But Guest had other ideas. Despite their misgivings about the diplomatic world—all those champagne toasts!—Guest's parents beamed with pride from the dais in the State Department's Diplomatic Reception Room when Secretary of State Colin Powell swore him in on September 18, 2001 as America's first openly gay ambassador confirmed by the Senate (James Hormel was a recess appointment of President Bill Clinton's). I was there as a guest, and witnessed Powell recognizing Guest's longtime partner, Alexander Nevarez, in his remarks, a gesture that inspired LGBT groups and infuriated conservatives.

"I don't think I was really aware of the history of that moment," Guest said. "But the responsibilities it placed on me soon became clear."

Guest assumed his post as the U.S. ambassador to Romania on September 24, sharing the official residence in Bucharest with Nevarez. A media frenzy erupted after the "gay ambassador and his boyfriend" arrived in the highly conservative, religiously orthodox country—only two months after it had repealed its law banning homosexuality. "I remember the hysteria in all the newspapers in Romania from the day after I arrived," said Guest. "They had glommed onto the fact that I was gay from the swearing-in ceremony where Alex was with me on the dais. A Romanian journalist read a little article in the *Washington Post* and picked up on it, and BOOM! It was big news."

The U.S. embassy didn't know what to do. "The press officer said we have to keep you under cover," Guest recalled. He refused. "I said you can't do that. The U.S. ambassador in a country like Romania is a big fish. You make public appearances, and a lot of times what you say is listened to as closely as any Romanian political leader." As plans emerged for a first press conference to introduce the new ambassador, the embassy's press person proposed to get Guest inside through a back door and limit the questions to only five trusted journalists. "I said I will go in the front door, shake hands, and answer every question they ask," said Guest.

After an hour of talking about NATO, adoption, and other Romanian interests, the questions petered out. Guest turned to the issue the gathered reporters, and really all of Romania, were most interested in. "At the end of the conference," he told me, "I asked if that was all the questions they had. No one raised a hand. And so I said I would have thought everyone would ask about my being gay, since every newspaper article the last few days has mentioned my being gay." A reporter raised his hand, rose slowly from his seat, and told Guest that he was the one raising the question. Guest said no, that reporters had mentioned it in every news article, whether it was relevant or not. "I said I was proud to come from a country where being gay is not an impediment to serving your country, even at high levels," said Guest. "But that was not why I was ambassador. And then I reiterated my agenda, my country's agenda in our bilateral relationship."

After they got that out of the way, Guest enjoyed an outstanding experience as ambassador to Romania. He became known for speaking out against public corruption, which he said had impeded Romania's development since the fall of communism. During his tenure, the United States and Romania enjoyed strong relations. Romania committed troops to support U.S.-led efforts in Afghanistan and Iraq, was admitted to NATO, and moved closer to joining the European Union. President George W. Bush visited Bucharest in 2002.

In his early days as ambassador, as he and Nevarez lived their lives openly, Guest noted that "bags and bags of hate mail" arrived from the States. "Most people in Romania saw that I was doing good things for the country and the bilateral relationships," said Guest. "What was harder was all the attacks from the U.S. The Family Research Council and Concerned Women for America were raising a stink back home, wanting me recalled. It was hard to face a pile of letters every night, in some cases calling me everything I would never say, words I would never use. One I remember called me everything possible and then at the bottom said 'P.S., Jesus loves you.' It was from Lynchburg, Virginia. It was at that point that I didn't want to look at mail from certain zip codes or parts of the country."

Nevarez asked one night whether they would be better off just returning to the States. "I said we would be better off," said Guest, "but it would make it harder for the next guy to be named as an openly gay ambassador." Although he doesn't consider himself religious, Guest said he drew on his faith to calm him in the face of the anti-gay attacks. He also credits his resilience in this challenging time to a sense of personal commitment. "I couldn't let down my community," he said. "I couldn't let down LGBT people in America who saw [my appointment] as an advance for LGBT people."

By the time he left Romania, Guest had become one of the country's most popular public figures. Before his departure from the country at the end of his duties in 2004, Romania's then-President Ion Iliescu awarded Guest the "Order for Faithful Service in the Rank of Grand Cross" in appreciation for his "high professionalism, dedication to his mission, and for his personal contribution to the strengthening of the Romanian-American partnership."[28]

Before serving in Romania, Guest already had been awarded the Department's Superior Honor Award five times, as well as the Meritorious Honor Award once. While in Romania, he was awarded the Department's prestigious Charles E. Cobb Award for Initiative and Success in Trade Development. Back in Washington after his posting, Guest served as dean of the State Department's Foreign Service Institute, and in 2006 he received the Christian A. Herter Award, given by the American Foreign Service Association to a senior foreign service officer in recognition of intellectual courage, initiative, and integrity in the context of constructive dissent.

That award was given for his determination to end the State Department's unequal treatment of American diplomats' same-sex partners. A year later, having failed to remedy that inequality, Guest ended his career. In the State Department's Treaty Room, Guest gave a farewell speech in which he shared his reason for leaving, expressing what the New York Times called "eloquent sadness, not anger."[29] "For the past three years," said Guest, "I've urged the Secretary [Condoleezza Rice] and her senior management team to redress policies that discriminate against gay and lesbian employees. Absolutely nothing has resulted from this. And so I've felt compelled to choose between obligations to my partner—who is my family—and service to my country. That anyone should have to make that choice is a stain on the Secretary's leadership and a shame for this institution and our country."

Guest pointed out that unlike heterosexual spouses, gay partners were not entitled to State Department–provided security training, medical care (paid or otherwise) at overseas posts, guaranteed evacuation in case of a medical emergency, transportation to overseas posts, or special living allowances when foreign service officers are assigned to places like Iraq, where diplomatic families were not permitted. Gay people comprised an estimated five percent of the twelve thousand foreign affairs officers, and there were about three hundred fifty same-sex partners, at the time.

"At first I looked at it through the lens of 'I can't leave my career over these issues, I love my career too much,'" Guest said in our interview. "Then it became 'I can't stay because I love my husband too much, and I love my country too much. It wasn't right or fair to us or anyone else when we had the same service obligations.'"[30]

The *New York Times* called it "foolhardy" for the State Department to lose a top diplomat and other LGBT employees because of its unequal treatment. "Treating gay public servants by different standards than apply to everyone else is unacceptable," said the *Times*, "especially when all American diplomats and military personnel are being called on to serve—sometimes repeatedly—in war zones like Iraq and Afghanistan." The newspaper concluded, "The government should be doing everything in its power to retain its best and brightest, beginning with treating them equally."[31]

In 2008, in part because of his public stance and sacrifice on this issue, Guest was invited to serve on President Barack Obama's State Department transition team. In that time, he sat down with Secretary-designate Hillary Clinton, outlining for her what the problems were and how they could be remedied. Even after Guest officially left the State Department, his impact there didn't end. "When I sat down with [then Secretary of State] Hillary Clinton and told her about what it was like to be a representative of a country without being an equal citizen in some ways, she got it," he said. The Obama administration announced changes in June 2009, giving fully equal treatment and benefits to same-sex couples as to heterosexual couples—its first action on behalf of America's LGBT community.

That year he also cofounded and remains senior advisor to the Council for Global Equality, a coalition of twenty-nine human rights and LGBT advocacy organizations that advocates "to make sure the U.S. government is standing fully and fairly for the equal treatment of LGBT people around the world," as Guest explained it in our interview. "It's a bit of a labor of love that keeps me focused on trying to make sure the ill treatment and ill consideration of LGBT people ends in our lifetime."[32]

After his retirement, Guest said he left it up to Nevarez as to where they would live. They looked around the country but kept coming back to Sonoma, California. Nevarez grew up in California, and it was about as far from Guest's world of politics and diplomacy in Washington as they could get. So they bought a house perched on a hill and forty acres amidst the rolling hills of Sonoma County. Nevarez teaches school. Guest spends a lot of time on conference calls and e-mail related to his work with the Council for Global Equality. "Then," he said, "I get on a plane and fly back to do meetings at senior levels with people I know, to push on policy issues that matter to our community."

In between those trips, he works around the house on the lavender field. "There is something, not just about the lavender," he said, "that frees your mind, allows you to think of other things, and allows you to grow." He's glad to be away from the pressure cooker of Washington. "It's really a blessing to be able to work on policy issues I care about, but to pull myself away from them long enough to go out to the field to hoe, plant, and do irrigation in the two acres of lavender. No pun intended with the lavender!" He laughed, acknowledging the association of that color with the LGBT community. "Sometimes I spend more time there than I want, but when I pull weeds I see the difference. You can weed, or hoe, and you are doing something to change the earth and seeing the difference in a short span of time. Then at the end of the season it's something beautiful: two acres of purple."

Reflecting on what had brought him here, to California and to this point in life, Guest said, "I'm so glad, feel so blessed, that I had the opportunity to work on an issue of such importance from the inside and then from outside in a way that resulted in its closure, and then to do the lavender farm." He thought a moment, then added, "It's very balanced."[33]

CHAPTER TWENTY-THREE

~

Doubly Different, Twice as Strong

*Gay Men of Color or Different Ability Show
How to Find Resilience in
All Their "Identities"*

In more than three decades of writing about HIV-AIDS, black, Latino, and Asian gay men have regularly told me they experienced the epidemic differently from urban white gay men. Unlike those migrants from small towns and disapproving families across America, many gay men of color frequently must find ways to be as "out" as they comfortably can be while still living in the same neighborhoods, even attending the same churches, as their families. Their experience is much like that of all gay men in the decades before Stonewall emphasized "coming out." The programs gay men of color created to serve their brothers in the early years of AIDS were the very model of "cultural appropriateness" as they reached deep into their shared culture and history, and claimed for themselves the bravery and resilience of the heroic men and women who came before them. Gay men of color drew on the heritage of survival they inherited from their families and communities to create organizations that understood that who they are, where they belong, is about *much* more than their sexuality.

Another group of gay men I call "doubly different, twice as strong" are those living with a disability. These men know a lot about needing to look to other sources of identity beyond their disability, beyond their sexual orientation, to find the strength and sustenance they need to live with—and not allow themselves to be defined by—their particular physical challenge. A visit to gaydisabilitydating.com or whisper4u.com, two dating sites for gay people with disabilities, turns up smiling faces and handsome men—who happen to be living with a prosthetic leg, or some other health condition that gives them their extra difference. It also makes one thing clear: These men are the first to say, "Don't pity me. Date me!"

Those of us living with HIV may not often think of ourselves as disabled, but in fact HIV infection is legally classified as a disability in the United States, under the Americans with Disabilities Act (ADA).[1] The Centers for Disease Control and Prevention (CDC) reports that at the end of 2013, 687,800 gay and bisexual men were living with HIV in the United States. Of those, an estimated 15 percent were unaware of their infection. The CDC says that if current diagnosis rates continue, *one in six* gay and bisexual men will be diagnosed with HIV in their lifetime, including 50 percent of black/African American gay and bisexual men, 25 percent of Hispanic/Latino gay and bisexual men, and one in eleven white gay and bisexual men.[2] Clearly, a *lot* of gay men already live with a disability, and potentially many more will do so at some point in their lives. Which is to say it's to our benefit to consider the experiences of gay men who have been down the roads we ourselves might travel in the years ahead.

Gay men of color in the AIDS years found—and showed us how we, too, can find—courage, hope, and resilience by mining the depths of their family and cultural past for the roots that kept them anchored. Gay men living with disabilities—"QueerCrips" is their preferred, cheeky, and empowered term—show what "gay pride" means when living in "differently abled" bodies necessitates finding other ways to identify and value themselves *and* their physicality when even sex itself is "different."

Among H. Alexander Satorie-Robinson's identities are African American; Baltimore, Maryland, resident; and longtime gay equality and AIDS activist. In an interview for my 2013 story for *The Atlantic* about gay men's resilience, we spoke about the first-ever HIV-AIDS prevention organization created by and for gay men of color—an exceptional example of black, Latino, and Asian gay men demonstrating how best to reach men like them in language and images that resonate with them. Satorie-Robinson was president of the National Task Force on AIDS Prevention when the nation's first prevention program targeting gay men of color was created in 1988. Lacking a full embrace in the mostly white gay community—and the AIDS service organizations it created—and not very welcome in the black, Latino, and Asian communities that reared the men it served, the Task Force "was a place of comfort," said Satorie-Robinson. "Just from an instinctual part of it, whatever culture or community we're from, or faith or religious belief we have, we often in times of trouble move back toward those places because they bring comfort and some sort of continuity."

Of course not all gay men of color had positive experiences in their home communities or with religion even before AIDS, so the group took what spoke to them and left the rest. "While we were going back to the black community," said Satorie-Robinson, "or the Latino or Christian culture, we weren't *literally* going back to our places of origin; we were *recreating* those places in our gay and bisexual image." Even without empirical data, Satorie-Robinson said the gay men who created the Task Force drew on their own cultural and survival instincts. "To the extent there was healing and healthy behaviors that were part of those cultures," he said, "we looked at what works, what doesn't work, and what's adaptable for us as gay men."

Looking at the numbers of gay men living with and still becoming infected with HIV today, Satorie-Robinson said, "The number of young gay men in particular becoming infected is disturbing. The number of black men becoming infected is disturbing." He sees it as an unfortunate side effect of successful HIV treatment. "It's kind of like 'we survived,' but now what's been the impact of the survival? What's the impact of being resilient? There is post-traumatic stress that goes along with that capacity to survive. There is that lack of urgency that comes with feeling like you made it through. I look at our culture, the number of places I see where there is acceptance of barebacking, places where people can say 'I'm negative so therefore I can have certain behaviors put me at risk.' The urgency has been taken away because the impact seems not as critical."

We learned in the AIDS years about the impossibility of sustaining rage and even grief indefinitely. But the challenge remains for the LGBT community, gay men in particular, to make sure the stories of our community's extraordinary courage and resilience are shared with young people. Satorie-Robinson pointed to the Jewish community as an example of how to keep alive a community's history not only of its people's suffering but, as importantly, their surviving and thriving in spite of it. His spouse, Greg, has worked for years with Jewish Community Services, educating young people in their schools. "I think there's a lesson there," said Satorie-Robinson. "There's a community that has a deep history of what it takes to survive, who have not diminished at all their education of their kids about these issues. A community that knows that if there is a threat and you take your eyes off of it because you think it's going away, you do it to your own detriment."

Looking back three decades to his experience with the Task Force and all that's happened since, Satorie-Robinson said, "We've got to remember what happened, how we responded and what the response was about, and we've got to keep it alive. That goes to resilience. To the extent that you can draw upon your history, your religious or cultural values, and apply those lessons to new and emerging threats, your ability to survive seems likely to be increased." On an unsettling note, he added, "When I talk to many out gay youth, they are so unaware of the history."[3]

Mauro Walden-Montoya was also marking three decades when I interviewed him for this book on the last day of February 2016. It was in February 1986 that Walden-Montoya, just out of law school, went to Whitman-Walker Clinic (today Whitman-Walker Health), in Washington, D.C., to volunteer his legal services. During those darkest of pretreatment AIDS years, the young lawyer had no idea what he was in for.

He had a call from the social worker at George Washington University Hospital a week after he started. She had a patient who needed legal documents. The man was sixty-eight, single, and had a brother with two daughters. "When I got there," recalled Walden-Montoya, "he was on a respirator and couldn't talk. I was thinking, 'How do I get information from him?' His brother said he didn't know his brother was gay, and now he has AIDS and is dying. The brother was in total shock, didn't know what to do. I had to find out what the guy wanted, how to get him to communicate. I figured out how to ask him yes and no questions by blinking once for yes, twice for no. I asked if he had stuff to leave someone? He said yes. I asked if it was to a family member? He said yes. Is it your brother? No. It was his niece." Walden-Montoya went back to the clinic and typed up the will. "I was back there within the hour," he said, "and he had died. I said, oh my god, I failed a client. The brother consoled me. I was so shaken up."

By the time the *Washington Post* in February 1988 ran "Advocates in the Realm of Sorrows," a story about him and some other D.C.-area lawyers working on behalf of people with AIDS, Walden-Montoya had written hundreds of wills and powers of attorney. Only two years after he started Whitman-Walker's legal services program, Walden-Montoya was burned out and would leave April 1. "It's just too much," he told the *Post*'s Elizabeth Kastor. He had no full-time secretary and only a part-time law school student assistant. But it wasn't just the overwhelming administrative responsibilities that weighed him down. He realized he couldn't continue when he saw the AIDS Memorial Quilt at its first national display a few months earlier. "I have never been the same since then," he told Kastor. "It was seeing the names of friends and all those people. I cried for forty-five minutes. I had thought at one point that I'd get used to people dying. You don't. It's impossible. I have seen nine hundred people die now and it just gets to be too difficult."[4]

In our interview for this book I asked Walden-Montoya how he was able to go on in spite of the tremendous burden of grief and loss. "It was hard," he said. "I kept going back into professional mode." In psychology, this detachment is called "dissociation." It's a common coping mechanism for responding to the stress of trauma. A ten-year-old boy raped by a priest, as Walden-Montoya was, probably learned how to dissociate early in life. Now it was hard for the grown man to see so many gay men in the hospital, dying horrible deaths. And then there were all the funerals. "After about fifty funerals I said I can't do it anymore," said Walden-Montoya. So how did he? "I found a strength I didn't know I had," he said. He leaned on his partner at the time. He also felt a strong sense of justice on behalf of the mostly gay men he was helping. "They were brothers," he said.

But it was a lesson Walden-Montoya learned from his AIDS clients in those years that personally helped him the most. "Back then," he told me, "one of the first things that hit me was when someone sitting across my desk would say 'I have AIDS and will be dead in a year, and I wish I could do this or that.' That made me think 'Wow! These guys are trying to live their lives as best they can, and they know they have a death sentence hanging over their heads.'" Since then he has focused not on *wishing*, but *doing*, and it has led to memorable experiences—including hiking naked in the Puerto Rico rain forest, and winning the 1996 Mr. Mid-Atlantic Leather competition five years after his own 1991 HIV diagnosis.

Walden-Montoya's father died in 1998, and his beloved mother followed in 2013. "If I didn't have Andy as my husband, I don't know what I would do," said Walden-Montoya of the man, twenty-two years his junior, who shares his life—and his positive HIV status. They met on Walden-Montoya's fifty-first birthday at a bar called the Albuquerque Social Club. Andy had moved to Albuquerque from Seattle about six months earlier, and heard people at the gay social club talking about Mauro. Back in Albuquerque, where he grew up, Walden-Montoya is president of the city's Gay and Lesbian Chamber of Commerce, on the boards of several other organizations, and active in a drag group called The Dolls. "I'm at the social club, with a twenty-one-year-old kid on my lap," he recalled. "Andy came up and said I've been told I should meet you. I looked up and said, 'Yes, you should!'" They became friends, and six months later, Andy told him he had found out he was HIV-positive the day they met. "I just took him in my arms and said I'm going to take care of you now," said Walden-Montoya. "It's ironic that HIV brought us together."

Walden-Montoya said his Latino heritage "definitely" factors into his resilience. "I was raised Catholic, and went to Catholic school through ninth grade," he said. "We have a serious sense of family. I still have that. I am very close to both sides of my family. All my cousins came to our wedding."

He is aware of the difference between his relationship with his family and Andy's relationship with his own family. "I see the difference between Andy and me," he said. "He talks with his family every couple of weeks. I used to talk with Mom every week or more. Being Latino, family has a serious connection for me."

At the center of Walden-Montoya's family is his husband. "What keeps me going now is I absolutely love being married to Andy," he said. "He has put me in such a good place in my life that I want to live as long as possible, spend as much time together as we can." He laughs remembering the discussions he had with Andy before they got married. Andy said he never wanted to get married because it was such a "hetero-normative institution." But the men talked about it and considered their options. "Then," said Walden-Montoya, "Andy said I guess there's no real reason we can't get married because I'm already going to spend my life with you." Walden-Montoya asked Andy to marry him five days later as same-sex marriage was becoming legal in New Mexico. He used a Dolls' play rehearsal to propose—as his fellow cast members sang the "Chapel of Love" song. As of this writing, they have been together nearly seven years.[5]

Sacramento native Steve Lew was liberated, and terrified, at the same time when he and his younger brother Brian came out to each other in their twenties. Brian had joined the gay and lesbian student union at Sacramento State, and was finding a place of belonging and leadership, while Steve was seeking ways to integrate his identities and activism in the Asian American, third world, and gay liberation movements in Los Angeles. Each of them was already living as an openly gay man in his own circles, but not in their family.

Both men were determined to come out to their parents, yet Steve was concerned how their parents would handle having two gay sons, considering the cultural values and expectations of Chinese sons. Their sister Elaine was supportive, and helped them "rehearse" coming out together. They also decided to get counsel from their grand uncle, their father's uncle and a gay man. Frank Eng was known as an iconoclast in the extended family, even beyond his homosexuality. He was an arts and culture critic for a Los Angeles newspaper in the 1950s McCarthy era, taking stances for which he was labeled a Communist sympathizer and had to leave the work. He managed one of the first multi-racial dance companies, Lester Horton Dance Theater, with his partner Lester, and held the groundbreaking company together for many years after Lester died. Uncle Frank had come out to his family in his early thirties after he served in the military and came home. As a young boy, Steve remembered watching Frank "work the room" during the big family dinners held in Oakland Chinatown, standing out in his sublime tie and sports jacket. Steve *knew* his uncle would have wise counsel about coming-out for his grand nephews.

The brothers drove up to see their uncle and his longtime partner Jim at Lake Tahoe. "I'm sure he thought about how he wanted to talk to us," said Lew in an interview for this book. "He told me and my brother in so many words, 'I think this is going to be a good thing for your family.'" He also told his nephews what he knew of their dad's growing up years, and how he was different from his own father, Hoy Lew, "the patriarch," as Steve Lew put it. "Frank described my dad's progression as a young man from being very involved in Baptist theology when my dad stayed with Frank to attend a Baptist university in Los Angeles, and how he moved away from fundamentalism. He also talked about his own sisters, and how he was able to become closer to them, including my grandmother, by being truly who he was." What really made a difference for Steve was hearing Frank say his dad had gone through similar struggles about who he wanted to be. "It made me think about my dad as more of a person with emotions and thoughts," he said. "I began to think that I could probably tell him this thing about myself."

Steve and Brian traveled back to Sacramento, where Steve said they had grown up "very Chinese American, middle class." Elaine was also there for support. It took about thirty minutes, and went well. "My dad was surprised, my mom wasn't, and they were both quite concerned for us and sad," said Steve. "At the end they told us they loved us and they wanted to learn more about our lives. I remember feeling quite relieved and close to my siblings and parents. It was summer and quite hot, and instead of going to a Chinese restaurant, as we usually did, we went to Folsom Lake and had a bucket of Kentucky Fried Chicken."

After assuring the sons of their parents' love, and before the picnic, their father wanted to know how they could explain having two gay sons. "Face" is a very Chinese concept, and even after several generations, saving face is a serious family concern. Their dad didn't think his father and mother, or brothers and sister, would be able to understand and accept it. Which made it all the more striking when, a couple of years later, both parents eventually joined a PFLAG-type group for Asian parents. They even spoke a couple of times at press conferences, their stories in English translated for the Chinese press, and they volunteered to speak to other Asian families.

His family's acceptance provided a solid foundation for Steve Lew to become highly visible in San Francisco's Asian gay community. In 1987 he helped organize the first West Coast conference for Asian and Pacific Islander gay men and lesbians. He cofounded the Gay Asian Pacific Alliance Community HIV Project, which grew into a national service organization, was renamed the Living Well Project, and eventually merged with the Asian AIDS Project to become the Asian and Pacific Islander Wellness Center in 1997. In 1995, he was appointed and served for four years as a member of the Presidential Advisory Council on HIV/AIDS.[6]

When Lew found out he himself was HIV-positive, more than thirty years ago, he hesitated to tell his parents for several years. He knew they were supportive of his HIV work in the Asian community, but he was concerned about creating emotional distress for them as they were aging. In Chinese culture there is another strong tradition of children, particularly the eldest son, caring for elderly parents. At the time of Lew's diagnosis, before effective treatment for HIV was available, it was unlikely this eldest son would live long enough to fulfill his duties to his parents. While Lew and his family were very "American" in many ways, he saw so many of the Asian men with AIDS he worked with, and their families, struggle to accept this flipping of social and familial roles. "Even though I felt a sense of loss and confusion about being a good son," said Lew, "I don't think they did or, if they did, this wasn't of primary concern. We lost one of my sisters in her early twenties and it was hard for them to know another child might die young. I think they got even clearer in their minds that they wanted to work on our relationship. They knew it was really important for it to be solid so I could share more about what was going on with me, rather than hiding, not sharing parts of my life."

Fortunately, after effective HIV treatment became available after 1996, Lew said his parents were able to see him living with a long-term chronic illness rather than declining steadily as HIV took its well-known devastating course. "I didn't think I would be able to take care of them, much less make it to forty," he said, "and now, in my late fifties, I feel fortunate to be able to take care of them in their mid-eighties, with my sister and brother."

Of course life itself in 2017 has its own issues irrespective of HIV status. "I have had my own challenges and victories in aging beyond HIV disease," Lew told me. "I still eat fast food, drink alcohol, exercise randomly, I don't meditate or read POZ magazine. Having a stable sense of community over the years—of longtime friends, co-workers, siblings, and parents—has made a positive difference in caring more consistently for and about myself." He attributes the strength and health of his relationships to an awareness of "how much oppressive systems and beliefs"—including, sometimes, traditions—can undermine relationships and keep people apart. For example, Lew said, that as a gay man and a firstborn son, he has considered the differences between his and his sister's experience of growing up. He sees the impact of sexism and a male-dominant culture in the family's expectations that she would carry more of their emotional and practical burdens. "Noticing how it can degrade our relationship, talking about the impact of sexism, has helped me to change my own expectations of myself as a care giver, of her, and of my parents," said Lew. "It's given me a different view of being a 'good son' and ways of being in my family."

Another resource Lew has found to be helpful is "re-evaluation counseling," a peer-to-peer program in which individuals pair up and alternate being the counselor and client with the aim of helping to process and "discharge" old hurts and traumas. "I did a lot of thinking and organizing as a young adult around claiming my Asian, and gay identity," he told me. "I was doing conscious work around that by organizing support groups and community organizations around those identities working toward liberation." When his partner introduced co-counseling to him ten years earlier, he was surprised what it opened up, "how much internalized homophobia I have carried from experiences of ridicule and stigma growing up. Facing these old hurts with a peer counselor, feeling the feelings and holding a different contradicting perspective is healing. The more that I have been able to emotionally heal from past experiences in my sessions, I can connect with other gay, queer men differently, in a closer way." Lew uses the tools of re-evaluation counseling with other co-counselors as a grounding practice, to take on bigger goals in his life and in his work as a leadership coach with nonprofit leaders and social justice activists.

Lew and his partner Steve Bromer had been together for fifteen years at the time of our 2016 interview. They'd done all the civil marriage paperwork and gone to City Hall. Lew said they did it "more as a rite of passage for rights" than to be "welcomed into a lot of the hetero norm traditions." But the surprising part of the civil service and getting married, said Lew, is that it has "a big impact on each of our ways of thinking about staying healthy and alive." Reflecting on his own and his partner's health, Lew said, "I think that's huge, having a partner there who can be vulnerable in sharing highs and lows, who can ask for support in his life, and is there to give you support. To maintain intimacy, we have to keep paying attention to this, tackling the issues in our relationship, what's important to him, what's important to me. I don't know how it is for others, but it's challenging for me as a gay man to stay vulnerable and strong, to keep trusting that we can be both for each other. Luckily both of our families embrace our relationship wholeheartedly and that makes a big difference. But it has been a lifelong project for me, to be both vulnerable and strong in community, family, relationships, and movements."[7]

Another lifelong project for every gay man who lived through the dark years of AIDS is to take away from the loss, rage, and sorrow the epidemic brought upon us the lessons it taught us about life and about ourselves. AIDS certainly showed John Killacky and Larry Connolly what resilience looks like. "We had lived through most of our generation dying," as Connolly put it in an interview for this book. We were talking in the barn outside of Burlington, Vermont, where he and Killacky board their Shetland pony, Raindrop. "So when we were faced with something that was catastrophic, but people knew what it was, I think part of our resilience came from coming through the AIDS crisis."

The catastrophe Connolly is talking about on this August afternoon is what happened to Killacky in 1996, about a month after they had moved in together in Minneapolis, where they lived at the time. "I had a tumor inside my spinal cord," Killacky explained to me in an earlier interview for *The Atlantic*. "Larry and I were going to sleep. I had this spastic attack. It seemed like an epileptic seizure or something. We went to the hospital, got an MRI, and they found a tumor inside the spinal cord. It was blocking 60 percent of the cord. They couldn't do a biopsy to see if it was malignant or benign, so took it out."[8] The result was something called Brown-Séquard syndrome, a loss of sensation and motor function more commonly caused by a puncture or gunshot wound. Before he went to the hospital, Killacky was a dancer and marathon runner. When he was discharged, weeks later, he was in a wheelchair, paralyzed from the neck down. More than two decades afterward, he still has no sensation on the right side or sense of location on the left side of what he calls his "bifurcated body."

To his utter delight, Killacky discovered that he didn't need functional legs to drive a pony-pulling cart. "With a horse," he explained, "you need to use your legs to ride them. With a cart, you don't need your legs at all. You drive the animal through the rein and the bit." Inside the vast barn, rain pattering on the roof, I ride in the little cart with Killacky about the indoor ring, my digital voice recorder catching the sounds of snorting horses, the leathery squeaks of the horse's tack, Killacky's lip-smacking command to spur her along, and the reflections of a man who suffered something terrible but hasn't let it stop him. "For me," he said, "here is what is beautiful about it: I have legs again in the world." He added, "If other horses are in here, we are literally dancing, and she loves that."

So does he. "This gives me a completely different space than my work place," said Killacky, whose day job is overseeing the $7 million, 275-employee Flynn Center for the Performing Arts in Burlington. "I have no gravitas in this barn," he said. "Larry and I are Raindrop's dads. The kids who work here know more than us. It's nice for me to be completely co-dependent in a very good way. It teaches me different skills."

Besides the skills, the ten years Killacky has had with Raindrop have provided a reconnection to an earlier time in his life, and an earlier pony, when he was growing up on the South Side of Chicago. His father was "a very angry Irish alcoholic," said Killacky. He worked selling cattle in the Chicago stockyards. John was the third child. "I think it was very complicated for him to have a sissy son," he said. "I was like the lightning rod for him. We had a very complex relationship." But there was one thing John loved to do with his dad. "He had to visit farms to convince farmers to sell their cattle, I would go with him. I was eight years old." One farm, in Milledgeville, Illinois, had beef cattle—and Shetland ponies. A Shetland mare gave birth in the rain, and the filly was named Raindrop. "That Raindrop became my best friend for years," said Killacky. "Whenever we were in Milledgeville, I would spend afternoons in the field with her. She became this mythic thing for me."[9]

Four months after Killacky came out of the hospital, he and Connolly moved to San Francisco, where Killacky became executive director of the Yerba Buena Center for the Arts. After an attempt at horseback riding proved a "disaster" for him, Killacky suggested finding Shetland ponies, which they did at Fog Ranch in Moss Landing, about ninety-five miles south of San Francisco. When Killacky saw the ponies pulling carts, he thought, "I could do that." So he did. When a Fog Ranch mare birthed a filly born in the pouring May rain, they named her Raindrop after Killacky's boyhood pony friend. When the couple decided to move from California to Vermont, the owners of Fog Ranch gave Killacky the new Raindrop as a gift. "She has been here seven years with us," he told me, "and it's done *wonders* for my physicality. Larry can tell you. He says I am a lot stronger here because I have to walk on this uneven dirt in the barn. In the office I just sit, mainly. I have no relationship to the ground that I walk on. I could step on glass and not feel it."

Learning to feel in new ways has been one of the big challenges since Killacky's life-changing moment. That goes for sex, too. "In your forties," he said, "you don't think, when you're very sexual, that things are going to change radically." The instructional sex tape at the rehab hospital that was provided in response to Killacky's questions turned out to be irrelevant, not merely because it showed a man and woman, but because spinal cord injuries don't permit things like thrusting and being tossed about "like a baby doll," as was the disabled man in the video. "Why don't you ask someone about *where* they feel something?" Killacky asked the people at the hospital who provided the tape. "Maybe it's above your chest that is your erotic zone. You can't think that the only normative practice is for the man to be on top."

Killacky and Connolly are one of three couples coping with the many issues that arise with disability interviewed in *Holding On*, a 2006 documentary that Killacky produced and Vermont and Twin Cities PBS broadcast. In the film Connolly says he and Killacky, like other couples in similar circumstances, "have to redefine what sex is, the spectrum of what you consider sex and how you find sex to be pleasurable, revivifying, and renewing." He adds, "I think most everybody in America runs from A to C in that you run from this to this, you cum, and you're done. What disability has done is really made us, forced us, to walk from A to Z and to see what is every part of the body capable of. We have to articulate what it is we want, how do we want it, what does this feel like—and not just what does it feel like, but what does it feel like *now*."[10]

In *Queer Crips: Disabled Gay Men and Their Stories*, an anthology he coedited, Killacky writes, "As someone who was quite phallocentric, I have been forced to reorient my sexuality. With almost no sensation in my genitals now, my only indication of an orgasm is violent spasticity in my left arm and leg. Reciprocating with my enfeebled fingers and locked-in neck is often very short lived. Yet the unconditional love of my husband has allowed new patterns to emerge: light massage and hugging are central to our relating."[11]

From the moment they knew of Killacky's paralysis, both men were well aware of the odds stacked against their relationship. Connolly remembered, "When we were in the hospital and moved out of ICU into the rehab part of the hospital, the woman who ran it happened to be a lesbian. We asked her to tell us John's prognosis. She said most people don't make it, don't get much improvement. She said first of all if you don't have a partner, you don't have much motivation because there's so much pain, trouble, and effort to go through. The other thing is that, even if you do have a partner—and she said this is true for any catastrophic event, such as stroke or death of a child—most couples don't make it. She said if you can pull through this together, your chances of improving are much better."

When I interviewed Killacky and Connolly in Vermont, they were about to celebrate their twenty-second anniversary. Of the three couples featured in *Holding On* a decade earlier, and the only gay couple, they were the only ones still together.

"How would someone do this without a partner?" asked Connolly, looking back on the years of slow-going rehab and the many adjustments each of them had to make—not only in their sex life but in their expectations of life itself. "How do old people suffer strokes, etc., when they have no partner? How does someone go through any chronic problem without any live-in support? You need community, however it's formed—whether it's a spouse, friends, or neighbors—because illness is not a piece of cake."[12]

For his part, Killacky said, "I have gotten my resilience from Larry's unconditional love." His dance and running experience as a younger man have helped, too. "I was so grateful that I danced and that I learned different ways to move in the world," he said. He's adjusted to not moving quite as fast anymore. "It's actually marvelous to move slowly in the world," he said. "I experience things more fully. It's almost like I had blinders on before and now they're off. I can see a much wider world. Now I don't have to be at the center, with the megaphone. I can be in the crowd. It's changed my M.O. in the world, and I'm grateful for it. It's really fantastic just 'to be.'" And, with Raindrop's assistance, Killacky said, "For three or four hours a week, I can still be dancing in the world."[13]

CHAPTER TWENTY-FOUR

~

To Our Health!

Building Upon Our Resilience Is the Key to Good Health

Chad Upham had been the kind of kid any parent would be proud of—an Eagle Scout, a model student who didn't cause problems in his fundamentalist Christian family. He didn't touch a beer until 1999, when he was twenty-one. Jump forward to an early Monday morning in July 2005. Upham, then twenty-seven, had been up all night after another weekend of drugs and sexual hookups with men, strangers, he met online.

But instead of pushing his limits for indulgence again, this time Upham made a different choice. Around 3 a.m., Upham sent an email to his friends and family with some unexpected news. "Over the past four months," he wrote, "I have become a regular user of crystal methamphetamine." He added, "I acknowledge, without shame, a concern for my mental, physical, and emotional health."

Chad was well on his way to addressing his meth addiction by the time I interviewed him about three months later for a *Washington Post* story about the impact of crystal meth on Washington, D.C.'s gay community. He told me that he depended mainly on Crystal Meth Anonymous groups and constructive activities with family and friends to support his recovery. Although he saw a doctor for a standard checkup, he—unlike some of his recovering friends—wasn't taking any medications to treat anxiety or depression.

He told me he was discovering that what gay men who use meth call "Tina" continued to tempt. "I am thinking desirously about the people, places and things that were associated with my using," he said. Running into

221

a person he knew from those "hot days and nights" revived thoughts of "all that fun."

But he pulled himself back to his new reality—denying the drug, listening to his family, co-workers, and new friends in the support groups he attended several nights a week. They have "embraced me in my weakness," said Upham, "continually saying that I am brave, courageous, and strong for taking the steps to get and stay healthy and live independent of drugs for satisfaction."[1]

Just over a decade after our interview for the *Washington Post*, I again interviewed Chad Upham for this book. About a year after we met, he moved to San Francisco, where he was Skyping with me from the Starbucks on Market Street across from the Twitter building on what in his time zone was an early mid-February morning. Catching up on ten years is tough to do, but we went for some important highlights germane to this book. He told me he'd recently started seeing a therapist for the first time as an adult. And he was about to move into a new apartment at Van Ness and Market, with lots of windows and stunning sunset views. "It's extremely expensive," he said, "but it's the result of all the work I've done over the last ten years, being responsible, and having clients who trust me."

Upham is understandably proud of his accomplishments. He is also aware that anyone who Googles his name will find out about his past with crystal meth, including the *Post* story with his color photo. "I have no problem talking with people about that experience," he said. "I'm proud of the work that I did in allowing you to use my story. In many ways, it kept me accountable and in check over the past ten years."

To go from where he was—"I found acceptance through drinking and drugs," he said of that time in his life—to where he is today took a tremendous amount of determination, discipline, support, and resilience. By this point he has sponsored thirty or forty others in twelve-step programs, sharing his experience, strength, and hope with other gay men struggling the way he did. "I see that crystal meth in 2016 is still just as prevalent in the community," he said. "A friend of mine died last week when his heart gave out after a crystal meth relapse. I've known a few people die on crystal meth relapses the last few years. It's not far away. I could get it if I wanted to."

For himself, though, Upham said crystal meth did to him what he's seen it do to others. "It brought people to their knees," he said. "As a result they lived sober lives at a younger age. For those who were able to find a different way to live without substances in their twenties and thirties, they have a way to live lives of resilience." Not only that, but they are farther along in the journey of creating—as Upham is doing, as we should all aim to create—lives of integrity, integration, and even intergenerational friendship.

"In San Francisco," said Upham, "I feel the sober community exists right at the corner of Eighteenth and Castro streets. There are dozens of people who look me in the eye, know my name, and know what's going on in my life and I know what's going on in theirs." All of us who have used twelve-step programs to help us address the effects of addiction, whether our own or a loved one's, know that "you are only as sick as your secrets"—secrecy and shame undermine recovery, while openness and honesty support it.

An important step in Upham's own recovery was his decision to integrate his Instagram feeds, erasing the formerly hard line between his work and off-time lives. "For me Instagram is a way I can share my point of view," he said. "I've always had this separation of my professional and personal life. I can set up myself in my work life as androgynous, very unexpressive—whereas I can run around in jockstraps and thongs and go to the gay beach." Last summer was a new phase, he said. "I connected my Instagram to my work feed. I certainly edit, and don't put risqué stuff on it." Opening this window into the "real" Chad Upham, no secrets and no substances to hide behind, has been a long time in coming. "It's been a ten-year journey for me," he said, "that I can put these two pieces together, that I can be a totally authentic person at work and outside of work."

Then there's the intergenerational component. "I have fond relationships with guys in their sixties, seventies, and eighties," said Upham. "The mentors I'm seeing these days are the men in their sixties and seventies who are burying their mothers. They are the ones who have years of sobriety, so they are able to show up for their mothers and care for them."

Of course he sees the flip side, too, the men in their fifties and sixties still struggling with addiction. "I had the last drink when I was twenty-eight, and I'm thirty-eight now," said Upham. "Seeing those older men who are still struggling, in the bathhouses and doing crystal meth, I don't want to be one of those men. I'm happy building my life and doing things I want to do at thirty-eight—whereas I could have been homeless."

In his first few years of sobriety, Upham didn't think too much about the twelve-step programs' concept of admitting a need for God or another "higher power" to support sobriety. He had long since stopped believing in the evangelical version of God he grew up with. But he has come to a different view that works well for him. "For me it's about not resisting the universe," he told me. "When we try to take everything into control, we end up creating a lot of trouble, and that self-centeredness makes us miserable people to live with. So a lot of the tools of spirituality are about trusting the universe to take care of me." Facing a big decision these days, Upham said he consciously chooses to let the universe take care of him. He choked up when he added, "So far it hasn't let me down."[2]

Unfortunately for so many gay men, we grew up being let down by the very people who were supposed to love and protect us. Too many of us didn't have anyone to tell us we are brave, courageous, and strong—as Chad Upham's family and friends did after he asked for their support to overcome addiction to crystal meth. Instead, most of us struggled on our own to deal with the wounding words and, too often, physical assaults by bullies who were sometimes even members of our own families. It doesn't take scientists telling us to convince us of something we gay men know all too well: being beaten up and put down leads to depression and other psychosocial problems—and can lead us to treat ourselves in ways that guarantee the bullies win.

"Something horrible is happening during adolescence to young gay men," said Ron Stall, PhD, director of the University of Pittsburgh's Center for LGBT Health Research in an interview we did for *The Atlantic*. "By the age of eighteen we can demonstrate that young men who have sex with men are far more likely to suffer from a long list of psychosocial health problems, which we believe are driven by marginalization and violence victimization at a very young age. These young men don't understand what's happening to themselves. There's no community. Sometimes if a boy who is beaten up by schoolyard bullies because he is perceived to be a sissy, goes to his dad to tell about getting beaten up on the playground, he risks also being beaten up by his dad." He added, "That kind of experience has got to be searing, and leaves scars on gay men. They learn at a tender age not to step out of gender lines or they will become violently assaulted. If you treated an adult the way a lot of boys who are identified as sissies are treated in schoolyards, you would get arrested."[3]

Clearly, there is real harm from the messages gay boys receive telling them they are somehow not normal, maybe not even fully human—from churches claiming the attraction they may feel to other boys, the exact same way straight boys feel toward girls, is an "objective disorder" that inclines them "toward an intrinsic moral evil," as the Catholic church has put it,[4] to their government telling them they are second-class citizens. But it has become equally clear that positive messages and role models can bolster younger gay men's self-esteem and thereby reduce their risk for substance abuse, HIV, and other self-destructive behaviors that disproportionately afflict gay men.

This new awareness is driving an entirely new approach to gay men's health. Instead of focusing on our "deficits," it builds on the resilience and strength virtually all gay men demonstrate simply by surviving to adulthood. It uses our strengths as its starting point, rather than assuming weaknesses simply because we're gay. And it offers examples of gay men who are successfully managing their challenges—whether it's grieving a loss, or anxiety, living with HIV, or any of a myriad of large and small traumas that can upset our balance and maybe even lead us to do something we could regret later. "Doesn't it make more sense," Ron Stall asked, "to look at the people who have thrived, who are resilient, and learn not from what went wrong but what went right? Look at the guys who went through horrible situations and learned and grew. Learn from *them* rather than holding up the guys who exemplify the societal stereotype of gay men as failures."[5]

Stall and his colleagues in their research have identified four interconnected "epidemics" of psychosocial health conditions that disproportionately afflict gay and bisexual men, each one making the others worse: childhood sexual abuse, partner violence, depression, and drug use. Together, their insidious effects are referred to as "syndemics." Men who are most strongly affected by any one of these tend to be at high risk for HIV and substance abuse. Those of us from lower income or culturally marginalized ethnic groups are especially vulnerable to syndemic effects. In one study, Stall found that 11 percent of 812 men who reported one problem—depression, for instance—had engaged in high-risk sex (defined as unprotected anal intercourse). Of 129 men who reported three or four problems, 23 percent said they had high-risk sex.[6]

The usual reaction to such numbers is a comment about "reckless" gay men. But look again. Framed another way, the numbers tell us something quite astonishing that can't be ignored: 89 percent of the men reporting one problem did *not* engage in high-risk sex. Likewise, more than three-quarters of the men with three or four problems did *not* engage in high-risk sex. The numbers make it abundantly clear: the overwhelming majority of gay men—even those of us dealing with multiple mental health challenges, when only one is enough to undermine us—actually *do* take care of, protect, and value ourselves. How can it be? In the face of overwhelming pressures and struggles that can give gay men all the reasons we might want to harm or medicate ourselves, or worse, how is it that most of us don't?

Ron Stall attributes the surprising findings to gay men's resilience. "We're so focused on risk factors to the point that we forget about resilience," he said. He believes "a smarter way to go" in thinking about HIV prevention, for example, would be to look at the guys who are thriving in spite of their adversities, how they pulled that off, see what lessons their experience offers, and apply it to the interventions aimed at supporting gay and bisexual men's health and mental health.[7] Stall and his colleagues describe gay men's resilience as "an untapped resource" in addressing the high rates of psychosocial health problems—such as depression, substance abuse, and victimization—that also drive HIV risk. "Harnessing these natural strengths and resiliencies," they write, "may enhance HIV prevention and intervention programs, thereby providing the additional effectiveness needed to reverse the trends in HIV infection among men who have sex with men."[8]

This is exactly in line with the recommendations of a 2013 report from the National Institutes of Health, in which NIH's LGBT Coordinating Committee said resilience should be studied to find out "how it develops, may protect health, and may buffer against the internalization of stigma and/or other negative experiences associated with sexual or gender minority status." Unfortunately, the report also provided ample evidence that the health of LGBT Americans has been a low priority in the United States for a very long time—despite the well-documented health disparities among us, including higher rates of alcoholism, cancer, depression, smoking, suicide, and violence. Witness: in fiscal 2010 (the most recent year for which data were available at the time of analysis), only 5 percent of the institutes' LGBT health projects were focused on alcoholism; 7.7 percent on cancer; 2.7 percent on depression; 1.4 percent on smoking and health; 1.4 percent on suicide; and 6.3 percent on violence. The overwhelming majority of projects, 81.5 percent, dealt with gay men and HIV-AIDS, particularly on ways to reduce transmission.[9]

Research suggests our journey toward being resilient gay men begins by accepting our sexual orientation. As Ron Stall put it in our interview, "Guys who do the best job of resolving internalized homophobia are the least likely to have current victimization, substance abuse, and compulsive sex." Put a bit differently, he said, "Getting a population of people not to hate themselves is good for their health. This is not rocket science."[10]

It's also not a new idea. Stephen F. Morin, PhD, a recently retired medical professor, chief of the prevention science division and now former director of the Center for AIDS Prevention Studies at the University of California San Francisco, pointed out in an interview that the new focus on gay men's mental health is a kind of "back to the future" situation. Before the AIDS epidemic, Morin said health researchers and political activists alike were looking for effective ways to promote gay men's self-esteem, fighting the stigma associated with being gay with messages of pride and resilience, and fighting back against the social and legal discrimination against gay people. "I was the first chair of the American Psychological Association's gay psychologists group in 1973," said Morin. "When we issued our first set of demands, our first demand was that professional associations commit themselves to fighting the stigma that had long been associated with homosexual orientation."[11]

Fighting the stigma *inside* ourselves, self-stigma, is the challenge facing every gay man. Ilan H. Meyer, coeditor with Mary E. Northridge of *The Health of Sexual Minorities*, is a Williams Distinguished Scholar of Public Policy at the Williams Institute for Sexual Orientation and Gender Identity Law and Public Policy at UCLA's School of Law. His research as a social psychologist and psychiatric epidemiologist has focused on the public health aspects of sexual minority health. One of his studies, the NIH-funded Project Stride, explored the impact of social stresses on the mental health of those of us with "disadvantaged identities" related to gender, race/identity, or sexual orientation. In an interview for this book, Meyer said that even using the word *resilience* is new in connection with the LGBT population. In research, he explained, a person can be described as resilient only in the presence of stress, such as losing a job. "Coping" implies an effort in the face of stress, but isn't necessarily positive or successful coping. How we cope with such traumas is what shows us to be resilient—or not. Drinking can be used to cope with stress, but no one would consider drinking oneself silly to be an effective way to cope with the situation. "Resilience implies you were successful in your effort," said Meyer. "Resilience more directly indicates the outcome was positive."

To illustrate the point, Meyer cited a common explanation for why black LGBT people don't have higher rates of mental disorders (depression, anxiety, and substance use) than what are seen in the white LGBT population. "One explanation," he said, "is that having that experience of race identity, and having learned to some extent to cope with that and overcome that, has been helpful in coping with homophobia." In fact, a study reported in *Health Psychology* found that higher levels of "racial centrality," the degree to which being black is central to one's identity, combined with perceptions of society's views of black Americans, predicted decreases in risky sexual behavior (total anal sex acts and unprotected anal sex acts).[12]

Intangible things also add to the resilience of LGBT people, Meyer said. He mentioned religious faith and the LGBT community's own norms and values, noting that as *they* change they are likewise changing our understanding of resilience. That makes it hard to compare someone today who is resilient to somebody from, say, the 1950s—when even gay people were advocating for homosexuality to be considered an illness because that was better than a crime or a sin. "Just yesterday," Meyer said, "I was talking with a room of younger gay men, and they all want kids. That is not something that would have been in the repertoire of the 1950s." Of course the biggest change from the 1950s was the emphasis, after the 1969 Stonewall riots, on coming out. "*That* is resilience," said Meyer. "Coming out in terms of gaining self-acceptance and rejecting antigay social values is about resilience. Homophobia and related social rejection and discrimination produce stressors for gay people. In the face of those kinds of experiences, to overcome social attitudes after you realize you are gay . . . that self-acceptance *is* resilience. That is the first step, but it is *resilience.*"[13]

Gregory M. Herek, a professor emeritus of psychology at the University of California at Davis, and an internationally recognized authority on prejudice against gay men and lesbians, hate crimes and antigay violence, and AIDS-related stigma, said in an interview, "Certainly in the past, nearly everyone was brought up with the attitude that homosexuality was wrong, a sickness, a sin, and that anyone who was gay or lesbian was a bad person. Being raised in an environment where those ideas were ubiquitous, it's almost inevitable that many people accepted or believed them." But today fewer than ever accept or believe them. "What I think is amazing," said Herek, "is how many people are doing fine and are mentally healthy, and leading whole and productive lives. How do they do it, given all they're up against? How did they manage to come out of it? The answer is resilience. Once they've overcome their internalized self-stigma, they have more social and psychological resources for responding adaptively to other forms of stress."[14]

Supporting gay men's healing and wholeness requires holistic approaches, as New York University psychology professor Perry N. Halkitis pointed out in a "call to action" for research and clinical psychologists in *American Psychologist*. He wrote, "A new framework for HIV prevention must give voice to gay men; must consider the totality of their lives; must delineate the underlying logic, which directs their relation to sex and HIV; and must concurrently respect their diverse life experiences. This approach should be rooted in a biopsychosocial paradigm, should be informed by both theory and practice, and should be directed by three theoretical lenses—a theory of syndemics, developmental theories, and contextual understandings of HIV disease."[15]

Halkitis said in an interview for this book, "Gay men's health cannot be HIV health." He explained, "HIV is more than about the transmission of a pathogen. It is as much, if not more so, a socially constructed phenomenon as it is a biological or psychological phenomenon. If it was a purely biological phenomenon, the epidemic would be over." Stigma and discrimination facilitate the behavior that leads to transmission of the virus—or smoking or using crystal meth—by undermining our ability to make healthy choices. "There is this syndemic of violence, STIs, HIV, mental health, and they all fuel each other," said Halkitis. "But at the end of the day the behaviors that lead to HIV infection or substance addiction all come because someone's social or psychological well-being is diminished. When things are wrong, you do things to medicate the pain." That goes for gay men, and many millions of people, regardless of their HIV status. In fact, Halkitis noted that data show that many gay men who use crystal meth begin using the drug *after* they seroconvert. "That gets to untreated mental health issues, especially depression," he said. "You will only eradicate HIV in this country if you address the social, biological, and psychological, all three. You use three classes of drugs to treat HIV. Why wouldn't you attack the epidemic from these three fronts?"[16]

At Boston's Fenway Health, the world's largest LGBT-focused medical, mental health, and research institution, Dr. Kenneth H. Mayer, a Harvard professor and medical research director of The Fenway Institute, said it's not enough to dichotomize by HIV status; that is, HIV prevention for the uninfected, or treatment for the infected person. We need instead to focus on the person who wants to avoid, or has to live with, the virus. "Some of the things affecting individuals are the same as for HIV-infected or uninfected people," said Mayer. "There are behavioral issues, whether for prevention or treatment adherence. How you have sex is behavioral. Whether you take your pills is behavioral." He described a particular intervention at Fenway, Project Thrive, aimed at gay men who have experienced bullying or childhood sexual abuse, common traumas for gay boys. Mayer said behavioral scientists had developed a cognitive intervention to "help people to reprogram how they respond to the world so they are better able to cope."[17]

One of those behavioral scientists is Conall O'Cleirigh, a staff clinical psychologist in the psychiatry department at Massachusetts General Hospital and an assistant professor of psychiatry at Harvard. O'Cleirigh specializes in the use of cognitive behavioral therapy (CBT) to treat depression and other mood disorders, post-traumatic stress disorder (PTSD), and anxiety disorders, particularly among sexual minorities. His research on gay men has found that the same mental health issues that can put someone at risk for HIV can also prevent someone living with the virus from adhering to his treatment. In a St. Patrick's Day 2016 interview for this book, O'Cleirigh said, "The mental health vulnerabilities that gay and bisexual men have seem to interfere with medical adherence and adherence to care. They are the same issues that enable gay men to keep themselves out of sexually risky situations." When you add substance abuse, it's even trickier. "Having a trauma history," said O'Cleirigh, "managing depression, seems to be as important and influential in managing sexual risk."

One particular disparity unique to gay men jumps off the page. It turns out that up to 46 percent of gay/bi men who report condomless anal sex also report childhood sexual abuse (CSA). "That is a *huge* number," said O'Cleirigh. Some of his research focuses on designing an intervention to address the impact of CSA on gay and bisexual men—one of the syndemics Ron Stall described, and one that hasn't received all the attention its startling prevalence and documented impact warrant. For example, in a national study of 1,552 black gay and bisexual men, O'Cleirigh and his colleagues found the men who experienced CSA—or physical or emotional abuse, or stalking, or being pressured or forced to have sex—when they were younger than twelve years old had more than three male partners in the past six months. The men who had been forced or pressured to have sex as boys were likely to have receptive anal sex.[18] In another study of 162 men with CSA histories, participants reporting sexual abuse by family members were 2.6 times more likely to abuse alcohol, twice as likely to have a substance use disorder, and 2.7 times more likely to report a sexually transmitted infection in the past year. Not only that, but men whose abuser penetrated them were more likely to have PTSD, recent HIV sexual risk behavior, and a greater number of casual sexual partners. Physical injury and intense fear increased the odds for PTSD even more.[19]

"Having that history is repeatedly associated in every sample of gay men with increased likelihood of being HIV-positive," said O'Cleirigh. He said that since childhood sexual abuse "is very, very common in gay/bi men" it appears to be one of the most significant vulnerabilities that accounts for the disproportionately high rate of HIV among gay men. As for intervening to prevent the trauma of abuse from turning into risky behavior, O'Cleirigh said, "We have the idea that we could help prevent new infections if we could identify gay men with a CSA history before they become infected with HIV, and try to address the vulnerability that has been created in them, and see if we can reduce their specific distress around having that trauma history and provide them with specific strategies for reducing their sexual risk."

In fact O'Cleirigh and his fellow researchers, including Ken Mayer, have recruited about five thousand gay and bisexual men who experienced childhood sexual abuse. Based at Fenway Health, Project Thrive divided the men into two groups, one that received counseling and the other a ten-session therapy component. "It had a good effect on sexual risk," said O'Cleirigh, "but a modest effect on reducing HIV seroconversion rates over time." There was very little difference between men who had either counseling or the "heavy" therapy. "We concluded that childhood sexual abuse interferes with your ability to use public health messaging and condom usage. We hypothesized that it was due to PTSD."

The effects of childhood sexual abuse can be as unconscious as they are pernicious. O'Cleirigh said people who experience CSA "tend to carry around issues in their head they aren't aware of, such as 'I'm not good-looking enough,' or 'This abuse happened because I'm weak, stupid, and no one is ever going to love me,' because they are abused sexually and those are the things they take away from it." Another effect is for people to "absent themselves in sexual situations so they can get their rocks off," he said. "They put themselves on automatic, and in automatic they are not going to ask questions like 'Does this guy care for me?' or 'Is he HIV-positive?'" Psychologists call it "dissociation," this detachment from reality or even from our own bodies. It's a well-known, though not always healthy, reaction to trauma. Poppers, pot, meth, and alcohol are only four agents of dissociation that are part of the sex lives of many gay men. A mere coincidence? "To give you an idea of the level at which this operates," said O'Cleirigh, "I've worked with a client who described to me during a session a Friday night of going home, showering, grooming, douching, putting poppers, weed, and lube in his pockets, and getting ready to go out for the evening. I said 'You're preparing for sex.' He said 'No, just getting ready to go out.' His preparations were not fully accessible to him." An effective risk-reduction/health-promotion intervention that addresses the effects of CSA could help make this man more conscious of what he was doing to get ready for a night out—and where it was coming from in his psyche.

When he updated me on Project Thrive in late January 2017, O'Cleirigh reported the therapy aspect was "very popular with the gay/bi men who received it." They treated more than two hundred fifty gay/bi men for PTSD related to childhood sexual abuse, helping to increase the men's coping skills, ability to be more present in their immediate situation, and specific skills to evaluate and reassess these situations.[20] "Treatments are geared toward giving the men a more realistic sense of the world," said O'Cleirigh, which is an important ingredient of resilience. "As we say to our clients, we can't change the fact that you were abused, but *you* can change."[21]

For HIV-negative men who want other prevention options, there is PrEP (pre-exposure prophylaxis), a daily dosage of the HIV medication Truvada. Taken as prescribed, PrEP has been found to reduce the risk of HIV infection by more than 90 percent.[22] PrEP is prescribed as part of a robust program that includes ongoing HIV and STD testing, medical monitoring, and sexual health counseling. Conall O'Cleirigh said, "For many gay/bi men who, for whatever mental health or substance abuse reason, cannot use condoms consistently, PrEP is a real winning strategy."[23] PrEP can also be a winning strategy for men who weren't abused as kids, don't have depression and don't abuse substances, and either don't like or don't consistently use condoms.

The walls of Jim Pickett's office at the AIDS Foundation of Chicago display the set of posters created for a new campaign aimed at promoting PrEP use by the gay men and women, including transgender individuals, who could benefit from it. In an interview on my October birthday in 2016 at his office on West Jackson Street, Pickett, the foundation's director of prevention advocacy and gay men's health, said the time has come to "focus on the good things that make us happy." As for gay men he explained, "We characterize gay men's problems all the time. Can we focus on resilience? Strength? It's not ignoring the problems. It's your frame. If you're a young African American gay man, honey, you *are* resilient!" The foundation's "PrEP for Love" campaign—created pro-bono by a coalition of gay and nongay organizations and ad agencies, and aimed at vulnerable African American communities— is about engaging the community in conversations about PrEP with popular individuals they know. The posters, with campaign taglines like "Transmit love," "Contract heat," and "Catch desire," feature men and women of various sizes and skin tones represented in sex- and body-positive images.

Pickett points out one of the key differences between the new PrEP campaign and past campaigns. "So many things have been negative, focused on fear," he said. "Let's focus on our strength and joy, not on 'risk.' This is a great example of resilience and taking a positive frame, not a loss frame." He said we need to focus on what keeps gay men negative. "What assets are in place that people are able to rely and thrive on?" he asked. "We want people to learn about PrEP, but we have to remember HIV prevention is not the only thing on people's list of challenges. It may not be at the top of their lists, either. If you don't address people that way, as myriad and complex, but only as potential vectors, you are not respecting them." It's far more effective, said Pickett, to start by talking about pleasure and intimacy, "things that make us juicy and warm and tingly." Showing an interest in someone's feelings, finding out what makes him tick, is a much better way to get to a conversation about his personal business. "When we tell people to have a good day, we don't necessarily say 'Be careful of the traffic,'" said Pickett. "It's about respecting people as beautiful and complex."[24]

John A. Schneider, MD, MPH, an associate professor of epidemiology and medicine at the University of Chicago, researches networks and how to use them to create positive, health-promoting change. "After thirty years," he told me in an interview for an *Atlantic* article about the LGBT health movement,[25] "we are moving away from individualized behavioral interventions toward things that can integrate those components. We are looking at networks and structural things that can drive HIV." His clinical work with largely young African American gay and bisexual men on the South Side of Chicago has yielded intriguing findings about how best to support those at greatest risk. Schneider has found, for example, that the more men there are involved in a young man's life—straight or gay, and especially male kin, fathers and also brothers or male cousins—the more inclined he is to protect himself if he is HIV-negative and adhere to treatment if he's positive. "Some of my very young guys have come in with their fathers," said Schneider. "There is something powerful about that."

In the ball community, where a good deal of Schneider's recent work has focused, "a lot of these guys have a gay father or gay mother," he said, suggesting that a more nuanced approach is needed in talking about "families of choice" and "chosen families." What is any functional family but a "network of mutual commitment," as Schneider puts it, and it can include relatives as well as trusted friends. With that in mind, Schneider said, "We found that having a greater proportion of family members in one's personal network is negatively associated with drug-use and group sex, and positively associated with having a regular primary care physician and with discouraging group sex and drug use among one's network of men who have sex with men."[26]

In the same Deco Arts Building on East Fifty-Fifth Street as Tooth Fairy World and Chaturanga Holistic Fitness, at the clinic where Schneider's research and clinical work come together, he told me in an interview it's hard to predict when someone tests HIV-positive how he will respond, whether with resilience or what Schneider called "nonresilience." Whether the man responds with shame or self-esteem depends largely on his sensitivity to stigma, "the threshold of resilience," Schneider said. He sees in the young black men he works with from the ball community the resilience they developed, too often, from having to fend for themselves and simply growing up black in a society preoccupied with skin color. "I think there are survival skills the young black guys develop even before they realize they are gay," he said. "So having a gay identity may be just another issue that comes up for them." The ball community itself is a source of resilience. "Vogueing and dance are very liberating and healing activities," said the doctor.[27]

It's not formally billed as "resilience building," but the Mpowerment Project does exactly that. Mpowerment, an HIV prevention intervention aimed at young urban gay and bisexual men, was originally developed and evaluated with funding from the National Institute of Mental Health. The CDC included it in its compendium of evidence-based interventions, and continues to fund organizations to implement it. Coprincipal investigator Greg Rebchook, an assistant professor at the University of California San Francisco's

Center for AIDS Prevention Studies, told me in an interview, "We don't start from a place where gay men are wounded, their wings are broken." Instead, Mpowerment uses outreach, drop-in centers, and community-building efforts to strengthen young gay men's self-esteem, positive relationships, social support, and healthy choices. Using a "whole-man" approach, Rebchook said, "It's not just about condoms, but about all the factors that come together to affect their lives."[28]

Mpowerment's focus on "upstream" issues that drive risk behavior is new territory for government HIV prevention funders. It has been extremely popular and well regarded. Since the first article about Mpowerment, in 1996,[29] Rebchook said the project has had "enormous reach" with fifty or sixty projects going at any one time, each one reaching between one hundred to three hundred guys, and twenty-five or so participants in each of the six to nine trainings a year for new project organizers. Despite the popularity of Mpowerment and resilience-building interventions, Rebchook said most federal research funding proposals continue to focus on health disparities even as people at the community level see plainly what works and do their best to make it work with available resources.

In an interview in his office at UCSF, Rebchook said, "The big new thing is trauma-informed therapy." Like the syndemics that Ron Stall identified, this approach focuses on adverse childhood events—such as childhood sexual abuse, parental incarceration, parental substance abuse, or substance abuse in youth. "You look at these childhood events and add them up, and you are more vulnerable to other outcomes in your life," said Rebchook. The goal is to avoid retraumatizing people and help them heal from their childhood trauma. "There are a lot of parallels with gay men, the trauma we grow up with," he added. "How that connects to resilience is we survive and flourish despite all that trauma in our lives."[30]

Rebchook put me in touch with another UCSF faculty member, a physician who calls his own adoption of trauma-informed care into his clinical work with patients an "epiphany." Edward Machtinger, MD, professor of medicine and director of UCSF's Women's HIV Program, told me in an interview for this book that addressing trauma has the potential to transform primary medical care. Instead of treating symptoms with medications, this new paradigm aims to address medical and mental health problems by getting to the root causes of so many of those problems—and thereby provide *genuine* healing. Addressing the trauma that underlies so much illness makes doctors "healers instead of treaters," said Machtinger. Unfortunately for patients living with HIV in particular, the dominant way of framing discussions of HIV are strictly biomedical. Speaking of federal agencies that fund HIV care and support for those with limited resources, Machtinger added, "They are addicted to the idea that their mission and focus has to be narrowly on controlling the virus, and not on the well-being of the patient."

Machtinger described a study at another clinic at UCSF, looking at older gay men. It found a rate of current PTSD of 12 percent, a rate dramatically higher than general rates of PTSD among men. "To me," said Machtinger, "HIV is a symptom, especially in new cases of HIV, of a far bigger problem: unaddressed trauma." For younger gay men, he said, "Their HIV seems to be a symptom or consequence of an underlying history of trauma or discrimination, toxic stress, or whatever else is going on in their lives that puts them at risk for HIV." Machtinger pointed out that many older gay men in San Francisco who have lived with HIV for years—like the men featured in the *San Francisco Chronicle*'s March 2016 story "Last Man Standing"[31]—struggle against depression, isolation, and thoughts of suicide. "These aren't consequences of their HIV medication or the HIV virus," he said, "they are related to underlying histories of trauma that are largely going unaddressed by simply treating their HIV with medication."

Describing an analysis of the causes of death in people with HIV in the city that he was doing with the San Francisco health department, Machtinger said it was clear "how inadequate our death statistics are." Referring to how the deaths are categorized when someone with HIV dies, he said it's irresponsible to report that approximately 40 percent of people living with HIV are dying of AIDS. "They are really dying from substance abuse, depression, PTSD and other consequences of trauma that lead people to stop taking their medications. It's like dying from a completely preventable condition," he said. Isolation, too, is a preventable and potentially deadly condition. Said Machtinger, "Reducing isolation is by far the most effective way I have found to help people develop coping mechanisms that are more healthy, that allow them to leave abusive partners, to forgive themselves, and ultimately to become leaders in their communities."

The power of trauma—and addressing it—became clear to Machtinger when he worked with The Medea Project, an expression-based theater group that brings together incarcerated women in small groups and gives them writing assignments on topics such as "What is love?" or "Why are you here?" or "When was the last time you experienced love?" The women would read their stories to one another and, as they developed trust in the group, they would disclose their traumatic experiences to more and more people through a public theatrical performance. Machtinger partnered with The Medea Project to work with his patients living with HIV. "I saw women who were addicted to cocaine, lost causes, develop a circle of friends and self-acceptance when they had an outlet to get out their own guilt and shame. The results were amazing." Machtinger added, "The single most effective intervention that we have, and that I have witnessed to help people heal from the impact of trauma, has been disclosure and community-building. Period."[32]

Bright sunshine pours through the floor-to-ceiling windows. Glass, steel, and wood abound in the architectural and design elements. Dance music pours out the door. Purple leather easy chairs splash color about the airy space. A gay man's fabulous city apartment? Guess again. This is Strut, the San Francisco AIDS Foundation's new health and wellness center for gay, bisexual, and transgendered men. Smack dab in the middle of what may be the gayest block in the world, on Castro Street between Market and Eighteenth streets, Strut was created to unite under one roof the foundation's sexual health services program called Magnet; the Stonewall Project's substance abuse and mental health services; Bridgemen, a program targeting gay men thirty to forty who want to help improve the community "through kindness and service"; the DREAAM Project's Drop-In Fridays for all lesbian, gay, bisexual, transgender, queer, questioning, and intersex (LGBTQQI) folks of color and their allies, ages thirty and under; the Elizabeth Taylor 50-Plus Network; and Positive Force, a peer support program to help HIV-positive guys live well with the virus.

Strut, its jaunty moniker intentionally chosen, is a sort of one-stop shopping center of health and wellness. All its services are free. Before it opened in early 2016, Strut's executive director Tim Patriarca said, "The new center will use a holistic approach to focus not on sickness and disease, but on health and wellness. We want to inspire and empower the gay and bisexual men in our community to take control of their health, and give them the tools, support, and knowledge to be able to do so." Integrating sexual health, primary care, substance use and other support services "is a major innovation, and it will extend the impact each is able to make," said Mike Discepola, the AIDS foundation's director of substance use services.[33]

This center for gay men's health and wellness in San Francisco can be traced to one man's vision of what "whole man" gay men's health and wellness services might look like. Steve Gibson, who created Magnet in 2003, told me in an interview for this book that from its inception, Magnet provided free sexual health services—but also offered a community space that hosted art receptions, massages, and acupuncture. The online San Francisco neighborhood news site *Hoodline*, reporting on Gibson's departure from Magnet in early 2016 after running it for thirteen years, quoted him as saying, "Magnet was conceived by a group of gay men and other community activists who wanted to redefine health beyond an HIV-positive or HIV-negative paradigm and look at our collective health in a broader context, including our health as a community."[34]

Chances are good those men knew another San Franciscan, and one of America's best-known gay activists until his untimely death in 2006, the late Eric Rofes. His book *Dry Bones Breathe: Gay Men Creating Post-AIDS Identities and Cultures*, was revolutionary at the time of its 1998 publication in reclaiming gay men's sexuality and health from under the dark, consuming shadow of HIV-AIDS. Rofes was realistic in his understanding that HIV would continue to plague gay men into the foreseeable future. But he also understood that life has to go on, and with it choices must be made about sex and love. He also knew that in our complex lives, these are only some of the many choices we make every day. Rofes championed the freedom of individual gay men to make their *own* choices, and rebuffed efforts to use fear and shame to compel us to practice anyone's list of acceptable behaviors.

"Prevention for gay men is at a turbulent crossroads," Rofes wrote, only two years after the drug "cocktail" finally made it possible to live with HIV rather than develop AIDS and die. "We can continue fine-tuning traditional interventions focused on providing individual gay men with information, motivation, and skills. Or we can acknowledge the complexity of sexuality and trust and support gay men truly to manage their own risk." What would that look like in practice? Rofes: "AIDS prevention efforts targeting gay men should be reconceptualized, restructured, and reinvented as multi-issue gay men's health programs that include strong components concerned with substance use, basic needs (food, housing, and clothing), and sexual health (broadly defined). They would no longer take as their central mission limiting the spread of HIV, but instead aim to improve the health and lives of gay men. AIDS should be seen as one of many challenges to gay men's health and our work should no longer position HIV prevention as the overarching focus. AIDS should join a list including suicide, substance abuse, hate crimes, other STDs, cancer, domestic violence, heart disease, and poverty as important threats to gay men's lives."[35]

Strut, like Fenway Health in Boston and other LGBT health and community centers across the country, is where inspiring visions of holistic gay men's health services, and of gay men as whole human beings, are brought to life. In these places created by and for LGBT people, the leading-edge behavioral research conducted by gay men at America's top universities—including Greg Herek, Perry Halkitis, Eddy Machtinger, Ken Mayer, Ilan Meyer, Conall O'Cleirigh, Greg Rebchook, and Ron Stall—is applied in the real world to support the health and well-being of other gay men. Thanks to their work, hope is stronger than ever that as more gay men heal from our childhood traumas—and future generations, we hope, can grow up far less traumatized—we will not only reduce the burden of HIV on gay men, but we will have altogether healthier gay men who make smart, informed choices that keep them well.

"The science has changed dramatically since Magnet opened," Gibson said in our interview. So has the way gay men have started to rethink HIV, what it "means" and doesn't mean. He noted that today, HIV-positive men with undetectable viral loads have little to no risk of transmitting HIV to their partners, and negative men using condoms or properly taking PrEP have little risk of becoming infected. He said this is having a tremendous impact in San Francisco on reducing new HIV infections—and transforming how gay men relate to one another across what has often been called the HIV "viral divide." Said Gibson, "What we're seeing in San Francisco now is very good public health attempts to encourage disclosure around serostatus. For the first time in my twenty-five years in public health, the conversation is changing around how positive and negative gay men are talking to each other about terms like 'clean' and 'dirty' and the stigma we internalized as a community. We know that viral suppression is highly effective and that PrEP is highly effective. So we can have a conversation about our *desires*."

Gibson described a UCSF study of PrEP that found an unexpected outcome of the changing conversation that has been made possible by effective medication for treatment and prevention: people are losing fear. "They were expressing sexual intimacy for the first time without feeling fear," he said. "Think about how powerful and scary that is, to pull back the layers of fear." Gibson said the gay community has to be involved in the conversation about what this means for us—just as it was after the advent of effective HIV treatment in 1996. "It was an historic marker in how gay men responded to the epidemic," said Gibson. "We went from being helpless in the 1980s—my own partner died in 1996—and then there was the 'Lazarus effect' where people started living. We as a community started changing because of that. From a community perspective it was like 'Wow! Things are different now.' The science and community are evolving, and you have to bring them together in conversation."[36]

As I walked down Castro Street after my visit to Strut, I noticed the bronze plaques embedded in the sidewalk along the street. The Rainbow Honor Walk[37] features twenty (with more to follow) three-by-three-foot plaques honoring the groundbreaking achievements of LGBT heroes—including the Castro District's former city supervisor and assassinated gay hero Harvey Milk, Mattachine Society and Radical Faeries founder Harry Hay, playwright and the world's most famously prosecuted homosexual Oscar

Wilde, and Randy Shilts, San Francisco's own famous chronicler of the early years of AIDS. The plaques in the sidewalk don't have anything obvious to do with "health." And yet they have *everything* to do with our community's efforts to build up one another by reminding us of a proud history of brave men and women to whom we can look back, and look up. Right there, under our feet, embedded in solid concrete, they show us the heroic legacy of courage, pride, and resilience. That legacy lives on in each of us who claims it for ourselves. It offers a solid foundation for what we call our gay pride—and, potentially *enormous* benefits for our health, too.

~

CHAPTER TWENTY-FIVE

Defining "Old" for Ourselves

The Open Secret Is That
Most of Us Already Do

All I knew of the next-door neighbor was that he was gay, a gardener, and a weaver of beautiful tapestry rugs. My friend Kitty, in Washington, had let me borrow her summer house to enjoy the solitude and Maine shoreline views out the windows as I worked on the book proposal I was contracted to write for the renowned microbiologist and HIV codiscoverer Robert C. Gallo. Kitty told me the neighbor's partner had died some years earlier. She also said I must see his gardens. Having something of a green thumb myself, I was intrigued. I Googled his name to find out about him whatever I could before picking up the phone to call. I learned he was born in 1937, the same year as my late father. I also learned that his work was currently on display at a gallery in nearby Rockland.

I left a message. A couple of hours later, the phone rang. A deep, resonant voice stated the caller's name. He asked if I liked food. Yes, and I love to cook, too. He suggested that we have dinner that night at Primo, the farm-restaurant in Rockland known for top-shelf quality (with prices to match). I was anxious about the prices. Back to being a "struggling writer" at the advanced age of fifty-three, expensive restaurants were no longer part of my usual fare.

I emailed a friend in Portland for advice. He said there could be an assumption that because I knew allegedly "fancy people" who had a summer home in "exclusive" Spruce Head, I might be taken for a fancy person (spelled "disposable income"), too. He said Dear Abby would advise candor, so I should simply say I can't afford dinner at a restaurant whose version of "surf and turf" goes for forty-two dollars.

By the time we toured his gardens and compared his view of the cove with the one I'd been enjoying just down the road, and certainly by the time we sat in his kitchen for a cup of tea and biscotti ("I like sweet things," he said), my anxiety was gone. This man was genuine and humble, too. It turned out Morrie's not a fancy person, either. Making lots of money hasn't been the driving force motivating his work.

I was eager to hear about his years in Provincetown, in the 1960s, long before I began going there in the 1980s. It's where he had met Bob and launched their thirty-two-year romance. Morrie had started as a dishwasher at Sal's Place, in the West End, before moving up his second year to waiter and, eventually, headwaiter. Like many painters, musicians, and writers, what he did for a living was very different from what he felt called to do.

"You're easy to talk to," he told me, a couple of times. So was he. Morrie took it in stride when I told him about the "real story" behind my stories, a key piece of my own recent biography: the big, unexpected bump in the road seven years earlier when my doctor said, "I have bad news on the HIV test." No judgments, no arched eyebrows like I've seen too often on my peers' self-assured faces. Morrie simply said I was fortunate to have been diagnosed when there was finally effective medical treatment. So many, so very many, of our brothers were not so fortunate.

I invited Morrie to join me and two friends I'd invited to dinner Friday night. One of them was Jim, the unrequited love object of my college years, who lived about twenty-five miles away. One of my favorite things in the world is to cook for friends. If they stay until midnight, I count my dinner party a success. This time they stayed until after midnight, having eaten every course despite the threat of burst belts and exploding bellies after each one.

Morrie was the hit of the party. I'm lucky to have friends who, as I do, revere our elders and soak up the drops of wisdom woven like pearls into the fabric of their stories. We agreed afterward that we had offered Morrie something, too: listening ears, real questions. How's it been since Bob died? Is there another love left in him? Most unlike the nurse at the hospital Morrie volunteers at, who asked, "Do you have children?" and asked nothing more when he said no.

Of all Morrie's stories that I've enjoyed so far, there was one about a long-ago visit to Puerto Vallarta that touched me deepest, choked me up, as we sat in the bright, plant-filled space of his living-work room near the huge wooden loom he imported from Scandinavia to weave his rugs. At the end of a two-week stay, about to leave the next day, Morrie said to a woman who had little in the way of money or material goods, whose daughter was joyfully feasting on a juicy ripe orange, "I'm so sad I have to leave tomorrow." She replied, "Why be sad? It's a beautiful day today."

In 2000, New York psychotherapist Harold Kooden and his coauthor Charles Flowers published a book that for many gay men, including me, was revolutionary in its candor and wisdom about growing older. *Golden Men: The Power of Gay Midlife* not only dared to say, loud and proud, there *is* life after thirty, and not only are a whole lot of gay men living it with great gusto, but you (young and not-as-young gay man) can, too. The book drew from Kooden's decades of work with gay men in his therapy practice, his own experience, and new behavioral research.

Kooden and Flowers—born on the same date, thirty years apart—provide what I personally found to be "the definitive book on the specific challenges gay men face at midlife," as the cover promises. Inside my own highlighted and underlined copy of *Golden Men*, the powerful truth unfolds. "[O]nly in speaking out do we have a chance of breaking out of the trap set by negative stereotypes about older gay men. We do have the power to age well. . . . our recent history suggests that gay men are on a journey toward power, both individually and collectively. In the last three decades, gay men have struggled to overcome the messages of shame, self-loathing, and homophobia inherited from the nongay world in order to create a community of love, pride, acceptance, joy, and power."

The authors continue:

> During the 1970s, gay men fought for and achieved liberation and set the foundation of a community of openly gay, self-loving men. In the 1980s, this fledgling community faced a life-threatening epidemic, and gay men and their allies devoted their time, energy, money, imagination, and lives toward saving one another. In the mid-1990s, the gay community came out of the despair and depression brought about by AIDS and began to fashion a new identity based on the lessons of the past and the promise of the present. The year 2000 heralds the approach of a new millennium, and gay men stand upon the threshold of liberation—not just sexual or political, but a liberation in all arenas of our lives: mind, body, and spirit. During our [now thirty-six year] battle against AIDS, we have taught the world that we know how to take care of our sick, honor and bury our dead. Now is the time to take our lessons and use them to live and to teach one another how to live. We owe it to ourselves, as well as to the generations to follow.[1]

It was raining cats and dogs when Harold Kooden buzzed me up to his and his husband John's Upper West Side apartment to do our interview for this book. The couple were recently back from a four-week trip to Iraq and Turkey. Kooden had been a gay activist inside the mental health field back in the 1960s, when gay men were still considered mentally ill for being gay. At seventy-eight, he said he was "still growing, still learning."

Kooden told me the impetus for *Golden Men* "was to write a book for gay men to celebrate aging." Gay men have a "wealth of experience where it comes to thriving and development," he said. "Successful aging means looking at one's history—pain, successes—and removing the false perceptions, the clouds, to look at the *reality* of our lives. It's about becoming conscious and aware. Unless you become aware of the negatives, you don't become aware of the positives."

We talked about one of our favorite gay male authors, John Rechy. His 1963 debut novel *City of Night* revealed the startling underworld of gay sex in several big U.S. cities in the 1950s, as seen through the eyes of a young hustler—a thinly veiled John Rechy himself. One of the book's, and Rechy's, themes was the dread of aging and the perceived lack of value attached to being an "older" gay man. I asked Rechy himself about it in the two interviews I've done with him over the years.

In 2003, I interviewed Rechy at his home in Los Angeles, hours before he and his longtime partner Michael were going to dinner to celebrate Rechy's seventy-second birthday. When I interviewed him again in 2014, he was eighty-three. Clearly the man who had been terrified of growing older when he was young had matured in wisdom as he advanced in years:

> J-MA: "In our 2003 interview, you said you were pleased with your appearance, accepted that the 'older' man in the mirror obviously wasn't the thirty-two-year-old John Rechy, and that was okay. How do you look now at 'the frantic running that, for me, was youth'? At some point you stopped 'running.' How did it affect you?"
>
> John Rechy: "I am still very much concerned with my appearance, to the extent that I continue to work out with weights, eat correctly, et cetera. But I am not obsessed with it as I was once. I am satisfied with how I have aged. I have, yes, stopped 'the frantic running,' and I am happy for that."[2]

Echoing Rechy's comments, Harold Kooden said that part of the process of aging well is "learning to accept the mirror, whether it's the wrinkles, gray hair, or paunch." He added, "It's about accepting what can't be changed and working at what can be. It's affirming to like what you look like *now*."

When I revealed that I have a large vegetable and flower garden, Kooden graciously showed me his roof garden, his and John's private oasis in the city. It's mainly all perennials, he explained. "Gardening teaches us so much of life," said Kooden, pointing out various plants and flowers. "Aging well is part of wisdom, like a garden. A garden is never done. With a garden you have to shift your focus to *now*." Another part of successful aging, he said, is rejecting society's stereotypes of "older." As Kooden put it, "I'm an 'old' man, but what I choose to do with that is *my* decision."[3]

Ken South was the president of Prime Timers of Washington, D.C., for fifteen years before moving to Fort Lauderdale in 2016. The social organization for older gay and bisexual men and their admirers brings together men with "like interests," as their website (primetimersdc.org) puts it, for social and recreational activities. In their monthly newsletter for January 2017, the hundred members of the D.C. chapter were celebrating three "birthday boys," recalling the annual "Zoolights" light show at the National Zoo in December, and smiling out from color photos of "Santa and the kids," men "of a certain age" sitting on the lap of Santa Claus.

"Prime Timers has been my living and aging workshop for gay men," South told me in an interview for this book as D.C. and the Northeast shoveled out from "Snowzilla," the January 22–24, 2016, blizzard that buried the city in upward of two feet of snow. "It has helped to destroy my own myths about being an old gay man," South said. Prime Timers World Wide was founded in 1987 by a retired professor, Woody Baldwin, from his awareness of the wide gap between generations and society's obsession with youth. Today the organization, really a brotherhood, has grown to a worldwide network including eighty-seven chapters in the United States. Palm Springs is the home of the largest Prime Timers chapter, with two thousand members.

South had just turned seventy a month before we spoke. One of the myths the group destroyed for him was the assumption that no younger man would be attracted to him or other older men. He mentioned he is also a member of Silver Daddies, a website for older gay men and their admirers. "God bless Silver Daddies," he said. "I have yet to contact somebody to set something up. Younger guys have contacted *me*!" He described one man in his thirties who came around the D.C. group. "We called him the gigolo," said South. "We all thought he was out to get someone's money. He sat me down one time and asked, 'Why are you older guys so judgmental?'"

Of course the other side of ageism, the way we more often think of it, is what the Prime Timers group sees every year at its Pride Day booth. "We experience the same things all day long," said South, "especially when young gay guys go by the booth. There's always a comment and usually a giggle or a laugh. They will walk wide of the booth—as if getting older was physically catching! Avoid the booth and they won't get old!"

It's only sometimes funny that South had such difficulty trying to find Prime Timers to ride in a car in the Pride parade. Some of the guys, older ones, "are living discreet lives away from work and their wives," South said. "But if it came down to it and the Results Gym had a float, they would be glad to be on the float with the gym bunnies! But the idea of a bunch of old guys? They weren't interested." South contrasted D.C.'s experience with Palm Springs's the time he was there for a national Prime Timers convention during Pride. "Palm Springs is smaller than D.C., more like a little town," he said. "We had a big contingent of guys, some on floats, some walking. The side of the road, Main Street in Palm Springs, was literally side-to-side beach chairs, filled with older guys. And here we were D.C. Prime Timers, and we were chicken!"

South reflected on his experience of aging as one of the men whose generation was hardest hit in the early years of the AIDS epidemic. He has worked professionally on HIV-AIDS since the darkest years of the epidemic in the early 1980s. "I never thought in my thirties, forties, and fifties I'd be looking at the obits in the paper," he said. "That's something that old people do, looking to see if their friends have passed away. Now that the epidemic has changed, people are dying of other things besides AIDS. I'm now in the senior cohort. In some ways it has helped me to be more self-reliant. It certainly has helped me appreciate the meaning of life, that life is very precious."

That view was reinforced at the weekly Prime Timers cocktails and dinner at DIK a few days before our interview. DIK is local gay shorthand for the popular Dupont Italian Kitchen restaurant at the corner of Seventeenth and Q streets, the heart of the Northwest D.C. gay neighborhood. "We had a couple who came to the Christmas party," South said. "They were very healthy. One had been through surgery. The partner was outgoing and effervescent. Two weeks ago they were dressing to go out to dinner and he falls over with a massive brain aneurism." He paused. "The shock of it is just incredible, realizing we literally don't know when our time is up."

Then there was South's own experience a day or two earlier. "I had fluttering going on in my heart," he said. He'd taken off a day from work because he thought he had a cold. "I had a type of tachycardia [irregular heartbeat] years ago. I kept thinking all day of whether to go to the emergency room. It was a male thing. Around six o'clock, when the flutterings got closer and closer, this voice in my head said 'Ken you are a seventy-year-old man and your heart is not working right. Get yourself to the ER!' Lucky I did: I had a thing called a VT, ventrical tachycardia. The doctor said 'You should have been here this morning.'" He sighed, then added, "I have to constantly remind myself of the phenomenon that I am an old guy."[4]

For those of us who experienced the HIV-AIDS epidemic most personally from our younger years forward—perhaps HIV-positive ourselves, having lost friends and partners, seen gay urban neighborhoods decimated—it's no surprise we carry the deepest scars of what for many of us were our life's greatest traumas. For too many of us the epidemic heaped yet *more* trauma in our adult lives on top of what we grew up with as gay boys. AIDS was all our collective bullies rolled into one big sucker punch to our hearts and psyches. Now, as we age, and face the inevitable changes that befall aging bodies, we face the challenge of not letting ourselves simply disappear from the gay community—or to diminish in our own internal assessments of our "market value" in the community.

As Ken South and the Prime Timers show so clearly, and Harold Kooden said so well: It's up to each one of us to choose what kind of older gay man we wish to be. We can choose to isolate ourselves, to buy the lie that age "means" anything more than that the calendar is turning, the seasons are changing. Or we can heed the wisdom of Walt Whitman, our renowned gray-bearded gay poet forbear, and consider older age to be life's very apex: "As the days take on a mellower light," Whitman wrote in *Leaves of Grass*, "and the apple at last hangs/really finish'd and indolent-ripe on the tree/ Then for the teeming quietest, happiest days of all! The brooding and blissful halcyon days!"[5]

Richard Wight is a researcher in the Department of Community Health Sciences at UCLA's Fielding School of Public Health focusing on how the people, places, social, and historical contexts in which people live affect their stress levels and health. In a 2012 study, Wight and his colleagues looked at data from the Los Angeles site of the Multicenter AIDS Cohort Study (MACS), the world's largest and longest ongoing study of gay and bisexual men's health. Since 1984, MACS has tracked nearly five thousand gay men, HIV-positive and -negative, with twice-yearly assessments and medical tests. They found that men between forty-four and seventy-five years of age were at high risk of poor mental health if they reported feeling stress because of *both* their sexual orientation *and* their age.[6] Wight found in a 2015 study that some midlife and older gay men experience what he and his colleagues termed "internalized gay ageism," which they define as "feeling denigrated or depreciated as they grow older within the context of a gay male culture in which youth and physical attractiveness are disproportionately valued." It's important to point out that most of the men in the study did *not* feel this way, but those who did were more likely to report symptoms of depression.

The good news is Wight has also found that for gay men who experience internalized gay ageism, a sense of *mattering* makes a tremendous difference.

Wight described mattering as "the degree to which people feel they are an important part of the world around them." His research also suggests that having a sense of control over one's life can mitigate the damage done by allowing others' stigmatizing attitudes to matter. He's also found that legal marriage may protect partners against poor mental health.[7]

Another weapon we can draw from our arsenal of internalized gay ageism-slayers is, interestingly enough, coming out—the experience of having worked through the issues we may have had in affirming our sexuality as a permanent and positive aspect of ourselves. Research suggests that by addressing and defanging homophobia and HIV-related stigma, we develop resilience that can protect us against the stigma attached to aging—and define aging and "old" on our own terms.

Brian de Vries, professor of gerontology at San Francisco State University and a fellow of the American Gerontological Society of America, writes in *The Lives of LGBT Older Adults: Understanding Challenges and Resilience*: "The psychological weight of lives at the margins exact a toll on mental health, in turn jeopardizing physical well-being in an oscillating fashion." But a concept referred to as "positive marginality" suggests that marginalized individuals, including gay men, "can find meaning in their experiences of stigma; these meanings promote a sense of agency and resilience and may allow individuals to thrive even in non-supportive conditions and circumstances. Positive marginality supports the reframing of one's stigmatized characteristics as ultimately positive aspects of one's identity."

De Vries referenced a number of studies that found the overwhelming majority of LGBT individuals felt they had become better people, and formed strong communities, precisely *because of* their experience of stigma. One 1978 study in particular, predating AIDS and all we learned about ourselves because of it, found that nearly three-quarters of the twelve hundred participants said that being LGBT had helped prepare them for aging. Although they said that living with the stigma attached to being LGBT had made their lives harder, when asked what about being LGBT prepared them for aging, they said it was the need to fight their way through life, forge their own paths, and form their own communities.[8]

In an interview for *The Atlantic*, de Vries told me, "We have been excluded, and there are huge costs of that exclusion. But as a result we've had to find our own way, to find ways of interacting and being that are unlike ways that were modeled by our [heterosexual] peers and elders. We've created ways that fit *us*." Besides redefining what "older" might look like or mean, de Vries said gay men of all ages can choose to frame our personal stories as stories of resilience and survival. "In the stories we tell of our lives," he said, "as gay men, as survivors, the *victims* story is one of discontinuity, how we're not what we 'should' be because of all these things. The *victory* story is one that sees the ways we can grow from them. It provides hope, direction, and allows you to learn from the experiences."[9]

The choice is each of ours to make. Really it's a lifelong series of choices, as de Vries made clear in an interview for this book. True to his academic roots, he described a flow chart. It starts with recognizing one's gayness or "otherness," then leads on a path that has no endpoint. Each juncture along the way—including whether to come out or not, and deciding what being out means in a social or political sense—is a decision point. "At each one we could choose to hide or move forward," said de Vries. "If you move forward you're going to encounter more of these points. Then later in life, you look back at those decision points and see the hardiness of your choices." Ideally you want to look back and see how you chose to move forward, even at the most challenging points along the path.

For himself, fifty-nine at the time of our interview, de Vries described a common enough experience for older gay men in his own life. "Many of my friends and I will talk about how the Castro has changed as a district of the city," he said. "It has changed really a lot, but so too have we. Part of the change is that we're older in an environment that still covets youth and beauty." That much is familiar. But there's the decision point. Said de Vries, "My personal experience is that, on the one hand, I feel sidelined within my community by virtue of being an older man, not a bodybuilder Adonis. And here is where the age kicks in: I don't begrudge that. I may wish it were different even as I don't wish I were younger. There is something freeing for me to be able to observe and not feel the need to play a certain role."

Therein lies the choice: whether to play a role, to be someone else's idea of an "older gay man"—or to be one's *own* man.

For older gay men who are also living with well-managed HIV, de Vries pointed out that there is a potentially even bigger payoff for successful aging. As de Vries put it in a nonacademic but precise observation, "My HIV-negative view of this is that by being HIV-positive and aging, it creates a 'fuck you' kind of script toward those who want to denigrate aging. We are all survivors at some level by virtue of making it this far, and HIV-positive survivors are at a whole other level."

What the gay community learned, and taught the world, from our collective experience of "living with HIV" is now providing models for elder care. "Some of the caregiving literature," said de Vries, "makes reference to the early years of HIV and government inattention and neglect, families, the medical environment, some friends turning their backs, and a community recognizing the need and developing these care environments and settings for care provision. People are looking at that now and thinking of how we might apply that in the aging of our own populations—especially gay men, aging alone, without children, afraid to present themselves as vulnerable. Gay men in particular are at high risk."

A 2011 report from New York–based SAGE (Services and Advocacy for GLBT Elders) showed the growing need for senior housing, particularly for low-income residents, where our elders can enjoy their halcyon days in comfort and safety, not going back into the closet to live in a senior community where they may feel isolated and vastly outnumbered. Based on a survey of more than twenty-five hundred LGBT adults between age fifty and ninety, SAGE reported that 80 percent of the respondents feared discrimination, three-quarters feared abuse and isolation, and 85 percent felt it would be unsafe to live in a typical nongay residence for elders. The report also found an exceptionally high level of resilience. "Among the LGBT older adult participants in our project," it said, "nearly 90 percent feel good about belonging to their communities, and many have at least moderate levels of social support. Most engage regularly in wellness activities (91 percent) and moderate physical activities (82 percent)." Another not-so-surprising finding: "While family members related by blood or marriage play a primary role in the support of older adults in the general population, most LGBT older adults care for one another."[10]

Brian de Vries noted that there is a "sort of wave moving across the nation" in LGBT-affirmative housing for older adults. Cities including New York, Chicago, San Francisco, and Seattle have either opened or are developing residences. The general sense in those communities is that, as de Vries put it in our interview, "We were there for each other before AIDS; we'll be there for each other now."[11]

In Los Angeles, the LGBT Center was about to open a new one-hundred-unit residence for low-income LGBT seniors. When I asked Lorri L. Jean, the center's CEO, what she sees as the LGBT community's "next big thing," she didn't miss a beat: "Seniors," she said. She explained, "This is the first generation of seniors who are out. So we are just now learning their needs and issues. We just had a tidal wave, like the rest of the population, coming our way. We are now learning—and this is new knowledge—that they are poorer than we ever imagined, and are going to need so much more help. The consequences of *not* providing it are very tragic."[12]

SAGE is working to prevent those tragedies. The organization began in New York City in 1978, when a small intergenerational group of LGBT people recognized that older people still needed a voice in the equality movement. In that first decade after Stonewall, the movement had grown and spread, but the community had overlooked its elders. Originally known as Senior Action in a Gay Environment, SAGE was formed to create a support network for older community members, first in New York City and then nationwide. Today SAGE offers supportive services and resources for, and advocates for supportive public policy that addresses the needs of, LGBT older adults and their caregivers. The national organization includes thirty local SAGE affiliates in twenty states and the District of Columbia.[13]

In an interview at SAGE's Seventh Avenue offices in Manhattan, Catherine Thurston, SAGE's senior director for programs at the time, described LGBT older people as "the last wave in our movement, the last frontier." And that is coming from a woman who has worked in geriatric and aging issues since age eighteen. Adding to what Thurston describes as some of the most innovative work she has seen in her career, SAGE is again pioneering with the first-anywhere senior center for LGBT elders. A hundred and ten people a day take their dinner there.

Thurston echoed Brian de Vries's observations about how programs originally created to serve people with AIDS have provided models for new elder services. Thurston said more gay men are using SAGE's services, and in LGBT service centers across the country, "opposite of typical senior centers, which are mostly women." Because one of its core values is "LGBT older voices come first," the word *queer* isn't used at SAGE. "It's painful for older people," said Thurston. Although SAGE employs a lot of young people—who mostly come here to work in an LGBT organization, she explained—it's hard to organize intergenerational programs. "People want to be people, not just older people," she said.[14]

SAGE's longest-serving staff member, Thomas Weber, came to the organization after fifteen years at Gay Men's Health Crisis, where his final position was directing the agency's large AIDS buddy program. Buddy programs like GMHC's, created in the early years of the epidemic, have been looked at as potential models for low-cost, home-based care and support for homebound elders. Although it predated AIDS, SAGE's own "Friendly Visitor" program is an example of a buddy-style program and the first of its kind for older adults. Volunteers are trained and assigned to one person whom they visit weekly. Weber said they will often stay with the person to the end of their lives. Most of the volunteers are in their thirties and forties. "Some of the forty-somethings and fifty-somethings," said Weber, "have in mind that someone will be there for them, too. Some are new to the city, so this will be part of plugging into the community. Some just like old people. Some had great relationships with their grandparents, and miss them. Some imagine what their grandparents would have been like if they were gay."

I wondered what his many years of working in LGBT social services, particularly with elders at SAGE, had taught Weber about his own resilience. The son of an alcoholic father, he mentioned his years in twelve-step programs that he said "helped me get sober and clean, and gave me new hope and community." He found additional support in therapy, repairing family relationships, supportive friends, and a partner who is a therapist and has been living with HIV a long time. As for how his experience at SAGE has contributed, Weber mentioned a few of the great experiences he said he wouldn't have enjoyed if he wasn't there. "I know Edie Windsor [namesake of the 2013 *United States v. Windsor* Supreme Court case overturning the Defense of Marriage Act], she came out of SAGE. I know Stonewall survivors. I know from people's experiences what things were like when they were young and coming up, and how much things have changed." Perhaps one of the biggest lessons Weber has learned at SAGE, from those who would know best, is simply this: "It takes *courage* to be yourself!" he said.[15]

When I asked Weber if he could put me in touch with a Stonewall survivor to interview for this book, he connected me with Mark Segal in Philadelphia. As noted earlier in this book, Segal was only eighteen years old at the time of the 1969 Stonewall raid and protests, and was one of the organizers of the Gay Liberation Front that followed and transformed the gay civil rights movement from "respectable" to in-your-face.

On a bright sunny and brisk prespring afternoon in Philadelphia, I am sitting with Segal—Stonewall veteran and founder in 1975, and still publisher, of *Philadelphia Gay News*—eating a chicken fajita salad at Copacabana, on bustling South Street. We're talking about his new memoir *And Then I Danced*, about his decades as a gay activist and much-awarded commentator on LGBT life in his column "Mark My Words." The word *joy* comes up a lot in Segal's side of our conversation. And I can only describe as joyful the way his eyes squint in merriment, what strikes me as his sheer zest for living. It's funny to picture this bouncing ball of energy "zapping" Walter Cronkite, America's most trusted newscaster, back in 1973. But that's what he did to *The Tonight Show Starring Johnny Carson*, *The Mike Douglas Show*, and in what *Straight News: Gays, Lesbians, and the Media* author Ed Alwood called his "last and most notorious zap," a live on-air *CBS Evening News with Walter Cronkite* broadcast on December 11, 1973. As Cronkite began a story about Secretary of State Henry Kissinger, Segal darted in front of the camera holding up a sign reading "Gays Protest CBS Prejudice." Segal sat on Cronkite's desk until crewmembers wrestled him to the ground and tied him up in wire—on camera.[16]

"Gay activism can be fun, and should be," Segal said. "It's possible to be radical and have fun at the same time." For good measure, he added, "If I were in D.C., I would zap the Republicans!" Meanwhile, here in Philly and really everywhere, he said, "Our job is to create a loving community that includes our most vulnerable, youth, trans, and seniors." Now qualifying for "senior" status himself at sixty-five, Segal told me he found a "new agenda": fighting ageism.

As one of the vanguard of what Segal calls "the first out generation," he saw a need in Philadelphia for low-cost housing where LGBT elders could feel comfortable and enjoy all the social and cultural benefits of living in Center City—not shoved off to another margin. He debunked the myth that all gay people are affluent in an interview with the *Philadelphia Inquirer*'s architecture critic, discussing the John C. Anderson Apartments, the city's first—and the nation's third—LGBT-friendly senior housing project built by and for the LGBT community in Pennsylvania. "A lot of gay people didn't get good jobs because of discrimination," Segal said.

In fact SAGE reports that poverty is at least as high, if not higher, among gay and lesbian elders than among the heterosexual population. Research from UCLA's Williams Institute found that 15 percent of gay and bisexual men are poor, compared to 13 percent of heterosexual men. The factors contributing to the "high and persistent levels of poverty among LGBT communities" include employment discrimination, lack of access to marriage, higher rates of being uninsured, gender and racial inequalities, less family support, and family conflict.[17]

The *Inquirer* critic noted the Anderson Apartments building, opened in early 2014, "happens to be a useful model for how to build urban-friendly, affordable housing in a rapidly gentrifying neighborhood."[18]

Mark Segal led the fundraising campaign for the $19.5 million, light-filled six-story building with fifty-six one-bedroom apartments in the heart of the area known in the City of Brotherly Love as the "Gayborhood." To qualify, prospective residents must have income between $8,000 and $30,000. The community is classified as "LGBT friendly" so no one feels excluded. There are nongay residents, many of whom have LGBT sons and daughters. The apartments are bright, and there is a common outdoor courtyard that community groups recognized quickly was a terrific space for fundraising events. Mark Segal's favorite feature is the "drag-queen closets" in each apartment. In the lobby is a life-size portrait of the building's namesake, John C. Anderson, a first-term city council member who died in 1983, at age forty-one, reportedly from AIDS. Every floor features framed black-and-white photographs of the 1969 Stonewall riots.[19] On the ground floor is a large, framed image of the first gay and lesbian march in front of Independence Hall in 1964.

John James is one of the young men featured in the image of that march all those years ago—as the Anderson Apartments resident points out to me.

Still tall and lanky at seventy-five, James left San Francisco after decades there because the cost of living got too high. I haven't seen him since I interviewed him in San Francisco, in 1995, for my book *Victory Deferred*. After more than two decades of publishing *AIDS Treatment News*, his pioneering and very popular newsletter that activists and doctors alike relied on for research updates, James has shifted coasts and his focus. He chose aging. "Ultimately we may be able to cure aging," he said over coffee in Square One Coffee, conveniently located on the ground floor of the Thirteenth Street apartment building. He said that compared to the vast amount of money spent on the diseases related to aging, not much is spent on aging itself. Such research, he said, "could have a tremendous impact on the medical bills related to aging." The main goal, said James, is to "extend the health span—not just the lifespan—so people have a longer period of health."[20]

While we work to make that happen, there's the Anderson Apartments and all it represents—for Philadelphia, for the LGBT community, for the future. "The whole city takes pride in the building," Mark Segal said. "It's not just the LGBT community, but the whole city of Philadelphia."[21]

For gay men who are "older," especially by gay male standards, but not yet ready to get on the lengthening waiting list of Anderson Apartments, there's the Bridgemen project—at least if you live in San Francisco, because it's the only project like it in the country. Because San Francisco's gay demographics skew older—due to the city's high cost of living—gay and bisexual men in their thirties and forties represent the leading edge of new HIV infections in the city. Drawing from the Mpowerment model of HIV prevention for young urban gay and bisexual men, Bridgemen doesn't "look like" prevention but instead focuses foremost on building up, and building upon, gay men's resilience—only these men are considerably older than Mpowerment's eighteen-to twenty-nine-year-old demographic.

Launched by the Stop AIDS Project in July 2011 and originally funded by the CDC before the San Francisco AIDS Foundation adopted it, Bridgemen reaches out to gay and bisexual men in what the project's founding director Frank Stenglein in an interview called our "third life." He explained that after a first stage of making friends and having fun in our twenties, then building careers and settling down, men in this third stage ask themselves such questions as "What comes next? What am I going to leave behind me?" Stenglein, forty-five at the time of our 2013 interview, said gay men at this point in our lives—particularly those who don't have a partner—are at risk for depression, isolation, and drug use. Through weekly and monthly meetings, events and community service projects, Bridgemen offers the chance to make new friends and talk about things in a safe space. "By men being involved in their community," said Stenglein, "they are more likely to take care of themselves, their brothers and their community." The HIV prevention aspect, he explained, lies in building "a happy, healthier community that embraces each other and men who are taking care of each other, being responsible for each other."[22]

Forty-two-year-old Jared Hemming, Stenglein's successor as Bridgemen director, told me in an interview at Strut, the group's Castro Street home, that Bridgemen has "grown incredibly" since its start. It now has a thousand members, four or five hundred of whom are active, mostly in their forties and fifties. One of the oldest and most active members is seventy. Hemming told me the most rewarding aspect of his job is "seeing guys come back to life." Many of the men, as happens to so many gay men as we age, had withdrawn themselves from the gay community. Bridgemen offers them a social bridge from their isolation, loneliness, and possibly risky behavior back into the community.

"It's remarkable to see how lives change," said Hemming. He offered an example. "One member, in his late forties, felt discontented with the community," he said. "He didn't feel he belonged, and was just living life but not engaged. He was on the shy side, and joined almost two years ago. He came to a group and was very interested in service projects, but not a lot of socializing. As he came back, we saw him open up. He brought in his outside friends. He has become the photographer for the group. He is *so* engaged now. He actually cried and said this has changed his life. He is dating one of the guys in the group, and has gone from being close to flickering out to being *very* active."

Hemming recalled a meeting of the fifty-plus group, another program at Strut. He explained that those groups are more focused on processing things, and the topic was resiliency. Hemming said it gave the gay men there a chance "to talk about what they've come through." A lot of pain and sorrow poured out of hearts that long ago had curled into fetal balls to keep from breaking one more time. But now, with the acceptance and safety of other gay men who understood because they had experienced the same thing, healing could happen. And they could move with greater comfort and confidence inside their new role as men who are older, wiser, and who embrace their own aging because they know, like Ken South, how precious life is. By helping gay men reconnect who had been withdrawing from the gay community, Bridgemen offers the sense of "mattering" that Richard Wight said helps drive out internalized gay ageism. "A lot of people isolated themselves," said Hemming, "and now there's this weird sense of re-engaging."

Maybe it's not so weird. Maybe it's one of life's cycles, like the seasons, for older gay men—especially those of us who lived through the dark years of AIDS—to reconnect to the community. Maybe we gay men are like the perennials in Morrie's gardens in Maine, or Harold Kooden's rooftop garden in Manhattan. In the ice and snow of winter these hardy plants look for all intents and purposes like dried dead husks, brown and curled upon themselves. But in the life-giving spring sunshine, a yearly miracle occurs. Irresistible light and warmth summon new life from the earth. Even the nobbiest old vines and trees burst into leaf and blossom, as if celebrating the irrepressible power of life itself. That's what strongly rooted, resilient perennials *do*.

CHAPTER TWENTY-SIX

~

Stonewall Strong

*Life Is Good When We Are the Heroes of Our
Own Life's Story, Standing Firmly on Our
Community's Proud History of Resilience*

Portland knows a *lot* about resilience.

The largest city in Maine, located on a peninsula in Casco Bay, was first settled by Europeans in 1632. The Native Americans already there didn't welcome them, but instead raided the settlement, twice, first in 1675 and then again, with French assistance, in 1690, when they wiped out the last of the white population. Major Samuel Moody in 1716 established a new port, which thrived—until the British bombarded and burned the city in 1775. It was rebuilt.

After Maine gained independence from Massachusetts, in 1820, Portland became the state capital until the capital was moved to Augusta in 1832. On June 26, 1863, a Confederate raiding party entered Portland's harbor, inciting the Battle of Portland Harbor, one of the northernmost battles of the Civil War.[1] And then, to top it all off, an Independence Day 1866 sparkler or flicked cigar ash ignited the greatest fire in American history to that point: eighteen hundred buildings burned to the ground, including most of the commercial buildings in the city, half the churches, and hundreds of homes. More than ten thousand were left homeless in the 1866 Great Fire of Portland, Maine.[2] Not long after the fire, poet Henry Wadsworth Longfellow described his old hometown in a letter to a friend: "Desolation! Desolation! Desolation! It reminds me of Pompeii; but has not so many walls left standing as that 'sepult city.'"[3]

Once again, Portland rebuilt.

In an old New England city like Portland, history matters. You might say it's a living thing here, because it's all around, in plaques and monuments, birthplaces and memorials. The red brick buildings and cobblestone streets of the Old Port evoke the charm and long history of Boston, just over a hundred miles to the south, and the buildings and streets of even older London that were the reference points for the people who built Boston and rebuilt Portland. Naturally the sea also is ever-present in this port city, from the briny smells of the Atlantic and the fish markets along the waterfront, to the local fishermen's tales of peril and survival as they pursue their treacherous livelihood.

Portland is a quintessential New England city, old, steeped in history, and yet wonderfully new and vibrant. The city is authentic in its architecture, doesn't pretend to be better or worse than it is. You might call it a very "real" place. Its people, like their forbears, display their fortitude every winter as they put shoulders to the wind and push through another Maine winter—proving once again why Yankees occupy a place in the American mythology as archetypes of resilience.

"Are you ready to come back yet?" John Preston said it was the question his big-city gay friends always asked him. They thought he was crazy when he moved from New York to Portland in 1979.

Preston had been editor of the *Advocate*, author of nearly fifty books including fiction (*Franny, the Queen of Provincetown*), essays (including *Hometowns: Gay Men Write About Where They Belong*), and what he proudly and unabashedly called pornography (including *I Once Had a Master and Other Tales of Erotic Love*). He had done his own "gay circuit" of big cities. Said Preston, "They were convinced that I, the quintessential modern urban fag, would be unable to live in Portland. I would have no leather bars, I would have to go to the theater, I would have to take part in the excitement of national politics. I certainly had to live in the big city to have sex."

Preston's friends couldn't understand how happy he really was in Maine. "But of course they had never met the men here," he wrote in an essay about the city. "My friends in New York were sure that one had to be able to carry off the costumes of the new gay life to be attractive. They had never seen my friend Brian who worked on the fishing piers here and who would come by my apartment after work wearing three layers of torn up thermal underwear underneath his yellow slicker. I kept telling Brian that if he packaged the concept and sold it on Christopher Street, he'd make a fortune."

It wasn't only the men's authentic work clothes Preston admired; he loved just to hear them speak. He had lost his own Massachusetts accent when he went to college at Lake Forest, where he felt humiliated into practicing an "acceptable" public television kind of spoken English. "Now," in Portland, he said, "I could hear the sounds of New England straight from the lips of the men I met, the same men who would kiss me." He added, "I used to seduce men into my bed and then, to their confusion, just ask them to speak, to let me hear their Maine accents."[4]

Community meant the world to John Preston, and he recognized from the time it appeared that AIDS could seriously damage not only gay men individually but also the community he so valued. In 1982, the year after the first cases were reported, Preston wrote, "If we can stand up and declare ourselves to be proud to be gay, we must also show some substance to our gayness. Our lives have been testaments that we will not allow the world to trivialize us. We have insisted that being gay is more than a sexual act. We have demanded that the world—and we ourselves—see gayness as a way of being, of relating, of loving. Now, faced with a monumental crisis, we are being challenged as we've never been challenged before. We have to respond with righteous anger, careful caution, thorough preparation, and, above, all, complete compassion."[5]

Preston learned in the late 1980s he himself was HIV-positive. His diagnosis fueled his activism like gasoline fuels a fire. He became a regular source on the epidemic for Maine news reporters, openly discussing his medical situation and the politics of the epidemic on TV and in newspapers. He also created a position for himself as writer-in-residence at The AIDS Project, in Portland. He worked with people with AIDS, mainly gay men, to record their stories. "As I've taken my tape recorder around the state and listened to people's stories," Preston wrote in an essay about his experience, "I've been most struck by the extent to which people are convinced they aren't important enough to be listened to. Who would care? What value would anyone find in the life of a waiter or a warehouse worker or a fisherman? Then, with the tape recorder running, the most dramatic and powerful stories would come out of these men. Here were novels of trust and betrayal, legends of reconciliation and the discovery of peace; poems of love and happiness."[6]

In Portland it was inevitable that John Preston and Frannie Peabody would cross paths. The literary leather man and the grande dame of Portland society became great friends because both of them cared passionately about AIDS and the injustices suffered by people with the misfortune of having it. Peabody's grandson Peter died from AIDS in November 1984. Her daughter Barbara Peabody, Peter's mother, wrote a book called *The Screaming Room*, about the devastating experience of caring for her son as he slowly succumbed to the illness.

Even before she cofounded The AIDS Project in Portland, Frannie Peabody was already visiting AIDS patients in the hospital, making a special point to speak with their parents—if they visited their sons, that is. "AIDS wasn't a chic disease in 1986, it was a frightening one," Preston wrote in a loving tribute to Frannie Peabody called "A Woman of a Certain Age." "But here, into the basement room of the downtown church, walked Mrs. Millard S. Peabody, the great matriarch of Portland society. Frannie was used to volunteer organizations. She'd been on the board of directors (often as president) of the Portland Museum of Art, the Maine Historical Society, the Portland Landmarks Commission, the Colonial Dames of America, and many more. The members of the AIDS support group weren't used to having society ladies in their midst. They were grassroots activists, committed to egalitarianism. They had no idea what to do with Frannie."

Frannie Peabody, of course, was undeterred. "She told the story of her grandson," Preston wrote, "and announced her intention to do something about the need for education, and the need for the compassion which she was convinced would come from that education. And with that first visit, Frannie took the nearly invisible movement of AIDS activism in Maine and made it instantly respectable. That's the power of a Yankee woman of a certain age and standing in the community."

Frannie Peabody was already in her eighties when she became Portland's most famous AIDS activist. Her daughter Barbara recalls her mother as "very puritanical" when she and her two sisters and gay brother were growing up. "Now, here she was," wrote Preston, "a grandmother, carrying bags of condoms to rural schools and distributing them."

"I couldn't believe that was *my mother!*" recalled Barbara Peabody in an interview at her home and art studio in Tucson.[7]

Indeed it was. In fact, Frannie Peabody never forgot who she was—and never missed an opportunity to use it to the advantage of Portland's efforts to address its local AIDS crisis. When the AIDS Project was in financial straits, Preston said, "Frannie convened a luncheon meeting in the Cumberland Club, the bastion of Portland's ruling circles. She strong-armed a dozen of the most powerful people in the city to come: the head of the local newspaper, a television station manager, the chairman of the board of one of the biggest banks. When all the power brokers had been seated, Frannie addressed her peers: 'My dears, I did not order the lobster roll,' she told them, 'because it's too expensive. I saved money on the menu, and I intend to give that money to the AIDS Project. Now, let's see what the rest of you are going to do.'"[8]

Frannie Peabody changed the landscape of HIV/AIDS education and services in Maine, helping to establish Maine's first AIDS hotline and The

AIDS Project in 1985, and cofounding (and funding) Peabody House, an AIDS hospice, in 1995. The two organizations merged in 2002 to form the Frannie Peabody Center—today the largest community-based HIV-AIDS organization in Maine, providing prevention services to those at risk and direct services for people living with HIV. In her final years, Frannie was the grand marshal for Portland's annual Gay Pride Parade, sporting her signature pink boa—a gift for her ninetieth birthday—while riding atop an antique yellow convertible as a representative of Peabody House.[9]

In the lobby of the Frannie Peabody Center hangs a large, framed blow-up of Frannie's photo that ran on the front page of the *Portland Press Herald* when she rode in her final Pride parade in 2001, only two weeks before her death at age ninety-eight. The diminutive, white-haired lady in the picture—"everybody's grandmother," as John Preston described her—is beaming from ear to ear, clearly right at home among the "gay boys" she had come to love, who loved her right back.

For thirty-three-year-old Katie Rutherford, a career in nonprofits and a determination to move to Maine led her to the Frannie Peabody Center. At twenty-four, she had founded Dollars for Change, a nonprofit in South Africa focused on social issues in the community, such as fetal alcohol syndrome and HIV, and teaching people how to do practical things like install solar heaters. The center offered her a chance to do what she was interested in for an organization with an awesome history, but she could still feel she was contributing to the global effort to address the HIV pandemic. Rutherford read John Preston's tribute to Frannie, and we laugh imagining the proper little lady and the gay pornographer.

The center is suffused with Frannie Peabody's spirit. Said Rutherford, the center's development director, "Every time we have a staff meeting, or the AIDS walk, or a board meeting, we sit in the conference room and there is a big picture of Frannie. Often we talk about client success stories or someone who has passed away, and honor their life. We talk about the person, the strides they made. We often ask ourselves, 'What would Frannie think of us now?' I think she would be proud that we carry her ideals."

One of the departed Colonial Dame's ideals was her reverence for history, evidenced by all the historic society and museum boards she served on. In that spirit, Rutherford said that at the Frannie Peabody Center the general feeling is it's important to "always remember where we came from" because a lot of the center's clients these days are long-term survivors. "Those early days are real for them," she said. "We have several clients who knew Frannie, including a client who went to Peabody House to die. He has a wonderful story about how Frannie brought him custard every day, and he would eat it just because Frannie brought it. He is alive today, and it's wonderful to hear his story."[10]

Not only is it wonderful to hear David Simpson's story, but it's positively awe inspiring.

"My story is a hard one to hear because I've been through a lot," Simpson told me in an interview for this book. He got his AIDS diagnosis in 1984, over the telephone, a dozen years before effective treatment finally became available. "I panicked for a couple of weeks because at that time it was a death sentence," he said. At first he drank to try coping with the devastating news. Then he started thinking about staying alive, and "snapped out of it." Simpson grew up in a poor Catholic family in Old Orchard Beach, the Maine beach resort town where my own parents took their honeymoon in 1957, when it was a "big drinking town with lots of bars," as Simpson put it. He was living in Old Orchard with his partner of fourteen years at the time of his diagnosis. "I was very promiscuous at the time, like everybody," he said. "There was one gay bar in Portland at the time, and we all gave [HIV] to each other."

That was before The AIDS Project existed. "We'd meet with Frannie in this one little dumpy room and just talk and have therapy," Simpson said. "That's where I got my support." It's also where he met John Preston. His parents never visited him when he was at Peabody House. "My parents didn't even come to see me when I was dying," he told me. "They were embarrassed." He had come out to them, but they denied up until their own deaths that he was gay. That didn't stop him from giving interviews to the local newspaper. "I knew I was dying anyway, and I wanted to get out my message," he said. Where did that gumption come from? "I think it came from me being out as a gay man and not caring what people think of me," he said. "I've gotten beaten up by people and even by a police officer, brutally."

While he was in hospice at Peabody House, expecting to die, Simpson went back to college, majoring in communication. He got an "A" for the class in which the professor interviewed him in front of his fellow students about living with AIDS. "Every weekend," he said, "you would see me at the Peabody House. I wouldn't go anyplace, just hang out doing my school work." Even while he was a resident himself, and "skinny, skinny, skinny," as he put it, Simpson also volunteered at Peabody House. "I used to read to the guys who were dying," he said. "Even though they were in a coma they could still hear you."

Simpson somehow managed to survive until protease inhibitors, beginning in 1996, began to change HIV from a fatal illness to a chronic, manageable one. The drugs were hard to take. Crixivan, for instance, was notorious for inducing diarrhea and projectile vomiting. When he first took it, he got sick and stopped, feeling death would be preferable to the way he was feeling from the drugs. The doctors finally convinced him to try again. Each new treatment advancement bought more time, more life, in Simpson's own Lazarus story.

He'd been living with HIV for thirty-two years by the time we spoke. At sixty, he goes to the gym every day. He's back to work and trying to get off of disability. Simpson said he feels like so many other long-term HIV survivors, "isolated, depressed, and poor—and very much by themselves." He lost his partner, the love of his life, ten years ago. "He was part of my happiness because he had met me in hospice," Simpson said. "He used to pick me up and take me away to his house in the country, just to get me out of the hospice."

As if his own miraculous survival weren't enough, Simpson recounts the times when he himself has been the caregiver for others, as if extraordinary acts of kindness are second nature to him—which I expect is the case. A few years ago he used his own money to fix meals for shut-in older people. It made him feel good, too. "It's selfish because it made me feel good about myself," he told me. He has taken care of other friends, too, even bringing morphine pumps to them. "I slept with one man who had KS [Kaposi's sarcoma] when he was dying," he said. "He came from a wealthy family that didn't want anything to do with him. I cuddled next to him just to keep him warm. He just wanted someone to keep him warm. I just held him; it wasn't sexual. I think just holding someone helps a lot."

Where does a man find the strength to face his own impending death and then not merely have the audacity to live, but to love so generously? "I felt in taking care of these people, it was my spirituality coming through," Simpson said. "I felt this loving outburst coming to me when I took care of these guys." He's now caring for a man, another long-term HIV survivor, who is blind from the CMV that stole his eyesight in the dark preprotease days. "Can you imagine losing your sight back then and being sick?" asked Simpson. "So I go and help him and take him to the store, help him clean his apartment. *He* has a wonderful story of resilience!"

So does David Simpson. "I'm a survivor," he told me. "It's just been hard. I take care of myself—you *have* to take care of yourself. You have to keep on going. You can't let anybody stop you. The older I get the more I realize it's just *me* that can change my life."[11]

When he let himself out of the hospital after a bout of pneumonia in May 1992, John Preston reflected on his adopted city. Just looking around him at Portland inspired him. "This was what I loved about living," he wrote, "the sheer sensuality of a New England summer, the soft breeze from the ocean, the explosion of color that came out of nowhere, out of the gray and bleak landscape of winter in Maine."[12] At his funeral, in 1994, Preston's longtime friend and editor Michael Denneny said of him, "He was one of the few people I have known for whom the need for community was an immediate and tangible reality. He spent years moving from city to city until he realized that at heart he was a New Englander and he came to Portland, to be near to his roots and his family."[13]

"Are you finally going to come back?" his New York friends had continued to ask Preston. "No. Life's good here," he answered. A year before he died of complications arising from AIDS, Preston penned an essay called "Portland: Life's good here."[14] In 2013, nearly two decades after John Preston's death, the city of Portland rolled out its new slogan: "Yes, life is good here."[15]

Life is good for thousands of gay men, and plenty of nongay folk, too, in and far beyond New York City because of Gay Men's Health Crisis. Since its 1982 formation in Larry Kramer's living room, the world's first and leading provider of HIV prevention, care, and advocacy has been a beacon of hope and one of the gay community's most impressive examples of "love in action." The agency today serves more than ten thousand clients a year, 59.9 percent of them gay and 29.7 percent nongay.[16]

In an interview at his office, I asked GMHC's CEO Kelsey Louie how his career in social work led him to focus on HIV. Partly, he said it was wanting to "do his part" for the gay community. His earlier work on foster care, homelessness, and substance abuse were certainly connected in ways to the epidemic. But Louie wanted something with a deeper personal connection. He wanted to give back to the LGBT community, too. "HIV is still the number-one issue that plagues this community, and I wanted to contribute and do my part," he said.

Born in 1975, Louie was too young even to have sex when the epidemic hit in the early 1980s. But he's seen more than enough of it in the years since. Now he is able to appreciate not only what the community suffered but also the awesome courage and resilience it took to achieve the things we did. He is also old enough to have an awareness of his own role in gay history. "We all stand on giants," he said. "As CEO of GMHC, I stand on the broadest shoulders of the biggest giant in the HIV field."

On the wall behind Louie's desk is a large framed photo of Larry Kramer. Louie said he draws resilience from Kramer. He said that when he saw the HBO film version of Kramer's 1985 play *The Normal Heart*, he "not only felt the impact of the work before me, but upholding the legacy." He continued, "There won't be another Larry Kramer. To be in the same room, on the same stage, in a conversation with Larry Kramer is so amazing and inspiring."

But it's not only the famous heroes like Kramer who inspire him. "Not everybody has Larry Kramer's platform or voice," he said, "but I see heroes and heroines here all the time. The men and women who work here are way more resilient than I am. I draw from them. There are heroes we know about, and others we don't know."[17]

On a crisp September morning in San Francisco, I'm sitting on a granite bench inside the National AIDS Memorial Grove. John Cunningham, the Grove's executive director, and longtime AIDS activist and Grove board chair Mike Shriver, are describing plans for a center that will give visitors "an epiphany," including young gay men who don't yet know how things like the Grove came about—or that homophobia continues to be a major factor worldwide in the ongoing pandemic. It will be a positive and hopeful place to be educated and contemplate history, much like the Grove itself. Life is evident everywhere in the Grove, amid the trees, flowers, and open lawns. An engraved stone bench reads "L'Chaim"—"To Life." The living memorial, marking twenty-five years since ground in Golden Gate Park was first broken in 1991 to build and plant it, is one way of helping to "carry the story along," as Shriver puts it.

In the Grove's Circle of Friends, a circle comprised of inlaid granite pavers engraved with names of the dearly departed, the words "Hope, Healing, and Remembrance" stand out. "We have the handle on healing," said Shriver. He pointed to the estimated two hundred thousand volunteer hours it took to make the Grove happen. As for hope, Shriver said, "What's exciting to me is it won't be done until the epidemic is done." The Grove's original vision was to provide a place people "could come in and just grieve," he said, adding, "Oddly enough, the next step is to get their hands in the dirt."[18]

From the Grove I'm off to Cafe Flore for a lunchtime interview with longtime HIV survivor and gay America's biggest champion of what he says is "the only status that matters," what he calls "HIV-resilient." Tez Anderson is developing a "simple, secular, and structured program" by that name. "HIV-Resilient" aims to strengthen the resiliencies of older adults living with HIV and those affected by HIV. "We want to help people living with HIV learn the skills to live a full, connected, independent life," says a flyer for the program. It points out that the Centers for Disease Control and Prevention (CDC) estimates that by 2020, 70 percent of people living with HIV in the United States will be fifty or older. In San Francisco, 84 percent of people living with HIV are over age forty.

The proverbial lightbulb came on for Anderson when he saw a news show about Iraqi veterans suffering from PTSD. "I had all the symptoms," he said. But he soon learned there was "no literature on trauma and survivorship" among gay men at that point. There were certainly no guidelines for anyone who, as had David Simpson, faced death—and then lived to die another day. "I did not prepare to be an old man with HIV; I planned to die," said Anderson. He was hardly the only one. When he called for a meeting of long-term HIV survivors in 2013, two hundred fifty showed up. The outcome was a group Anderson calls Let's Kick ASS (for AIDS Survivor Syndrome). "I would like to get people to tell their stories of survival," he said, "lessons we've learned as elders of our community." One of the most important lessons, he pointed out, was "Yes, it was awful but it also forged our community. We fought with a community spirit we had not seen since Stonewall."

As an elder of the community, his Walt Whitmanesque beard and masculine gentleness underscoring his words, Anderson said, "Most of us had the fortitude and courage to come out. That is resilience." He pointed out that even pansies, the pejorative slang used since at least the 1920s to describe and dismiss femme gay men, are actually quite hardy cool-weather flowers.

After he pulled himself out of the funk that had threatened to envelop him early on in his life as an HIV-positive gay man, Anderson told me he "began to focus on the times I got back up again." The man who at fifty-seven savors life and "looks for the *amazing* in everyday life" offers up the hard-earned wisdom that comes of going through the mill of life. "I have come to understand that resilience is something you develop and choose," he said. "Then it must be something you can teach, to help people *not* to be victims."[19]

It's hard to end my conversation with Tez Anderson, but I am due at the GLBT Historical Society—a fitting follow on, it seems to me—to interview its executive director, longtime AIDS activist Terry Beswick. He is a walking history book of San Francisco's AIDS epidemic since it began in 1981, the year he arrived in the city to study theater at San Francisco State University. He became the first national organizer for ACT NOW, the coalition of ACT UP chapters that formed in the wake of the Second March on Washington for Lesbian and Gay Rights on October 11, 1987. His office, along with other small LGBT organizations, was in the attic of John James's house on Church Street. That was just the beginning of his own career in HIV-AIDS. "It was crazy," he told me, "to go from the street corner to two years later running this multi-site research treatment effort—with a theater degree! But I had about the same credentials as others."

Through his activism, Beswick learned a lot about living in a diverse community. He called it a "profound education" around cultural awareness and sensitivity, as he learned about the impact of HIV-AIDS on other hard-hit communities besides gay men, including prisoners and sex workers. He called it "good preparation for where I'm at today." When he gets together with other gay men who lived through the worst of AIDS in San Francisco—he mentions the Grove's John Cunningham and Mike Shriver—Beswick said, "We're like old soldiers sharing war stories."

Helping to preserve those stories is part of what the GLBT Historical Society offers the fifteen thousand annual visitors to its GLBT History Museum, fittingly located on Eighteenth Street in the Castro district. "By telling the specific anecdotes from my and other people's stories, people grab on and identify with them," Beswick said. "I see my role and the organization's role as being facilitators to equip people with the tools to learn and see their history. The power of our stories goes *beyond* our stories. When young people come in, they find it mind-blowing that the museum exists. They feel validated to know their community has a history, and that people struggled to have the things we have today."[20]

The question, and challenge, facing the historical society, the Grove, and even individual gay men is, "How do you carry a story along?" as Mike Shriver put it in our interview earlier in the day. "Post-Stonewall, post-AIDS, what is *your* cause?" John Cunningham asked at the Grove, "To use your own voice to improve the society you live in? What happens when AIDS is gone?"[21]

I asked John D'Emilio, one of the country's best-known gay historians, recently retired from the University of Illinois at Chicago, his thoughts about how gay history could best be shared among LGBT people, especially young people. For the first half of his career, D'Emilio said he taught "mainstream history." From 1999 until his retirement he was able to teach primarily LGBT-related courses. Two things in particular struck him as never changing from the time he began teaching those courses. "Except for a very small number of activist types who were in the class," he said, "all of the students, whatever their identity, knew nothing. The best example I can give: A large number of my students would either go to, or knew about, the Pride parade each year in June in Chicago. It's a *huge* event. But almost none of them knew the parade had any relation to this thing called Stonewall." The second thing that surprised D'Emilio was "the mixture of excitement, shock, surprise, and anger about the things they were learning in class." After looking at *The Times of Harvey Milk*, the documentary about Harvey Milk, he said "they would be shocked and outraged that something like this [Milk's 1978 assassination] happened, and outraged that no one told them about it."

As for conveying to young people their part in a long heroic history, D'Emilio said that creating an LGBT studies course is one option. He suggested three other "layered" approaches for making sure our history is included in general discussions of history. "At the simplest level," he said, "you can include it biographically, by taking the story of a person who had a significant life, as historians measure significance, and tell their story." Another option is to include LGBT topics and stories in the curriculum so that when you teach the United States in the 1960s, Stonewall and gay liberation is also part of how you teach the history. Still a third, deeper approach, is "making LGBT materials part of the mainstream topics," so that discussions of the Cold War or McCarthyism and the Communist witch hunts also includes talking about people who were targeted for their sexuality.

How had studying and working as a professional historian affected D'Emilio's own sense of belonging and resilience? "In the seventies and eighties," he said, "there were a small number of us doing LGBT history and research. We knew each other, met in conferences, corresponded, became friends, shared our research. We would use events like a march on Washington to gather in Washington that weekend. So even apart from what I was researching and learning, the project of finding our history was a very inspiring and activating one. In some ways, I feel nostalgic for the old days when we felt like we were on the cutting edge of something new. It profoundly changed my life and my sense of myself going back a generation now." More recently, he said, it has been his students who most inspired him. "What has been exciting is watching my students get so excited or outraged about what they're learning in their classroom. They tell me no one has ever told them this; they had no idea."[22]

Tim McFeeley was director of the Human Rights Campaign from June 1989 to January 1995, handing off the reins to Elizabeth Birch. McFeeley had been interested in politics since he was a kid. He got involved in Democratic politics in Boston before moving into gay politics. He used to joke with Barney Frank, when Frank was his state representative, that one of the first projects they worked on together was closing down a couple of seedy gay bars. When AIDS came about, McFeeley said it became more important to move in the direction of focusing on gay issues. "It was pretty clear this was *the* transcendent issue for gay men, and we had to use our political skills to do that," he said.

McFeeley recalled an essay based on the Magnificat that he wrote in his "somewhat spiritual/religiosity phase." In it he described coming out as a gay man as a spiritual revelation. "So coming out as who you are as a gay person magnifies God. It shows that after you think you've characterized all the species of flowers, there's another one. It magnifies creation." He laughs his warm laugh, his churchy language not his usual way of speaking. "But it comes back to my feelings about being empowered," he said. "I wouldn't go so far as to say that means I have a mission, but I think there's a little of that. And it's a counter-narrative to the narrative that I hate, which is the victim narrative." He much prefers the narrative that AIDS created. "There was a whole different narrative coming up because of people like Larry Kramer, screaming at people and saying we're not going to be ignored. Suddenly we became respected." That took us through the nineties and beyond, to same-sex marriage. "I don't think any other group has done that," McFeeley said.

In a recent panel he was on at Harvard, McFeeley said a young person during the questions-and-answers said, "I hate HRC." The organization's reputation as being controlled by white gay and lesbian elitists who love to play black-tie dress-up produces a lot of comments like that. But McFeeley sees it differently. "I took that moment," he told me, "and in my softest voice I said, 'You have no idea what it was like to put on a tuxedo and go to the Ritz Carlton ballroom in 1981, and have the mayor speak to you—when before that we were kept in a dark bar where your feet stick to the floor. You can keep doing that, or you can put on a tuxedo and go to the Ritz ballroom, and that makes you *powerful*.'"[23]

There are many ways to express our power and political awareness. Retired Representative Barney Frank said that of course, most people aren't going to hold elective office. "But having that political awareness is helpful. It gives you a sense of dealing with the frustration and bitterness. It makes you angry to be so unfairly treated by this [anti-gay] prejudice." He said it's hard in many ways to fight the prejudice, but that being aware, supporting organizations, and voting for supportive political candidates are ways individuals can fight back.[24]

At a time in America's history when "alternative facts" are regularly offered by the Trump White House in its apparent determination to keep George Orwell's *1984* on the best-seller lists, Americans of both sexes and all colors, creeds, and orientations are fighting back, resisting—just as gay Americans fought back and resisted at Stonewall and throughout the HIV-AIDS epidemic.

"We absolutely changed the world through AIDS, fighting back," says Tracy Baim, publisher and executive editor of Chicago's *Windy City Times* and *Outlines* LGBT community newspapers. "AIDS changed politics, the way the medical community operates, and sped up marriage by two decades. It brought so many out of the closet and showed them why AIDS mattered." What does Baim see as the role of the LGBT media, including her newspapers, in this new era? "I absolutely believe, and certainly pre-Internet, our community media have been and continue to be a vital voice for individuals and our community," she said. She thinks again about all the years of AIDS activism—fighting back, challenging the CDC and health departments, lobbying and protesting. "That is resilience at its best," Baim said. "It saved lives."[25]

Something else that has saved the lives of gay men, and played a central role in our resilience, is humor. Since the days of subverting the dominant heterosexual culture with "inside" slang, and inverting traditional gender roles in drag shows, gay men have always relied on our sense of humor to carry us through whatever we need to get through.

Being a careful journalist, I wanted to check my source on that. I went to a man who happened to be a former member of the Funny Gay Males comedy troupe, the first openly gay comedian to appear on *The Tonight Show*, and one of the first to get his own half-hour HBO comedy special. Bob Smith's 1997 book of biographical essays, *Openly Bob*, received a Lambda Literary Award for best humor book, followed by *Way to Go, Smith!* in 1999, nominated for a 2000 Lambda Literary Award in the same category. Smith published his first novel, *Selfish and Perverse*, in 2007, and *Remembrance of Things I Forgot* in 2011.

Beyond Facebook, I hadn't been in touch with Bob Smith since we were together on the "Hot Stuff, Hookers, and Humor" panel at the 2001 Tennessee Williams Literary Festival, in New Orleans. In the years since then, Smith has suffered one of the most devastating medical catastrophes anyone could get, ALS. "When I was diagnosed," he told me in an email interview—a telephone interview was out because the disease has stolen his voice—"I was with my friend and a brilliant stand-up and writer, Eddie Sarfaty. Eddie claims I said, 'Lou Gehrig's disease? I don't even like baseball.'"

Smith's first symptoms affected his voice. "I sounded like a drunk when I did standup," he said. "I opened my sets with humor explaining I wasn't drunk, but had a neurological problem. I also told my standup friends Eddie and Judie Gold that I was going to do a one-man show called 'I'm Dying Up Here.' Dying is a term stand-ups use when they bomb." His friends preface any complaint they might have with "I know this isn't as rough as ALS . . ." In the years since his diagnosis, Smith has written three books—most recently, *Treehab: Tales from My Natural Wild Life* in 2016. The essays cover subjects from his love of nature to his experience with ALS. "As I've grown older, I'm not afraid to mix the very unfunny with the very funny," said Smith. In fact, he said *Treehab* may be his funniest book yet.[26]

Originally from North Carolina, by way of fourteen years in D.C., and now San Francisco–based, Sampson McCormick was one of the first, and is still one of the few, young black LGBT comedians to gain national recognition. OUT.com named him "One of the 12 Queer Comics That Every One Must Know," and the *Bay Area Reporter* in 2016 nominated him for Best Male Comic in the San Francisco Bay Area. Sampson, as he bills himself, described in an interview how he used humor as a way to handle the hard stuff he grew up with—including homelessness and trying to kill himself. It comes with survival. "Where I came from we had roaches," he said. "We had this and that. We made fun of it and learned how to work it. That is the reason now I'm able to get through some serious situations."

Flipping painful or embarrassing situations on their head is the stand-up's art. It's also an essential skill for anyone, gay or not, who wants not only to survive his ordeals but to thrive as well. "Human beings are a lot like cars," said Sampson. "When a car is made, it has fog lights, windshield wipers. Sometimes it requires a tune-up or premium gas. That premium gas may be meditation or a therapist. Sometimes you need new windshield wipers. You make those little adjustments. But we are made to get through *storms*."27

Storms, adversity, and trauma come to every one of us—multiple times over our lifetimes. But instead of being bent and bowed by them, we have the power to choose how we will respond to them. "We all must face difficult events in our lives," writes Stephen Joseph in his book *What Doesn't Kill Us: The New Psychology of Posttraumatic Growth*. "What has happened cannot be undone. Our only choice is how to live with what has happened." Joseph, a professor and codirector at the University of Nottingham (UK) of the Center for Trauma, Resilience, and Growth, writes, "When adversity strikes, people often feel that at least some part of them—their views of the world, their sense of themselves, their relationships—has been smashed." This is where choice comes in. "Those who try to put their lives back together exactly as they were remain fractured and vulnerable. But those who accept the breakage and build themselves anew become more resilient and open to new ways of living."28

I asked Professor Joseph via email about his emphasis on personal responsibility with respect to trauma. Gay men abused and bullied as children certainly weren't responsible for the traumas they suffered. He hastened to point out he wasn't suggesting this means we are responsible for the tragedies that befall us, or in control of the overwhelming emotions that we might feel, but in "whether we adopt a growthful attitude to life and its challenges is our choice."

"We all have a choice about how we respond to events in our lives," he said. "This was a point made so eloquently by Viktor Frankl in his description of his experiences in the concentration camps, and subsequently by the humanistic psychologists who have emphasized the importance of taking responsibility for our own lives. The choice ultimately comes down to the story we tell ourselves about our suffering. "A lot of the time we might not recognize it as a story," said Joseph, "but really so much of it *is* a story in which we are the hero, the victim, or whatever, and we can reframe it very differently if we choose."[29]

Viktor Frankl, the renowned German psychiatrist Joseph referenced, described his soul-crushing experience at Auschwitz during the Nazi regime in his famous book *Man's Search for Meaning*. He wasn't writing about gay men, or even Americans, but about human beings stretched beyond what anyone ever imagined was their ability to survive excruciating circumstances—the back-breaking work, the starvation, the capricious murders of prisoners, the horrific odors from the crematoria.

"Man *can* preserve a vestige of spiritual freedom, of independence of mind, even in such terrible circumstances of psychic and physical stress," Frankl wrote. "We who lived in concentration camps can remember the men who walked through the huts comforting others, giving away their last piece of bread. They may have been few in number, but they offer sufficient proof that everything can be taken from a man but one thing: the last of the human freedoms—to choose one's attitude in any given set of circumstances, to choose one's own way."[30]

Notes

Chapter One

1. John-Manuel Andriote, "AIDS," *Washington Post*, May 14, 2006, at http://www.washingtonpost.com/wp-dyn/content/article/2006/05/13/AR2006051300033.html, accessed February 1, 2016.

2. Centers for Disease Control and Prevention (CDC), *HIV in the United States: At a Glance*, at www.cdc.gov/hiv/statistics/overview/ataglance.html, accessed January 18, 2016.

3. Centers for Disease Control and Prevention, "About HIV/AIDS," http://www.cdc.gov/hiv/basics/whatishiv.html, accessed February 1, 2016. In 2014 CDC classified three stages of HIV infection. Stage 3, what was known as AIDS, is now defined by having a so-called Stage 3–defining opportunistic infection *besides* the low CD4 count. At http://www.cdc.gov/mmwr/preview/mmwrhtml/rr6303a1.htm?s_cid=rr6303a1_e, accessed June 12, 2016.

4. Tom Ashbrook, "AIDS at 25," *On Point*, May 24, 2006, at http://onpoint.wbur.org/2006/05/24/aids-at-25, accessed February 1, 2016.

Chapter Three

1. John Boswell, *Christianity, Social Tolerance, and Homosexuality* (Chicago: University of Chicago Press, 1980).

Chapter Five

1. Janet Geringer Woititz, *Adult Children of Alcoholics* (Pompano Beach, FL: Health Communications, Inc., 1983).

2. John-Manuel Andriote, "AIDSweek," *Washington City Paper*, June 12, 1987, 6.

Chapter Eight

1. Alice Miller, *The Drama of the Gifted Child: The Search for the True Self* (New York: Basic Books, revised edition, 1997).

2. John-Manuel Andriote, "Healing the 'Broken Places' After 18 Years of Loss," *Provincetown Banner*, September 23, 1999, 9.

Chapter Nine

1. Centers for Disease Control and Prevention, *Human Papilloma Virus (HPV): What Is HPV?* at https://www.cdc.gov/hpv/parents/whatishpv.html, accessed October 30, 2016.

Chapter Eleven

1. Charles Kaiser, *The Gay Metropolis: 1910–1996* (New York: Houghton Mifflin Company, 1997), 188.

2. Peter Filichia, "Bring on the Men!" *Theater Mania*, October 17, 2002, at http://www.theatermania.com/new-york-city-theater/news/10-2002/bring-on-the -men_2682.html, accessed November 5, 2016.

3. George Chauncey, *Gay New York: Gender, Urban Culture, and the Making of the Gay Male World, 1890–1940* (Chicago: University of Chicago Press, 1997), 273.

4. Chauncey, *Gay New York*, 188.

5. Chauncey, *Gay New York*, 187.

6. Chauncey, *Gay New York*, 163.

7. Chauncey, *Gay New York*, 182.

8. Chauncey, *Gay New York*, 183.

9. Chauncey, *Gay New York*, 224.

10. Chauncey, *Gay New York*, 277.

11. Chauncey, *Gay New York*, 281.

12. Chauncey, *Gay New York*, 283.

13. Chauncey, *Gay New York*, 290.

14. Chauncey, *Gay New York*, 249.

15. Chauncey, *Gay New York*, 297–99.

16. Chauncey, *Gay New York*, 17, 19.

17. John Clum, *Something for the Boys: Musical Theater and Gay Culture* (New York: St. Martin's Press, 1999), 168.

18. John Clum, interview with author via Skype, January 25, 2016.

Chapter Twelve

1. Harry Hay, "A Separate People Whose Time Has Come," in *Gay Spirit: Myth and Meaning*, ed. Mark Thompson (New York: St. Martin's Press, 1987), 279–91.

2. Stuart Timmons, *The Trouble with Harry Hay, Founder of the Modern Gay Movement* (Boston: Alyson Publication, 1990), 292.

3. Harry Hay, "A Separate People Whose Time Has Come."

4. Radical Faeries, *Wikipedia*, at https://en.wikipedia.org/wiki/Radical_Faeries, accessed November 17, 2016.

5. John-Manuel Andriote, "Mattachine Society Founder Harry Hay Is Still a Dreamer," *The Washington Blade*, October 19, 1990, 1.

6. Douglass Shand-Tucci, *The Crimson Letter: Harvard, Homosexuality, and the Shaping of American Culture* (New York: St. Martin's Press, 2003), 268.

7. Charles Kaiser, *The Gay Metropolis: 1910–1996* (New York: Houghton Mifflin Company, 1997), 139.

8. John D'Emilio, *Sexual Politics, Sexual Communities: The Making of a Homosexual Minority in the United States, 1940–1970* (Chicago: University of Chicago Press, 1983), 163.

9. Cited in D'Emilio, *Sexual Politics, Sexual Communities*, 164.

10. Kaiser, *The Gay Metropolis*, 148.

11. Rev. Troy Perry, interview via Skype with the author, January 27, 2016.

12. Mark Segal, *And Then I Danced: Traveling the Road to LGBT Equality* (Philadelphia: Akashic Books, 2015), 29.

13. *Village Voice*, July 3, 1969, 18; cited in D'Emilio, *Sexual Politics, Sexual Communities*, 232.

14. Segal, *And Then I Danced*, 30.

15. Segal, *And Then I Danced*, 30.

16. *Village Voice*, July 3, 1969, 18, cited in D'Emilio, *Sexual Politics, Sexual Communities*, 232.

Chapter Thirteen

1. Arnie Kantrowitz, *Under the Rainbow: Growing Up Gay* (New York: St. Martin's Press, 1977; Stonewall Edition paperback 1996), 72.

2. "Homosexuals Hold Protest in 'Village' After Raid Nets 167," *New York Times*, March 8, 1970, 29, at https://www.instagram.com/p/BCu9WsJMM60/, accessed November 17, 2016.

3. Kantrowitz, *Under the Rainbow*, 94.

4. Kantrowitz, *Under the Rainbow*, 100.

5. Kantrowitz, *Under the Rainbow*, 107.

6. Kantrowitz, *Under the Rainbow*, 108.

7. Mark Segal, *And Then I Danced: Traveling the Road to LGBT Equality* (Philadelphia: Akashic Books, 2015), 31.

8. Segal, *And Then I Danced*, 31.

9. Segal, *And Then I Danced*, 35.

10. Barbara Gittings, telephone interview with author, April 8, 1993.

11. John-Manuel Andriote, "Shrinking Opposition," *10 Percent* (Fall 1993).

12. Robert L. Spitzer, MD, "The Homosexuality Decision—A Background Paper," *Psychiatric News*, January 16, 1974, 11.

13. Charles Hite, "APA Rules Homosexuality Not Necessarily a Disorder," *Psychiatric News*, January 2, 1974, 11.

14. John-Manuel Andriote, *Victory Deferred: How AIDS Changed Gay Life in America* (Chicago: University of Chicago Press, 1999), 28.

15. Marcia Chambers, "Ex-City Official Says He's Homosexual," *New York Times*, October 3, 1973, 1, at http://www.nytimes.com/1973/10/03/archives/excity-official-says-hes-homosexual-excity-official-says-hes.html, accessed November 16, 2016.

16. Howard Brown, MD, *Familiar Faces, Hidden Lives: The Story of Homosexual Men in America Today* (New York: Harcourt Brace Jovanovich, 1976), 204, 201.

17. Richard Pillard, MD, telephone interview with author, October 27, 2015.

Chapter Fourteen

1. Larry Kramer, *Reports from the holocaust: The Making of an AIDS Activist* (New York: St. Martin's Press, 1989), 9.

2. Kelsey Louie, "It's Been 35 Years Since Gay Men's Health Crisis Began in Larry Kramer's Living Room," August 11, 2016, at http://www.gmhc.org/content/its-been-35-years-gay-mens-health-crisis-began-larry-kramers-living-room, accessed November 21, 2016.

3. Larry Kramer, interview with author, New York City, March 4, 1995. Cited in John-Manuel Andriote, *Victory Deferred: How AIDS Changed Gay Life in America* (Chicago: University of Chicago Press, 1999), 87.

4. Kramer, *Reports from the holocaust*, 30.

5. Marcus Conant, MD, interview with author, Washington, D.C., July 13, 1995. Cited in Andriote, *Victory Deferred*, 90.

6. Cleve Jones, interview with the author, San Francisco, February 2, 1995. Cited in Andriote, *Victory Deferred*, 90.

7. Jim Graham, interview with the author, Washington, D.C., March 29, 1995. Cited in Andriote, *Victory Deferred*, 93.

8. Eric Rofes, telephone interview with author, July 7, 1995. Cited in Andriote, *Victory Deferred*, 95.

9. Rev. Carl Bean, telephone interview with author, December 12, 2015.

10. Rev. Carl Bean, interview with author, Washington, D.C., November 16, 1995. Cited in Andriote, *Victory Deferred*, 102–4.

Chapter Fifteen

1. Larry Kramer, "1,112 and Counting," *New York Native*, March 14–27, 1983, in *Reports from the holocaust: The Making of an AIDS Activist* (New York: St. Martin's Press, 1989), 33–51.

2. Randy Shilts, *And the Band Played On* (New York: St. Martin's Press, 1987), 131.

3. Paul Boneberg, interview with author, Washington, D.C., August 17, 1995. Cited in Andriote, *Victory Deferred*, 357.

4. Larry Kramer, "The Beginning of ACTing Up/1987," in *Reports from the holocaust*, 128, 135.

5. Hank Wilson, interview with author, San Francisco, January 30, 1995. Cited in Andriote, *Victory Deferred*, 218.

6. Larry Kramer, interview with author, New York City, March 4, 1995. Cited in Andriote, *Victory Deferred*, 216.

7. White Night Riots, *Wikipedia*, at https://en.wikipedia.org/wiki/White_Night_riots, accessed November 22, 2016.

8. Peter Staley, telephone interview with author, June 10, 2016.

9. Avram Finkelstein, Skype interview with author, August 16, 2016.

10. Staley interview.

11. Michael Callen and Dan Turner, "A History of the People with AIDS Self-Empowerment Movement," in *The Sourcebook on Lesbian/Gay Health Care*, eds. Michael Shernoff and William A. Scott (Washington, D.C.: National Lesbian/Gay Health Foundation, 1988), 187–92.

12. Sean Strub, interview with author, Milford, Pennsylvania, June 20, 2016.

13. Staley interview.

14. Paul Boneberg, interview with author, San Francisco, September 8, 2016.

15. Larry Kramer (March 4, 1995, interview), cited in Andriote, *Victory Deferred*, 254.

16. Larry Kramer, interview with author, New York City, July 29, 2015.

Chapter Sixteen

1. Evan Wolfson, "Samesex Marriage and Morality: The Human Rights Vision of the Constitution" (Harvard Law School, April 1983), at http://freemarry.3cdn.net/73aab4141a80237ddf_kxm62r3er.pdf, accessed December 1, 2016.

2. Evan Wolfson, telephone interview with author, November 28, 2016.

3. Wolfson interview.

4. Wolfson interview.

5. Freedom to Marry, "Winning the Freedom to Marry Nationwide: The Inside Story of a Transformative Campaign," 23, at http://www.freedomtomarry.org/pages/how-it-happened, accessed December 1, 2016.

6. Evan Wolfson, "Marriage Equality and Some Lessons for the Scary Work of Winning" (2004), at http://archive-freedomtomarry.org/evan_wolfson/speeches/scary_work_of_winning.php, accessed December 2, 2016.

7. Same-sex marriage in Connecticut, *Wikipedia*, at https://en.wikipedia.org/wiki/Same-sex_marriage_in_Connecticut, accessed December 2, 2016.

8. Maura Dolan, "Judge Strikes Down Prop. 8, Allows Gay Marriage in California [Updated]," *Los Angeles Times*, August 4, 2010, at http://latimesblogs.latimes.com/lanow/2010/08/prop8-gay-marriage.html, accessed December 2, 2016.

9. Freedom to Marry, "Winning the Freedom to Marry Nationwide: The Inside Story of a Transformative Campaign," 78.

10. Michael Barbaro, "A Scramble as Biden Backs Same-Sex Marriage," *New York Times*, May 6, 2012, at http://www.nytimes.com/2012/05/07/us/politics/biden-expresses-support-for-same-sex-marriages.html, accessed December 2, 2016.

11. Jackie Calmes and Peter Baker, "Obama Says Same-Sex Marriage Should Be Legal," *New York Times*, May 9, 2012, at http://www.nytimes.com/2012/05/10/us/politics/obama-says-same-sex-marriage-should-be-legal.html, accessed December 2, 2016.

12. California Proposition 8 (2008), *Wikipedia*, at https://en.wikipedia.org/wiki/California_Proposition_8_(2008), accessed December 2, 2016.

13. Defense of Marriage Act, *Wikipedia*, at https://en.wikipedia.org/wiki/Defense_of_Marriage_Act, accessed December 2, 2016.

14. *United States v. Windsor*, *Wikipedia*, at https://en.wikipedia.org/wiki/United_States_v._Windsor#cite_note-84, accessed December 2, 2016.

15. Freedom to Marry, "Winning the Freedom to Marry Nationwide: The Inside Story of a Transformative Campaign," 91.

16. Roberta Kaplan, "Gay Rights: Change Is Gonna Come. The Torah Says So," *Tablet*, November 23, 2016, at http://www.tabletmag.com/scroll/218446/gay-rights change-is-gonna-come-the-torah-says-so, accessed December 2, 2016.

17. Mary Bruce, "DOMA Ruling: 'Victory for American Democracy,' Obama Says," *ABC News*, June 27, 2013.

18. The White House, Obama Administration Statements on the Supreme Court's DOMA Ruling, June 27, 2013, at https://www.whitehouse.gov/blog/2013/06/27/obama-administration-statements-supreme-court-s-doma-ruling, accessed December 2, 2016.

19. Freedom to Marry, "Winning the Freedom to Marry Nationwide: The Inside Story of a Transformative Campaign," 96.

20. Freedom to Marry, "Winning the Freedom to Marry Nationwide: The Inside Story of a Transformative Campaign," 104.

21. Freedom to Marry, "Winning the Freedom to Marry Nationwide: The Inside Story of a Transformative Campaign," 108.

22. The Supreme Court of the United States, *Obergefell v. Hodges*, at https://s3-us-west-2.amazonaws.com/ftm-assets/ftm/archive/files/pdfs/SCOTUSObergefell Opinion.pdf, accessed December 1, 2016.

23. Evan Wolfson, "What's Next in the Fight for Gay Equality?" *New York Times*, June 26, 2015, at http://www.nytimes.com/2015/06/27/opinion/evan-wolfson-whats -next-in-the-fight-for-gay-equality.html, accessed December 2, 2016.

24. Wolfson interview.

Overview: Part III

1. Peter M. Nardi, *Gay Men's Friendships: Invincible Communities* (Chicago: University of Chicago Press, 1999), 206.

Chapter Seventeen

1. Sean Duggan, interview with author, New York City, July 31, 2015.

2. Barbara Althen, interview with author, Norwich, Connecticut, September 3, 2015.

3. PFLAG, "Our Story," at https://www.pflag.org/our-story, accessed December 14, 2016.

4. GLSEN, *2015 State Snapshot: School Climate in Connecticut*, at https://www .glsen.org/sites/default/files/Connecticut%20State%20Snapshot%20-%20NSCS .pdf, accessed January 12, 2017.

5. Charles Lynch, interview with author, Norwich, Connecticut, November 8, 2010.

6. Kathy and Tim Duggan, interview with author, Norwich, Connecticut, August 3, 2015.

7. Sean Duggan interview, 2015.

Chapter Eighteen

1. Interview with author, Burlington, Vermont, August 11, 2016.

2. Stephen Cadwell and Joe Levine, interview with author, Concord, Massachusetts, March 14, 2016.

3. John-Manuel Andriote, "For Pride Month, Daring to Be Wild and Precious in a New One-Man Show," *Huffington Post*, June 13, 2014, at http://www.huffington post.com/johnmanuel-andriote/for-pride-month-daring-to_b_5492213.html, accessed December 18, 2016.

Chapter Nineteen

1. Samuel Medina, interview with author, Willimantic, Connecticut, February 15, 2016.

2. Kamora Herrington, telephone interview with author, January 6, 2016.

3. William Pollack, *Real Boys: Rescuing Our Sons from the Myths of Boyhood* (New York: Random House, 1998), 23–24.

4. GLSEN, *2015 National School Climate Survey*, at https://www.glsen.org/article/2015-national-school-climate-survey, accessed December 26, 2016.

5. Pollack, *Real Boys*, 226.

6. Thomas Krever, interview with author, New York City, July 30, 2015.

7. Carl Siciliano, interview with author, New York City, July 30, 2015.

8. L. E. Durso, and G. J. Gates. *Serving Our Youth: Findings from a National Survey of Service Providers Working with Lesbian, Gay, Bisexual, and Transgender Youth Who Are Homeless or at Risk of Becoming Homeless.* Los Angeles: The Williams Institute with True Colors Fund and The Palette Fund (2012), at http://williamsinstitute.law.ucla.edu/wp-content/uploads/Durso-Gates-LGBT-Homeless-Youth-Survey-July-2012.pdf, accessed December 30, 2016.

9. B. Mustanski, M. Newcomb, and R. Garofalo, "Mental Health of Lesbian, Gay, and Bisexual Youth: A Developmental Resiliency Perspective," *Journal of Gay and Lesbian Social Services* 23, no. 2 (January 1, 2011): 204–25.

10. C. Ryan, D. Huebner, R. M. Diaz, and J. Sanchez. "Family Rejection as a Predictor of Negative Health Outcomes in White and Latino Lesbian, Gay, and Bisexual Young Adults," *Pediatrics* 1 (January 2009): 346–52.

11. Substance Abuse and Mental Health Services Administration, *A Practitioner's Resource Guide: Helping Families to Support Their LGBT Children.* HHS Publication No. PEP14-LGBTKIDS (Rockville, MD: Substance Abuse and Mental Health Services Administration, 2014).

12. Caitlin Ryan, telephone interview with author, February 1, 2013.

13. Caitlin Ryan, *Supportive Families, Healthy Children* (San Francisco: Family Acceptance Project, San Francisco State University, 2009).

14. Ryan interview, February 1, 2013.

15. Caitlin Conor Ryan, interview with author, Boston, Massachusetts, October 21, 2016.

16. Ryan, 2013 interview.

Chapter Twenty

1. John Riley, "Pride and Mourning," *MetroWeekly* (Washington, D.C.), June 16, 2016, 34–35.

2. President Obama addresses the nation after Orlando shooting, at https://www.youtube.com/watch?v=gOH7F0XCqpw, accessed January 4, 2017.

3. Kevin Naff, "A Tribute to Gay Bars," *Washington Blade* 47, no. 25 (June 14, 2016): 32.

4. Megan Rosenfeld, "At Ziegfeld's, Queen for a Night," *Washington Post*, August 2, 2001, 32, at https://www.washingtonpost.com/archive/lifestyle/2001/08/02/at-ziegfelds-queens-for-a-night/395ad8ff-4be8-4968-90fb-d61afc37f2bf/?utm_term=.1bcaeac62d8f, accessed January 4, 2016.

5. Christina Aguilera, "Change," at https://www.youtube.com/watch?v=OBSghlH0JgM, accessed January 4, 2017.

6. Rosenfeld, "At Ziegfeld's, Queen for a Night."

7. Lou Chibbaro Jr., "Academy Drag Group Disbands after 54-Year Run," *Washington Blade*, October 28, 2015, at http://www.washingtonblade.com/2015/10/28/academy-drag-group-disbands-after-54-year-run/, accessed January 5, 2016.

8. Donnell Robinson, telephone interview with author, February 10, 2016; interview with author, Arlington, Virginia, June 19, 2016.

9. Jennie Livingston, producer and director, *Paris Is Burning* (1990), at https://www.youtube.com/watch?v=hedJer7I1vI, accessed January 5, 2017.

10. Katrina Kubicek, Miles McNeeley, Ian W. Holloway, George Weiss, and Michele Kipke, "'It's Like Our Own Little World': Resilience as a Factor of Participation in the Ballroom Community Subculture," *AIDS Behavior* 17, no. 4 (May 2013): 1524–39.

11. CenterLink, *History of the LGBT Center Movement*, at http://www.lgbtcenters org/centerlink-history.aspx, accessed January 6, 2017.

12. Terry Stone, telephone interview with author, January 5, 2016.

13. Los Angeles LGBT Center, "About the Center: Anita May Rosenstein Campus," at https://lalgbtcenter.org/about-the-center/anita-may-rosenstein-campus, accessed January 6, 2017.

14. Lorri L. Jean, telephone interview with author, May 11, 2016.

Chapter Twenty-One

1. Rev. Carl Bean, telephone interview with author, December 12, 2015.

2. GLAAD in conjunction with the University of Missouri Center on Religion & the Professions, *Missing Voices: A Study of Religious Voices in Mainstream Media Reports about LGBT Equality* (April 2012), at glaad.org/missingvoices, accessed January 9, 2017.

3. Pew Research Center, *America's Changing Religious Landscape* (May 12, 2015), at http://www.pewforum.org/2015/05/12/americas-changing-religious-landscape/, accessed January 9, 2017.

4. Eliel Cruz, "LGBT People of Faith: Why Are They Staying?" Advocate.com, September 17, 2015, at http://www.advocate.com/religion/2015/9/17/lgbt-people -faith-why-are-they-staying, accessed January 9, 2017.

5. Rev. Troy Perry, Skype interview with author, January 27, 2016.

6. Rev. Dr. Mel White: Clergyman, Author, Activist, *Mel & Gary's Story*, at http://melwhite.org/mel-garys-story.

7. Rev. Dr. Mel White, telephone interview with author, December 10, 2015.

8. Rev. Dr. Mel White, email to author, March 1, 2017.

9. Mel White, *How to Resist Extremism!: A Pocket Guide to the Practice of Relentless Nonviolent Resistance*, at http://melwhite.org/wp-content/uploads/2016/05/Resist -Extremism.pdf, accessed January 10, 2017.

10. Rabbi Sharon Kleinbaum, interview with author, New York City, May 10, 2016.

11. Congregation Beit Simchat Torah, Dedication (official program), April 3, 2016.

12. Azmat Khan, "Meet America's First Openly Gay Imam," Aljazeera America, at http://america.aljazeera.com/watch/shows/america-tonight/america-tonight-blog/2013/12/20/meet-america-s-firstopenlygayimam.html, accessed January 10, 2017.

13. Imam Daayiee Abdullah, interview with author, Washington, D.C., June 16, 2016.

14. Kimberly Wreston, "Episcopal Church Suspended from Full Participation in Anglican Communion," Religion News Service, January 14, 2016, at http://religionnews.com/2016/01/14/episcopal-church-suspended-anglican-communion/, accessed January 11, 2017.

15. Gene Robinson, Wikipedia, at https://en.wikipedia.org/wiki/Gene_Robinson, accessed January 11, 2017.

16. Rt. Rev. V. Gene Robinson, telephone interview with author, April 14, 2016.

Chapter Twenty-Two

1. Richard A. Rasi and Lourdes Rodríguez-Nogués, eds., *Out in the Workplace: The Pleasures and Perils of Coming Out on the Job* (Los Angeles: Alyson Publications, 1995). Note that all quotations attributed to Rasi are from his essay "Dis-Integration" in this book.

2. Rodríguez-Nogués, interview with author, Boston, Massachusetts, August 6, 2015.

3. Brian McNaught, *Gay Issues in the Workplace* (New York: St. Martin's Press, 1993; first paperback edition 1995), 35.

4. Brian McNaught, telephone interview with author, October 29, 2015.

5. Todd Sears, telephone interview with author, November 6, 2015.

6. Stephen Snyder-Hill, *Soldier of Change: From the Closet to the Forefront of the Gay Rights Movement* (Lincoln: Potomac Books/University of Nebraska Press, 2014), 28–29.

7. Stephen Snyder-Hill, "Trust the Power of Your Voice," TED talk at Ohio State University, February 14, 2015, at https://www.youtube.com/watch?v=RPN_GnN027g, accessed January 17, 2017.

8. Stephen Snyder-Hill, TED talk (2015).

9. Stephen Snyder-Hill, TED talk (2015).

10. Leonard Matlovich, *Wikipedia*, at https://en.wikipedia.org/wiki/Leonard_Matlovich, accessed January 17, 2017.

11. GOP Debate Question Booed Soldier, at https://www.youtube.com/watch?v=ZvIittOP5r8, accessed January 18, 2017.

12. George Takei, in Stephen Snyder-Hill, *Soldier of Change*, ix–x.

13. Stephen Snyder-Hill, TED talk (2015).

14. Stephen and Joshua Snyder-Hill, telephone interview with author, February 23, 2016.

15. Stephen Snyder-Hill, 2016 interview.

16. Stephen Snyder-Hill, 2016 interview.

17. Barney Frank, *Frank: A Life in Politics from the Great Society to Same-Sex Marriage* (New York: Farrar, Straus and Giroux, 2015), 151.

18. Frank, *Frank*, 51.

19. Barney Frank, *Wikipedia*, at https://en.wikipedia.org/wiki/Barney_Frank, accessed January 18, 2017.

20. Barney Frank, telephone interview with author, October 13, 2016.

21. Michael Oreskes, "Representative Frank Asks for Full Inquiry by Ethics Panel," *New York Times*, August 29, 1989, at http://www.nytimes.com/1989/08/29/us/rep-frank-asks-for-full-inquiry-by-ethics-panel.html, accessed January 18, 2017.

22. Associated Press, "Barney Frank Calls Craig a 'Hypocrite,'" EdgeMediaNetwork.com, August 30, 2007, at http://boston.edgemedianetwork.com/index php?id=36258&pf=1, accessed January 18, 2017.

23. Barney Frank, *Frank*, 245.

24. Barney Frank, *Frank*, 246.

25. Frank interview.

26. Frank interview.

27. Michael Guest, telephone interview with author, June 29, 2016.

28. Michael Guest, Wikipedia, at https://en.wikipedia.org/wiki/Michael_Guest, accessed January 19, 2017.

29. *New York Times* Editorial Board, "Unequal Treatment at the State Department," *New York Times*, December 3, 2007, at https://theboard.blogs.nytimes.com/2007/12/03/unequal-treatment-at-the-state-department/, accessed January 19, 2017.

30. Michael Guest interview.

31. *New York Times* Editorial Board (December 3, 2007).

32. Michael Guest interview.

33. Michael Guest interview.

Chapter Twenty-Three

1. U.S. Department of Justice, Civil Rights Division, Disability Rights Section, Questions and Answers: The Americans with Disabilities Act and Persons with HIV/AIDS, at https://www.ada.gov/hiv/ada_q&a_aids.htm, accessed January 23, 2017.

2. Centers for Disease Control and Prevention, Fast Facts: HIV Among Gay and Bisexual Men, at https://www.cdc.gov/hiv/group/msm/, accessed January 22, 2017.

3. H. Alexander Satorie-Robinson, telephone interview with author, January 30, 2013.

4. Elizabeth Kastor, "Advocates in the Realm of Sorrows," *Washington Post*, February 23, 1988, at https://www.washingtonpost.com/archive/lifestyle/1988/02/23/advocates-in-the-realm-of-sorrows/47af4e93-b56e-470a-9f16-0153931e84af/?utm_term=.7a7acb952d5a, accessed January 27, 2017.

5. Mauro Walden-Montoya, telephone interview with author, February 28, 2016.

6. Steve Lew, *Wikipedia*, at https://en.wikipedia.org/wiki/Steve_Lew, accessed January 23, 2017.

7. Steve Lew, telephone interview with author, May 12, 2016.

8. John Killacky, telephone interview with author, January 25, 2013.

9. John Killacky and Larry Connolly, interview with author, Burlington, Vermont, August 12, 2016.

10. John Killacky, producer, *Holding On* (2006), at https://www.youtube.com/watch?v=RVwAHT5_lc8, accessed January 24, 2017.

11. John Killacky, "Careening Toward Kensho: Ruminations on Disability and Community," in *Queer Crips: Disabled Gay Men and Their Stories*, eds. Bob Guter and John R. Killacky (New York: Routledge, 2004), 58–59.

12. Larry Connolly, telephone interview with author, January 30, 2013.

13. Killacky, 2013 interview.

Chapter Twenty-Four

1. John-Manuel Andriote, "Meth Comes Out of the Closet," *Washington Post*, November 8, 2005, at http://www.washingtonpost.com/wp-dyn/content/article/2005/11/04/AR2005110402178.html, accessed January 24, 2017.

2. Chad Upham, Skype interview with author, February 17, 2016.

3. Ronald D. Stall, telephone interview with author, June 8, 2010.

4. Congregation for the Doctrine of the Faith, "Letter to the Bishops of the Catholic Church on the Pastoral Care of Homosexual Persons" (The Vatican, 1986), at http://www.vatican.va/roman_curia/congregations/cfaith/documents/rc_con_cfaith_doc_19861001_homosexual-persons_en.html, accessed January 26, 2017.

5. Stall interview, June 8, 2010.

6. R. Stall, T. C. Mills, J. Williamson, T. Hart, C. Greenwood, and J. Paul et al. "Association of Co-occurring Psychosocial Health Problems and Increased Vulnerability to HIV/AIDS among Urban Men Who Have Sex with Men," *American Journal of Public Health* 93, no. 6 (2003): 939–42.

7. Ronald Stall, telephone interview with author, January 28, 2013.

8. A. L. Herrick, S. H. Lim, C. Wei, H. Smith, T. Guadamuz, M. S. Friedman, and R. Stall, "Resilience as an Untapped Resource in Behavioral Intervention Design for Gay Men," *AIDS and Behavior* 15 Suppl. (April 2011): S25–29. doi: 10.1007/s10461-011-9895-0.

9. NIH LGBT Research Coordinating Committee, *Consideration of the Institute of Medicine (IOM) Report on the Health of Lesbian, Gay, Bisexual, and Transgender (LGBT) Individuals* (January 2013), at https://report.nih.gov/UploadDocs/LGBT%20Health%20Report_FINAL_2013-01-03-508%20compliant.pdf, accessed January 26, 2017.

10. Ron Stall, January 28, 2013, interview.

11. Stephen F. Morin, telephone interview with author, January 30, 2013.

12. J. J. Walker, B. Longmire-Avital, and S. Golub, "Racial and Sexual Identities as Potential Buffers to Risky Sexual Behavior for Black Gay and Bisexual

Emerging Adult Men," *Health Psychology* 34, no. 8 (August 2015): 841–46. doi: 10.1037/hea0000187, epub December 22, 2014, at https://www.ncbi.nlm.nih.gov/pubmed/25528178, accessed January 26, 2017.

13. Ilan H. Meyer, telephone interview with author, November 20, 2015.

14. Gregory M. Herek, telephone interview with author, February 2, 2013.

15. P. N. Halkitis, "Reframing HIV Prevention for Gay Men in the United States," *American Psychologist* 65, no. 8 (November 2010): 752–63. doi: 10.1037/0003-066X.65.8.752.

16. Perry N. Halkitis, telephone interview with author, February 19, 2016.

17. Kenneth H. Mayer, MD, telephone interview with author, February 12, 2016.

18. J. K. Williams, L. Wilton, and M. Magnus et al. "Relation of Childhood Sexual Abuse, Intimate Partner Violence, and Depression to Risk Factors for HIV among Black Men Who Have Sex with Men in 6 US Cities," *American Journal of Public Health* 105, no. 12 (December 2015): 2473–81. doi: 10.2105/AJPH.2015.3028/8.

19. M. S. Boroughs, S. E. Valentine, G. H. Ironson, J. C. Shipherd, S. A. Safren, S. W. Taylor, S. K. Dale, J. S. Baker, J. G. Wilner, and C. O'Cleirigh, "Complexity of Childhood Sexual Abuse: Predictors of Current Post-Traumatic Stress Disorder, Mood Disorders, Substance Use, and Sexual Risk Behavior among Adult Men Who Have Sex with Men," *Archives of Sexual Behavior* 44, no. 7 (October 2015): 1891–902. doi: 10.1007/s10508-015-0546-9.

20. Conall O'Cleirigh, email to author, January 25, 2017.

21. Conall O'Cleirigh, telephone interview with author, March 17, 2016.

22. Centers for Disease Control and Prevention, Pre-Exposure Prophylaxis (PrEP), at https://www.cdc.gov/hiv/risk/prep/, accessed January 28, 2017.

23. O'Cleirigh, email, January 25, 2017.

24. Jim Pickett, interview with author, Chicago, October 6, 2016.

25. John-Manuel Andriote, "The LGBT Health Movement, 40 Years Since Homosexuality Was a Mental Illness," *The Atlantic*, June 26, 2013, at http://www.theatlantic.com/health/archive/2013/06/the-lgbt-health-movement-40-years-since-homosexuality-was-a-mental-illness/277154/, accessed January 30, 2017.

26. John A. Schneider, MD, telephone interview with author, June 10, 2013.

27. John A. Schneider, MD, interview with author, Chicago, October 7, 2016.

28. Gregory Rebchook, telephone interview with author, January 29, 2013.

29. S. M. Kegeles, R. B. Hays, and T. J. Coates, "The Mpowerment Project: A Community-Level HIV Prevention Intervention for Young Gay Men," *American Journal of Public Health* 86 (Pt. 1) (August 1996): 1129–36.

30. Gregory Rebchook, interview with author, San Francisco, September 6, 2016.

31. Erin Allday, "Last Man Standing," *San Francisco Chronicle*, March 2016, at http://projects.sfchronicle.com/2016/living-with-aids/story/, accessed January 28, 2017.

32. Edward Machtinger, MD, telephone interview with author, November 4, 2016.

33. Emily Newman, "Strut: A New Home for Health & Wellness in San Francisco," *Beta*, September 25, 2015, at http://betablog.org/strut-a-new-home-for-health-wellness-in-san-francisco/, accessed January 28, 2017.

34. Steven Bracko, "After 13 Years, Magnet Founder Steve Gibson Moves On," *Hoodline*, April 19, 2016, at http://hoodline.com/2016/04/after-13-years-magnet -founder-steve-gibson-moves-on, accessed January 29, 2017.

35. Eric Rofes, *Dry Bones Breathe: Gay Men Creating Post-AIDS Identities and Culture* (New York: Harrington Park Press, 1998), 219, 231–32.

36. Steve Gibson, telephone interview with author, September 19, 2016.

37. Rainbow Honor Walk, at http://rainbowhonorwalk.org/?page_id=77, accessed January 28, 2017.

Chapter Twenty-Five

1. Harold Kooden with Charles Flowers, *Golden Men: The Power of Gay Midlife* (New York: William Morrow Paperbacks, 2000), back cover, 3.

2. John-Manuel Andriote and Tom Lutz, "John Rechy: An Interview," *Los Angeles Review of Books* (Fall 2014), at https://lareviewofbooks.org/article/john-rechy -interview/, accessed January 29, 2017.

3. Harold Kooden, interview with author, New York City, July 30, 2015.

4. Ken South, Skype interview with author, January 24, 2016.

5. Walt Whitman, "Halcyon Days," in *Leaves of Grass*. (Originally published 1855; Walt Whitman Archive, at http://whitmanarchive.org/published/LG/1891/ poems/324, accessed January 29, 2017.)

6. Richard G. Wight, Allen J. LeBlanc, Brian de Vries, and Roger Detels, "Stress and Mental Health among Midlife and Older Gay-Identified Men," *American Journal of Public Health* 102 (2012): 503–10.

7. Richard G. Wight, Allen J. LeBlanc, Ilan H. Meyer, and Frederick Harig, "Internalized Gay Ageism, Mattering, and Depressive Symptoms among Midlife and Older Gay-Identified Men," *Social Science & Medicine* 147 (2015): 200–8.

8. Brian de Vries, "Stigma and LGBT Aging: Negative and Positive Marginality," in *The Lives of LGBT Older Adults: Understanding the Challenges and Resilience*, ed. N. A. Orel and C. A Fruhauf (p. 63) (Washington, D.C.: The American Psychological Association, 2015).

9. Brian de Vries, telephone interview with author, February 1, 2013.

10. Karen I. Frederiksen-Goldsen et al., *The Aging and Health Report: Disparities and Resilience Among Lesbian, Gay, Bisexual, and Transgender Older Adults* (New York: SAGE, 2011), at http://depts.washington.edu/agepride/wordpress/wp-content/ uploads/2011/05/Full-Report-FINAL-11-16-11.pdf, accessed January 30, 2017.

11. Brian de Vries, telephone interview with author, April 18, 2016.

12. Lorri L. Jean, telephone interview with author, May 11, 2016.

13. SAGE, Mission and History, at sageusa.org, accessed January 30, 2017.

14. Catherine Thurston, interview with author, New York City, July 31, 2015.

15. Thomas Weber, telephone interview with author, January 28, 2016.

16. Edward Alwood, "Walter Cronkite and the Gay Rights Movement," *Washington Post*, July 26, 2009, at http://www.washingtonpost.com/wp-dyn/content/ article/2009/07/24/AR2009072402084.html, accessed January 30, 2017.

17. SAGE, Economic Security, at https://www.sageusa.org/issues/economic.cfm, accessed January 31, 2017.

18. Inga Saffron, "Changing Skyline: John C. Anderson Apartments, LGBT-Friendly and Urban-Friendly," *Philadelphia Inquirer*, January 18, 2014, at http://www.philly.com/philly/columnists/inga_saffron/20140117_Changing_Skyline__John_C__Anderson_Apartments__LGBT-friendly_and_urban-friendly.html, accessed January 31, 2017.

19. Emily Wax-Thibodeaux, "A Philadelphia Apartment Building May Be a National Model for Low-Income LGBT Seniors," *Washington Post*, September 12, 2014, at https://www.washingtonpost.com/politics/a-philadelphia-apartment-building-may-be-a-national-model-for-low-income-lgbt-seniors/2014/09/12/f64e06bc-352d-11e4-8f02-03c644b2d7d0_story.html?utm_term=.83ced0ec6d38, accessed January 30, 2017.

20. John James, interview with author, Philadelphia, March 9, 2016.

21. Mark Segal, interview with author, Philadelphia, March 9, 2016.

22. Frank Stenglein, telephone interview with author, February 3, 2013.

Chapter Twenty-Six

1. Portland, Maine, *Wikipedia*, at https://en.wikipedia.org/wiki/Portland,_Maine, accessed January 31, 2017.

2. 1866 Great Fire of Portland, Maine, *Wikipedia*, at https://en.wikipedia.org/wiki/1866_Great_fire_of_Portland,_Maine, accessed January 31, 2017.

3. Henry Wadsworth Longfellow, "Letter to George Washington Greene," in *The Letters of Henry Wadsworth Longfellow*, ed. Andrew R. Hilen (Cambridge: Harvard University Press, 1982), 66.

4. John Preston (Michael Lowenthal, ed.), *Winter's Light: Reflections of a Yankee Queer* (Hanover, NH: University Press of New England, 1995), 28–29.

5. Preston, *Winter's Light*, 101.

6. Preston, *Winter's Light*, 106.

7. Barbara Peabody, interview with author, Tucson, Arizona, December 28, 2016.

8. Preston, *Winter's Light*, 115–24.

9. Frannie Peabody (biographical sketch), Frannie Peabody Center, at http://peabodycenter.org/wp-content/uploads/2013/07/Frannie-Peabody.Bio-Sum.kmills.4-07.pdf, accessed February 1, 2017.

10. Katie Rutherford, telephone interview with author, September 1, 2016.

11. David Simpson, telephone interview with author, September 30, 2016.

12. Preston, *Winter's Light*, 133.

13. Preston, *Winter's Light*, xix.

14. Preston, *Winter's Light*, 30.

15. Bill Nemitz, "Backstory Makes 'Good' Portland Slogan Even Better," *Portland Press Herald*, June 19, 2013, at http://www.pressherald.com/2013/06/19/why-yes_-lifes-good-here-gets-better-still-_2013-06-19/, accessed February 1, 2017.

16. Gay Men's Health Crisis, at http://gmhc.org/about-us/about-us, accessed February 1, 2017.

17. Kelsey Louie, interview with author, New York City, May 9, 2016.

18. John Cunningham and Mike Shriver, interview with author, San Francisco, September 8, 2016.

19. Tez Anderson, interview with author, San Francisco, September 8, 2016.

20. Terry Beswick, interview with author, San Francisco, September 8, 2016.

21. Cunningham and Shriver interview.

22. John D'Emilio, telephone interview with author, October 28, 2015.

23. Timothy McFeeley, Skype interview with author, February 14, 2016.

24. Barney Frank, telephone interview with author, October 13, 2016.

25. Tracy Baim, interview with author, Chicago, October 7, 2016.

26. Bob Smith, email to author, December 29, 2015.

27. Sampson McCormick, Skype interview with author, February 9, 2016.

28. Stephen Joseph, *What Doesn't Kill Us: The Psychology of Posttraumatic Growth* (New York: Basic Books, 2011), xii, xiv.

29. Stephen Joseph, email to author, January 19, 2016.

30. Viktor E. Frankl, *Man's Search for Meaning* (Boston: Beacon Press, 2006), 65–66.

Bibliography

Aguilera, Christina. "Change." https://www.youtube.com/watch?v=OBSghlH0JgM (accessed January 4, 2017).

Allday, Erin. "Last Man Standing." *San Francisco Chronicle*, March 2016. http://projects.sfchronicle.com/2016/living-with-aids/story/ (accessed January 28, 2017).

Alwood, Edward. "Walter Cronkite and the Gay Rights Movement." *Washington Post*, July 26, 2009. http://www.washingtonpost.com/wp-dyn/content/article/2009/07/24/AR2009072402084.html (accessed January 30, 2017).

Andriote, John-Manuel. "AIDSweek." *Washington City Paper*, June 12, 1987, 6.

Andriote, John-Manuel. "Mattachine Society Founder Harry Hay Is Still a Dreamer." *Washington Blade*, October 19, 1990, 1.

Andriote, John-Manuel. *Victory Deferred: How AIDS Changed Gay Life in America.* Chicago: University of Chicago Press, 1999.

Andriote, John-Manuel. "Healing the 'Broken Places' After 18 Years of Loss." *Provincetown Banner*, September 23, 1999, 9.

Andriote, John-Manuel. "Meth Comes Out of the Closet." *Washington Post*, November 8, 2005. http://www.washingtonpost.com/wp-dyn/content/article/2005/11/04/AR2005110402178.html (accessed January 24, 2017).

Andriote, John-Manuel. "AIDS." *Washington Post*, May 14, 2006. http://www.washingtonpost.com/wp-dyn/content/article/2006/05/13/AR2006051300033.html (accessed February 1, 2016).

Andriote, John-Manuel. "The LGBT Health Movement, 40 Years Since Homosexuality Was a Mental Illness." The Atlantic.com, June 26, 2013. http://www.theatlantic.com/health/archive/2013/06/the-lgbt-health-movement-40-years-since-homosexuality-was-a-mental-illness/277154/ (accessed January 30, 2017).

Andriote, John-Manuel, "For Pride Month, Daring to Be Wild and Precious in a New One-Man Show." *Huffington Post*, June 13, 2014. http://www.huffingtonpost.com/johnmanuel-andriote/for-pride-month-daring-to_b_5492213.html (accessed December 18, 2016).

Andriote, John-Manuel, and Tom Lutz. "John Rechy: An Interview." *Los Angeles Review of Books*, Fall 2014. https://lareviewofbooks.org/article/john-rechy-interview/ (accessed January 29, 2017).

Ashbrook, Tom. "AIDS at 25." *On Point*. May 24, 2006. http://onpoint.wbur.org/2006/05/24/aids-at-25 (accessed February 1, 2016).

Associated Press. "Barney Frank Calls Craig a 'Hypocrite.'" EdgeMediaNetwork.com, August 30, 2007. http://boston.edgemedianetwork.com/index.php?id=36258&pf=1 (accessed January 18, 2017).

Barbaro, Michael. "A Scramble as Biden Backs Same-Sex Marriage." *New York Times*, May 6, 2012. http://www.nytimes.com/2012/05/07/us/politics/biden-expresses-support-for-same-sex-marriages.html (accessed December 2, 2016).

Boroughs M. S., S. E. Valentine, G. H. Ironson, J. C. Shipherd, S. A. Safren, S. W. Taylor, S. K. Dale, J. S. Baker, J. G. Wilner, and C. O'Cleirigh. "Complexity of Childhood Sexual Abuse: Predictors of Current Post-Traumatic Stress Disorder, Mood Disorders, Substance Use, and Sexual Risk Behavior Among Adult Men Who Have Sex with Men." *Archives of Sexual Behavior* 44, no. 7 (October 2015): 1891–1902.

Boswell, John. *Christianity, Social Tolerance, and Homosexuality*. Chicago: University of Chicago Press, 1980.

Bracko, Steven. "After 13 Years, Magnet Founder Steve Gibson Moves On." *Hoodline*, April 19, 2016. http://hoodline.com/2016/04/after-13-years-magnet-founder-steve-gibson-moves-on (accessed January 29, 2017).

Brown, Howard. *Familiar Faces, Hidden Lives: The Story of Homosexual Men in America Today*. New York: Harcourt Brace Jovanovich, 1976.

Bruce, Mary. "DOMA Ruling: 'Victory for American Democracy,' Obama Says." *ABC News*, June 27, 2013.

California Proposition 8 (2008). *Wikipedia*. https://en.wikipedia.org/wiki/California_Proposition_8_(2008) (accessed December 2, 2016).

Callen, Michael, and Dan Turner. "A History of the People with AIDS Self-Empowerment Movement." In *The Sourcebook on Lesbian/Gay Health Care*, eds. Michael Shernoff and William A. Scott (pp. 187–92). Washington, D.C.: National Lesbian/Gay Health Foundation, 1988.

Calmes, Jackie, and Peter Baker. "Obama Says Same-Sex Marriage Should Be Legal." *New York Times*, May 9, 2012. http://www.nytimes.com/2012/05/10/us/politics/obama-says-same-sex-marriage-should-be-legal.html (accessed December 2, 2016).

CenterLink. *History of the LGBT Center Movement*. http://www.lgbtcenters.org/centerlink-history.aspx (accessed January 6, 2017).

Centers for Disease Control and Prevention. Fast Facts: HIV Among Gay and Bisexual Men. https://www.cdc.gov/hiv/group/msm/ (accessed January 22, 2017).

Centers for Disease Control and Prevention. *HIV in the United States: At a Glance.* www.cdc.gov/hiv/statistics/overview/ataglance.html (accessed January 18, 2016).

Centers for Disease Control and Prevention. "About HIV-AIDS." http://www.cdc.gov/ hiv/basics/whatishiv.html (accessed February 1, 2016). http://www.cdc.gov/mmwr/ preview/mmwrhtml/rr6303a1.htm?s_cid=rr6303a1_e (accessed June 12, 2016).

Centers for Disease Control and Prevention. *Human Papilloma Virus (HPV): What Is HPV?* https://www.cdc.gov/hpv/parents/whatishpv.html (accessed October 30, 2016).

Centers for Disease Control and Prevention. Pre-Exposure Prophylaxis (PrEP). https://www.cdc.gov/hiv/risk/prep/ (accessed January 28, 2017).

Chambers, Marcia. "Ex-City Official Says He's Homosexual." *New York Times,* October 3, 1973, 1. http://www.nytimes.com/1973/10/03/archives/excity-official -says-hes-homosexual-excity-official-says-hes.html (accessed November 16, 2016).

Chauncey, George. *Gay New York: Gender, Urban Culture, and the Making of the Gay Male World, 1890–1940.* Chicago: University of Chicago Press, 1997.

Chibbaro, Jr., Lou. "Academy Drag Group Disbands After 54-Year Run." *Washington Blade,* October 28, 2015. http://www.washingtonblade.com/2015/10/28/academy -drag-group-disbands-after-54-year-run/ (accessed January 5, 2016).

Clum, John. *Something for the Boys: Musical Theater and Gay Culture.* New York: St. Martin's Press, 1999.

Congregation for the Doctrine of the Faith. "Letter to the Bishops of the Catholic Church on the Pastoral Care of Homosexual Persons." The Vatican, 1986. http:// www.vatican.va/roman_curia/congregations/cfaith/documents/rc_con_cfaith_ doc_19861001_homosexual-persons_en.html (accessed January 26, 2017).

Cruz, Eliel. "LGBT People of Faith: Why Are They Staying?" *Advocate.com,* September 17, 2015. http://www.advocate.com/religion/2015/9/17/lgbt-people-faith-why -are-they-staying (accessed January 9, 2017).

Defense of Marriage Act. *Wikipedia.* https://en.wikipedia.org/wiki/Defense_of_Mar riage_Act (accessed December 2, 2016).

D'Emilio, John. *Sexual Politics, Sexual Communities: The Making of a Homosexual Minority in the United States, 1940–1970.* Chicago: University of Chicago Press, 1983.

De Vries, Brian. "Stigma and LGBT Aging: Negative and Positive Marginality." *The Lives of LGBT Older Adults: Understanding Challenges and Resilience,* ed. N. A. Orel and C. A. Fruhauf (p. 63). Washington, D.C.: The American Psychological Association, 2015.

Dolan, Maura. "Judge Strikes Down Prop. 8, Allows Gay Marriage in California [Updated]." *Los Angeles Times,* August 4, 2010. http://latimesblogs.latimes.com/ lanow/2010/08/prop8-gay-marriage.html (accessed December 2, 2016).

Durso, L. E., and G. J. Gates. *Serving Our Youth: Findings from a National Survey of Service Providers Working with Lesbian, Gay, Bisexual, and Transgender Youth Who Are Homeless or at Risk of Becoming Homeless.* Los Angeles: The Williams Institute with True Colors Fund and The Palette Fund, 2012. http://williamsinstitute. law.ucla.edu/wp-content/uploads/Durso-Gates-LGBT-Homeless-Youth-Survey -July-2012.pdf (accessed December 30, 2016).

Filichia, Peter. "Bring on the Men!" *Theater Mania*, October 17, 2002. http://www
.theatermania.com/new-york-city-theater/news/10-2002/bring-on-the-men_2682
.html (accessed November 5, 2016).

Frank, Barney. *Frank: A Life in Politics from the Great Society to Same-Sex Marriage.*
New York: Farrar, Straus and Giroux, 2015.

Frank, Barney. *Wikipedia.* https://en.wikipedia.org/wiki/Barney_Frank (accessed January 18, 2017).

Frankl, Viktor E. *Man's Search for Meaning.* Boston: Beacon Press, 2006.

Frederiksen-Goldsen, Karen I., et al. *The Aging and Health Report: Disparities and
Resilience among Lesbian, Gay, Bisexual, and Transgender Older Adults.* New
York: SAGE, 2011. http://depts.washington.edu/agepride/wordpress/wp-content/
uploads/2011/05/Full-Report-FINAL-11-16-11.pdf (accessed January 30, 2017).

Freedom to Marry. "Winning the Freedom to Marry Nationwide: The Inside Story
of a Transformative Campaign." http://www.freedomtomarry.org/pages/how-it
-happened (accessed December 1, 2016).

GLAAD in conjunction with the University of Missouri Center on Religion & the Professions. *Missing Voices: A Study of Religious Voices in Mainstream Media Reports about
LGBT Equality*, April 2012. http://glaad.org/missingvoices (accessed January 9, 2017).

GLSEN. *2015 State Snapshot: School Climate in Connecticut*, at https://www.glsen.org/
sites/default/files/Connecticut%20State%20Snapshot%20-%20NSCS.pdf (accessed January 12, 2017).

GOP Debate Question Booed Soldier. https://www.youtube.com/watch?v=ZvIittOP
5r8 (accessed January 18, 2017).

Guest, Michael. *Wikipedia.* https://en.wikipedia.org/wiki/Michael_Guest (accessed
January 19, 2017).

Halkitis, P. N. "Reframing HIV Prevention for Gay Men in the United States."
American Psychologist 65, no. 8 (November 2010): 752–63.

Hay, Harry. "A Separate People Whose Time Has Come," in *Gay Spirit: Myth and
Meaning*, ed. Mark Thompson (pp. 279–91). New York: St. Martin's Press, 1987.

Herrick, A. L., S. H. Lim, C. Wei, H. Smith, T. Guadamuz, M. S. Friedman, and R.
Stall. "Resilience as an Untapped Resource in Behavioral Intervention Design for
Gay Men." *AIDS Behavior* 15 Suppl. (April 2011): S25–29.

Hite, Charles. "APA Rules Homosexuality Not Necessarily a Disorder." *Psychiatric
News*, January 2, 1974, 11.

"Homosexuals Lead Protest After 'Village' Raid Nets 167." *New York Times*, March 8,
1970, 29. https://www.instagram.com/p/BCu9WsJMM60/ (accessed November 17,
2016).

Joseph, Stephen. *What Doesn't Kill Us: The Psychology of Posttraumatic Growth.* New
York: Basic Books, 2011.

Kaiser, Charles. *The Gay Metropolis: 1910–1996.* New York: Houghton Mifflin
Company, 1997.

Kantrowitz, Arnie. *Under the Rainbow: Growing Up Gay.* Stonewall Edition paperback, New York: St. Martin's Press, 1977.

Kaplan, Roberta. "Gay Rights: Change Is Gonna Come. The Torah Says So." *Tablet*, November 23, 2016. http://www.tabletmag.com/scroll/218446/gay-rights-change -is-gonna-come-the-torah-says-so (accessed December 2, 2016).

Kastor, Elizabeth. "Advocates in the Realm of Sorrows." *Washington Post*, February 23, 1988. https://www.washingtonpost.com/archive/lifestyle/1988/02/23/advo cates-in-the-realm-of-sorrows/47af4e93-b56e-470a-9f16-0153931e84af/?utm_ term=.7a7acb952d5a (accessed January 27, 2017).

Kegeles, S. M., R. B. Hayes, and T. J. Coates. "The Mpowerment Project: A Community-Level HIV Prevention Intervention for Young Gay Men." *American Journal of Public Health* 86, no. 8 (Pt. 1) (August 1996): 1129–36.

Khan, Azmat. "Meet America's First Openly Gay Imam." *Aljazeera America*. http://america.aljazeera.com/watch/shows/america-tonight/america-tonight-blog/ 2013/12/20/meet-america-s-firstopenlygayimam.html (accessed January 20, 2017).

Killacky, John. "Careening Toward Kensho: Ruminations on Disability and Community." In *Queer Crips: Disabled Gay Men and Their Stories*, ed. Bob Guter and John R. Killacky (pp. 58–59). New York: Routledge, 2004.

Killacky, John. *Holding On* (2006). https://www.youtube.com/watch?v=RVwAHT5_ lc8 (accessed January 24, 2017).

Kooden, Harold, with Charles Flowers. *Golden Men: The Power of Gay Midlife*. New York: William Morrow Paperbacks, 2000.

Kramer, Larry. *Reports from the holocaust: The Making of an AIDS Activist*. New York: St. Martin's Press, 1989.

Kubicek, Katrina, Miles McNeeley, Ian W. Holloway, George Weiss, and Michele Kipke. "'It's Like Our Own Little World': Resilience as a Factor of Participation in the Ballroom Community Subculture." *AIDS Behavior* 17, no. 4 (May 2013): 1524–39.

Lew, Steve. *Wikipedia*. https://en.wikipedia.org/wiki/Steve_Lew (accessed January 23, 2017).

Livingston, Jennie. *Paris Is Burning* (1990). https://www.youtube.com/watch?v=hedJer 7I1vI (accessed January 5, 2017).

Longfellow, Henry Wadsworth. "Letter to George Washington Greene." In *The Letters of Henry Wadsworth Longfellow*, ed. Andrew R. Hilen (p. 66). Cambridge: Harvard University Press, 1982.

Los Angeles LGBT Center. About the Center: Anita May Rosenstein Campus. https://lalgbtcenter.org/about-the-center/anita-may-rosenstein-campus (accessed January 6, 2017).

Louie, Kelsey. "It's Been 35 Years Since Gay Men's Health Crisis Began in Larry Kramer's Living Room." New York: Gay Men's Health Crisis, August 11, 2016. http://www.gmhc.org/content/its-been-35-years-gay-mens-health-crisis-began -larry-kramers-living-room (accessed November 21, 2016).

Matlovich, Leonard. *Wikipedia*. https://en.wikipedia.org/wiki/Leonard_Matlovich (accessed January 17, 2017).

McNaught, Brian. *Gay Issues in the Workplace*. First paperback ed. New York: St. Martin's Press, 1995.

Miller, Alice. *The Drama of the Gifted Child: The Search for the True Self*, revised edition. New York: Basic Books, 1997.

Mustanski, B., M. Newcomb, and R. Garofalo. "Mental Health of Lesbian, Gay, and Bisexual Youth: A Developmental Resiliency Perspective." *Journal of Gay and Lesbian Social Services* 23, no. 2 (January 1, 2011): 204–25.

Naff, Kevin. "A Tribute to Gay Bars," *Washington Blade* 47, no. 25 (June 14, 2016): 32.

Nardi, Peter M. *Gay Men's Friendships: Invincible Communities*. Chicago: University of Chicago Press, 1999.

Nemitz, Bill. "Backstory Makes 'Good' Portland Slogan Even Better." *Portland Press Herald*, June 19, 2013. http://www.pressherald.com/2013/06/19/why-yes_-lifes-good-here-gets-better-still-_2013-06-19/, accessed February 1, 2017.

Newman, Emily. "Strut: A New Home for Health and Wellness in San Francisco." *Beta*, September 25, 2015. http://betablog.org/strut-a-new-home-for-health-wellness-in-san-francisco/ (accessed January 28, 2017).

New York Times Editorial Board. "Unequal Treatment at the State Department." *New York Times*, December 3, 2007. https://theboard.blogs.nytimes.com/2007/12/03/unequal-treatment-at-the-state-department/ (accessed January 19, 2017).

NIH LGBT Research Coordinating Committee. *Consideration of the Institute of Medicine (IOM) Report on the Health of Lesbian, Gay, Bisexual, and Transgender (LGBT) Individuals* (January 2013). https://report.nih.gov/UploadDocs/LGBT%20Health%20Report_FINAL_2013-01-03-508%20compliant.pdf (accessed January 26, 2017).

Oreskes, Michael. "Representative Frank Asks for Full Inquiry by Ethics Panel." *New York Times*, August 29, 1989. http://www.nytimes.com/1989/08/29/us/rep-frank-asks-for-full-inquiry-by-ethics-panel.html (accessed January 18, 2017).

Peabody, Frannie (biographical sketch). Frannie Peabody Center. http://peabody center.org/wp-content/uploads/2013/07/Frannie-Peabody.Bio-Sum.kmills.4-07.pdf (accessed February 1, 2017).

Pew Research Center. *America's Changing Religious Landscape*, May 12, 2015. http://www.pewforum.org/2015/05/12/americas-changing-religious-landscape/ (accessed January 9, 2017).

PFLAG. "Our Story." https://www.pflag.org/our-story (accessed December 14, 2016).

Pollack, William, *Real Boys: Rescuing Our Sons from the Myths of Boyhood*. New York: Random House, 1998.

Portland, Maine. *Wikipedia*. https://en.wikipedia.org/wiki/Portland,_Maine (accessed January 31, 2017).

1866 Great Fire of Portland, Maine. *Wikipedia*. https://en.wikipedia.org/wiki/1866_Great_fire_of_Portland,_Maine (accessed January 31, 2017).

President Obama addresses the nation after Orlando shooting. https://www.youtube.com/watch?v=gOH7F0XCqpw (accessed January 4, 2017).

Preston, John. *Winter's Light: Reflections of a Yankee Queer*, ed. Michael Lowenthal. Hanover, NH: University Press of New England, 1995.

Radical Faeries. *Wikipedia*. https://en.wikipedia.org/wiki/Radical_Faeries (accessed November 17, 2016).

Rainbow Honor Walk. http://rainbowhonorwalk.org/?page_id=77 (accessed January 28, 2017).

Rasi, Richard A., and Lourdes Rodríguez-Nogués, eds. *Out in the Workplace: The Pleasures and Perils of Coming Out on the Job*. Los Angeles: Alyson Publications, 1995.

Re-evaluation Counseling. *Wikipedia*. https://en.wikipedia.org/wiki/Re-evaluation_Counseling (accessed January 23, 2017).

Riley, John. "Pride and Mourning." *MetroWeekly* (Washington, D.C.), June 16, 2016, 34–35.

Robinson, Gene. *Wikipedia*. https://en.wikipedia.org/wiki/Gene_Robinson (accessed January 11, 2017).

Rofes, Eric. *Dry Bones Breathe: Gay Men Creating Post-AIDS Identities and Culture*. New York: Harrington Park Press, 1998.

Rosenfeld, Megan. "At Ziegfeld's, Queen for a Night." *Washington Post*, August 2, 2001, 32. https://www.washingtonpost.com/archive/lifestyle/2001/08/02/at-ziegfelds-queens-for-a-night/395ad8ff-4be8-4968-90fb-d61afc37f2bf/?utm_term=.1bcaeac62d8f (accessed January 4, 2016).

Ryan, C., D. Huebner, R. Diaz, and J. Sanchez. "Family Rejection as a Predictor of Negative Health Outcomes in White and Latino Lesbian, Gay, and Bisexual Young Adults," *Pediatrics* 1 (January 2009): 346–52.

Ryan, Caitlin. *Supportive Families, Healthy Children*. San Francisco: Family Acceptance Project, San Francisco State University, 2009.

Saffron, Inga. "Changing Skyline: John C. Anderson Apartments, LGBT-Friendly and Urban-Friendly." *Philadelphia Inquirer*, January 18, 2014. http://www.philly.com/philly/columnists/inga_saffron/20140117_Changing_Skyline__John_C__Anderson_Apartments__LGBT-friendly_and_urban-friendly.html (accessed January 31, 2017).

SAGE. Mission and history. http://sageusa.org (accessed January 30, 2017).

Same-sex marriage in Connecticut. *Wikipedia*. https://en.wikipedia.org/wiki/Same-sex_marriage_in_Connecticut (accessed December 2, 2016).

Segal, Mark. *And Then I Danced: Traveling the Road to LGBT Equality*. Philadelphia: Akashic Books, 2015.

Shand-Tucci, Douglass. *The Crimson Letter: Harvard, Homosexuality, and the Shaping of American Culture*. New York: St. Martin's Press, 2003.

Shilts, Randy. *And the Band Played On*. New York: St. Martin's Press, 1987.

Snyder-Hill, Stephen. *Soldier of Change: From the Closet to the Forefront of the Gay Rights Movement*. Lincoln: Potomac Books/University of Nebraska Press, 2014.

Snyder-Hill, Stephen. "Trust the Power of Your Voice," TED talk at Ohio State University. February 14, 2015. https://www.youtube.com/watch?v=RPN_GnN027g (accessed January 17, 2017).

Spitzer, Robert L. "The Homosexuality Decision—A Background Paper." *Psychiatric News*, January 16, 1974, 11.

Stall, R., T. C. Mills, J. Williamson, T. Hart, C. Greenwood, J. Paul et al. "Association of Co-Occurring Psychosocial Health Problems and Increased Vulnerability to HIV/AIDS Among Urban Men Who Have Sex with Men." *American Journal of Public Health* 93, no. 6 (2003): 939–42.

Substance Abuse and Mental Health Services Administration. *A Practitioner's Resource Guide: Helping Families to Support Their LGBT Children.* HHS Publication No. PEP14-LGBTKIDS. Rockville, MD: Substance Abuse and Mental Health Services Administration, 2014.

The Supreme Court of the United States. *Obergefell v. Hodges.* https://s3-us-west-2 .amazonaws.com/ftm-assets/ftm/archive/files/pdfs/SCOTUSObergefellOpinion. pdf (accessed December 1, 2016).

Timmons, Stuart. *The Trouble with Harry Hay, Founder of the Modern Gay Movement.* Boston: Alyson Publication, 1990.

U.S. Department of Justice, Civil Rights Division, Disability Rights Section. Questions and Answers: The Americans with Disabilities Act and Persons with HIV/ AIDS. https://www.ada.gov/hiv/ada_q&a_aids.htm (accessed January 23, 2017).

United States v. Windsor. Wikipedia. https://en.wikipedia.org/wiki/United_States_v._ Windsor#cite_note-84 (accessed December 2, 2016).

Walker, J. J., B. Longmire-Avital, and S. Golub. "Racial and Sexual Identities as Potential Buffers to Risky Sexual Behavior for Black Gay and Bisexual Emerging Adult Men." *Health Psychology* 34, no. 8 (August 2015): 841–46. https://www.ncbi .nlm.nih.gov/pubmed/25528178 (accessed January 26, 2017).

Wax-Thibodeaux, Emily. "A Philadelphia Apartment Building May Be a National Model for Low-Income LGBT Seniors." *Washington Post*, September 12, 2014. https://www.washingtonpost.com/politics/a-philadelphia-apartment-build ing-may-be-a-national-model-for-low-income-lgbt-seniors/2014/09/12/f64e06bc -352d-11e4-8f02-03c644b2d7d0_story.html?utm_term=.83ced0ec6d38 (accessed January 30, 2017).

The White House. Obama Administration Statements on the Supreme Court's DOMA Ruling (June 27, 2013). https://www.whitehouse.gov/blog/2013/06/27/ obama-administration-statements-supreme-court-s-doma-ruling (accessed December 2, 2016).

White, Mel. *How to Resist Extremism!: A Pocket Guide to the Practice of Relentless Nonviolent Resistance.* http://melwhite.org/wp-content/uploads/2016/05/Resist -Extremism.pdf (accessed January 10, 2017).

White, Rev. Dr. Mel. *Mel & Gary's Story.* http://melwhite.org/mel-garys-story (accessed February 1, 2017).

White Night Riots. *Wikipedia.* https://en.wikipedia.org/wiki/White_Night_riots (accessed November 22, 2016).

Whitman, Walt. "Halcyon Days." *Leaves of Grass* (1855). Walt Whitman Archive. http://whitmanarchive.org/published/LG/1891/poems/324 (accessed January 29, 2017).

Wight, Richard G., Allen J. LeBlanc, Brian de Vries, and Roger Detels. "Stress and Mental Health Among Midlife and Older Gay-Identified Men." *American Journal of Public Health* 102 (2012): 503–10.

Wight, Richard G., Allen J. LeBlanc, Ilan H. Meyer, and Frederick Harig. "Internalized Gay Ageism, Mattering, and Depressive Symptoms Among Midlife and Older Gay-Identified Men." *Social Science & Medicine* 147 (2015): 200–8.

Williams, J. K., L. Wilton, and M. Magnus et al. "Relation of Childhood Sexual Abuse, Intimate Partner Violence, and Depression to Risk Factors for HIV among Black Men Who Have Sex with Men in 6 U.S. Cities." *American Journal of Public Health* 105, no. 12 (December 2015): 2473–81.

Woititz, Janet Geringer. *Adult Children of Alcoholics*. Pompano Beach, FL: Health Communications, Inc., 1983.

Wolfson, Evan. "Samesex Marriage and Morality: The Human Rights Vision of the Constitution." Cambridge: Harvard Law School, April 1983. http://freemarry.3cdn.net/73aab4141a80237ddf_kxm62r3er.pdf (accessed December 1, 2016).

Wolfson, Evan. "Marriage Equality and Some Lessons for the Scary Work of Winning" (2004). http://archive-freedomtomarry.org/evan_wolfson/speeches/scary_work_of_winning.php (accessed December 2, 2016).

Wolfson, Evan. "What's Next in the Fight for Gay Equality?" *New York Times*, June 26, 2015. http://www.nytimes.com/2015/06/27/opinion/evan-wolfson-whats-next-in-the-fight-for-gay-equality.html (accessed December 2, 2016).

Wreston, Kimberly. "Episcopal Church Suspended from Full Participation in Anglican Communion." Religion News Service, January 14, 2016. http://religionnews.com/2016/01/14/episcopal-church-suspended-anglican-communion/ (accessed January 11, 2017).

Index

~

About the Author

John-Manuel Andriote has written about LGBT, HIV-AIDS, and other health and medical subjects since the early 1980s, for publications ranging from the *Advocate* to the *Washington Post*. He is the author of *Victory Deferred: How AIDS Changed Gay Life in America*; *Hot Stuff: A Brief History of Disco/Dance Music*; *Tough Love: A Washington Reporter Finds Resilience, Ruin, and Zombies in His 'Other Connecticut' Hometown*; and a "fable for kids ages 5 to 105" called *Wilhelmina Goes Wandering*. His articles have appeared in the *Washington Post*, *The Atlantic*, the *Huffington Post*, and leading LGBT publications across America. The interviews and research materials for *Victory Deferred* are part of a special collection curated by the Smithsonian's National Museum of American History. Andriote regularly speaks to audiences at conferences and universities, is interviewed and profiled by print and broadcast media, and has been an adjunct communication professor at Eastern Connecticut State University.